10 0486845 8

KU-279-673

WITHDRAWN

D   OR RETU

A Guide to
Radiological
Procedures

Commissioning Editor: Timothy Horne
Project Development Manager: Siân Jarman
Designer: Erik Bigland
Project Manager: Nancy Arnott
Illustrator: David Gardner

A Guide to
Radiological Procedures

Edited by

Stephen Chapman

MBBS, MRCS, FRCP, FRCPCH, FRCR
Consultant Paediatric Radiologist
Diana, Princess of Wales Children's Hospital
Birmingham Children's Hospital NHS Trust, Birmingham
Honorary Senior Clinical Lecturer, University of Birmingham

Richard Nakielny

MA, BM, BCh, FRCR
Consultant Radiologist (CT Scanning)
Royal Hallamshire Hospital, Sheffield
Honorary Clinical Lecturer, University of Sheffield

FOURTH EDITION

SAUNDERS

EDINBURGH • LONDON • NEW YORK • OXFORD • PHILADELPHIA • ST LOUIS
SYDNEY • TORONTO   2001

SAUNDERS

An imprint of Elsevier Limited

1004868458

© Elsevier Limited 2001. All rights reserved.

The rights of Stephen Chapman and Richard Nakielny to be identified as editors of this work have been asserted by them in accordance with the Copyright, Designs and Patents Act 1988

No part of this publication may be reproduced, stored in a retrieval system, or transmitted in any form or by any means, electronic, mechanical, photocopying, recording or otherwise, without either the prior permission of the publishers or a licence permitting restricted copying in the United Kingdom issued by the Copyright Licensing Agency, 90 Tottenham Court Road, London W1T 4LP. Permissions may be sought directly from Elsevier's Health Sciences Rights Department in Philadelphia, USA: phone: (+1) 215 238 7869, fax: (+1) 215 238 2239, e-mail: healthpermissions@elsevier.com. You may also complete your request on-line via the Elsevier homepage (http://www.elsevier.com), by selecting 'Customer Support' and then 'Obtaining Permissions'.

First published in 1981
Second edition 1986
Third edition 1993
Fourth edition 2001
   Reprinted 2002, 2003, 2004, 2005, 2006

ISBN 0 7020 2565 8

British Library Cataloguing in Publication Data
A catalogue record for this book is available from the British Library

Library of Congress Cataloguing in Publication Data
A catalogue record for this book is available from the Library of Congress

Note
Medical knowledge is constantly changing. As new information becomes available, changes in treatment, procedures, equipment and the use of drugs become necessary. The editors, contributor and the publishers have taken care to ensure that the information given in this text is accurate and up to date. However, readers are strongly advised to confirm that the information, especially with regard to drug usage, complies with the latest legislation and standards of practice.

ELSEVIER
your source for books,
journals and multimedia
in the health sciences

www.elsevierhealth.com

Working together to grow
libraries in developing countries
www.elsevier.com | www.bookaid.org | www.sabre.org

ELSEVIER   BOOK AID International   Sabre Foundation

The
publisher's
policy is to use
paper manufactured
from sustainable forest

Printed in China
C/07

MEDICAL LIBRARY
QUEENS MEDICAL CENTRE

At this stage in the life of this book the time was right to cast a careful and critical eye over all the contents to ensure that what is retained reflects up to date radiology practice. To this end we have welcomed Dr Amaka Mbamali who has just finished her radiology training and is consequently in a good position to act as a filter to achieve this. Consequently, we trust that what has been produced will continue to reflect contemporary radiology practice in as concise and helpful a manner as possible. There has been some reorganization of the chapters and the whole book has been redesigned to reflect modern publishing practice.

Our thanks go to those who contributed to previous editions and helped make the book what it is today, to those who contributed their time and knowledge to the current edition and to the team at Harcourt, particularly Siân Jarman, who encouraged us when our spirits were waning.

Birmingham and Sheffield   S. C.
2001   R. N.

CONTENTS

The numbers in brackets refer to the chapters written or co-written by the contributor.

C. M. Boivin BSc, MPhil
(1–5, 7–14, 16, 17)
Senior Computer Scientist and Deputy
Head of Nuclear Medicine
Queen Elizabeth Hospital
Birmingham

V. Cassar-Pullicino FRCR
(13, 14)
Consultant Radiologist
Robert Jones and Agnes Hunt
Orthopaedic Hospital
Oswestry
Senior Clinical Lecturer
University of Birmingham

A. Mbamali BSc, MRCP, FRCR
Specialist Registrar
Radiology Department
Royal Hallamshire Hospital
Sheffield

J. F. C. Olliff MRCP, FRCR
(3–6, 10, 17)
Consultant Radiologist
Queen Elizabeth Hospital
Birmingham
Senior Clinical Lecturer
University of Birmingham

S. Olliff MRCP, FRCR
(3–6, 10, 17)
Consultant Radiologist
Queen Elizabeth Hospital
Birmingham
Senior Clinical Lecturer
University of Birmingham

T. Powell FRCP, DMRD, FRCR
Formerly Consultant Radiologist
Royal Hallamshire Hospital
Sheffield

ABBREVIATIONS

The following is a list of common abbreviations used throughout the text.

AP	anteroposterior
CT	computerized tomography
ECG	electrocardiogram
HOCM	high-osmolar contrast media
LAO	left anterior oblique
LOCM (370)	low-osmolar contrast media (containing 370 mg ml^{-1} iodine)
LPO	left posterior oblique
MRI	magnetic resonance imaging
PA	posteroanterior
RAO	right anterior oblique
RPO	right posterior oblique

General notes

RADIOLOGY

The procedures are laid out under a number of sub-headings, which follow a standard sequence. The general order is outlined below, together with certain points that are omitted from the discussion of each procedure to avoid repetition. Minor deviations from this sequence will be found in the text where this is felt to be more appropriate.

Methods

Indications

Contraindications

All radiological procedures carry a risk. The risk incurred from undertaking the procedure must be balanced against the benefit to the patient from the information obtained. Contraindications may, therefore, be relative (the majority) or absolute. Factors that increase the risk to the patient can be considered under three headings: due to radiation; due to the contrast medium; due to the technique.

Due to radiation

Radiation effects on humans may be hereditary, i.e. revealed in the offspring of the exposed individual, or somatic. Somatic injuries fall into two groups: stochastic and deterministic. The latter, e.g. skin erythema and cataracts, occur when a critical threshold has been reached and are rarely relevant to diagnostic radiology. Stochastic effects are 'all or none'.[1] The cancer produced by a small dose is the same as the cancer produced by a large dose but the frequency of its appearance is less with the smaller dose. It is obviously impossible to avoid some radiation exposure to staff and patients and stochastic effects cannot be completely eliminated. There is an excess of cancers following diagnostic levels of irradiation to the fetus[2] and the female breast,[3] and trends of increasing rates of cancer are seen in workers in the nuclear power industry exposed to low doses.[4] The total collective population dose from medical X-rays could be responsible for between 200 and 500 of the 160 000 cancer deaths each year in the United Kingdom.[5] A number of principles guide the use of diagnostic radiation:

1. *Justification* that a proposed examination is of net benefit to the patient.[6]
2. *ALARP* – doses should be kept *As Low As Reasonably Practicable*, economic and social factors being taken into account.[7]

Justification is particularly important when considering the irradiation of women of reproductive age because of the risks to the developing fetus. In addition to the tumour risk from diagnostic levels of radiation and the risks that have been extrapolated from atomic bomb survivors,[8] Otake and Schull[9] have shown that irradiation of the maternal abdomen between 8 and 15 weeks post-conception also results in an increased incidence of arrested forebrain development and mental subnormality. Earlier advice by national and international bodies aimed at confining less urgent radiological examinations of the lower abdomen and pelvis on females of child-bearing age to the 10 days following the start of menstruation – the 'ten-day rule'.[10,11] This would be a time when there is the least likelihood of harm to any possible developing fetus because conception is unlikely to have occurred. Patients exempted from this rule were:

1. Women who denied recent sexual intercourse.
2. Women who were menstruating at the time.
3. Women who had been taking an oral contraceptive pill for no fewer than 3 months and were satisfied that it was effective.
4. Women who had an intrauterine contraceptive device for no fewer than 3 months and had found it effective.
5. Women who had been sterilized.

The arguments against the 'ten-day rule' have been summarized under four headings:[12]

1. *Timing.* Organogenesis occurs during the fourth to eighth week after conception. Thus, irradiation after the tenth day of the menstrual cycle but before the next menstrual cycle will not result in radiation damage to organogenesis.
2. *Irradiation of the unfertilized ovum.* There is no evidence that

irradiation of the conceptus is any more dangerous than irradiation of the unfertilized ovum.

3. *Magnitude of the hazard.* The risks are extremely small and are greatly outweighed by the likely benefits to the mother or fetus of an earlier diagnosis. Irradiation of a fetus during the first few weeks of gestation will, if it has any detrimental effect, induce a spontaneous abortion. This is unlikely to be of serious personal or social concern unless the couple is subfertile.[13]

4. *Cost-effectiveness.* The cost of implementing the ten-day rule appeared to be 100 times greater than the value of the possible benefit derived from it, assuming a benefit existed.

More recent advice[14] has superseded the earlier ten-day rule recommendation and is based on a statement by the International Commission on Radiological Protection[15] which reads 'During the first ten days following the onset of a menstrual period there can be no risk to any conceptus, since no conception will have occurred. The risk to a child who had previously been irradiated in utero during the remainder of a four week period following the onset of menstruation is likely to be so small that there need be no special limitation on exposures required within these four weeks.'

The chain of responsibility for ensuring that the fetus is not exposed to ionizing radiation is:

1. The patient
2. The referring clinician
3. The radiologist
4. The radiographer.

Clinicians and radiologists should regard any woman as pregnant if her period is overdue or missed unless she is definitely known not to be pregnant. A pregnancy test may be helpful. It may be possible to defer the answer to a clinical question until it is known that she is not pregnant or it may be possible to answer the question using a safer technique such as ultrasonography. If the examination is necessary, a technique that minimizes the number of films and the absorbed dose per film should be utilized. However, the quality of the examination should not be reduced to the level where its diagnostic value is impaired. The risk to the patient of an incorrect diagnosis may be greater than the risk of irradiating the fetus. Radiography of areas remote from the pelvis and abdomen may be safely performed at any time during pregnancy with good collimation and lead protection.

Due to the contrast medium

The following are high risk factors associated with the administration of intravascular contrast medium:

1. *A previous severe adverse reaction to contrast medium.* With HOCM this carries a 20% risk of a similar reaction on a subsequent occasion. The risk is decreased to 5% with LOCM.[16] Radioisotopes, ultrasound, CT or MRI may provide an alternative means of investigation.
2. *Asthma or a significant allergic history.*
3. *Proven or suspected hypersensitivity to iodine.*
4. *β-blockers.*
5. *Heart disease.* Cardiac failure and arrhythmias can be precipitated. The risk is less with LOCM but if only HOCM are available, meglumine-containing salts are preferable to those containing sodium.
6. *Infants and small children.*
7. *Hepatic failure.*
8. *Moderate to severe impairment of renal function*, especially when associated with diabetes. A deterioration in renal function may follow but can be minimized if the patient is well hydrated.
9. *Myelomatosis.* Bence Jones protein may be precipitated in renal tubules. The risk is diminished by ensuring good hydration.
10. *Poor hydration.*
11. *Sickle-cell anaemia.* The risk of precipitating a sickle-cell crisis is less with LOCM.
12. *Co-administration of Metformin (glucophage).* The administration of intravenous (i.v.) iodinated contrast medium to diabetic patients receiving Metformin may lead to acute alteration of renal function and lactic acidosis. The Royal College of Radiologists gives the following advice:[17]
    a. The referring clinician should take responsibility for assessing the patient's renal function. The Radiology Department should inform the referring clinician of the timing of the investigation to enable this to occur.
    b. There are, as yet, no reports of Metformin-induced lactic acidosis in patients with normal renal function after i.v. contrast agents, but there is a theoretical risk of interaction. Metformin should, therefore, be discontinued at the time of the investigation and withheld for the subsequent 48 h.

  c. For those patients with abnormal renal function,
   Metformin should also be discontinued, but not reinstated
   until renal function has been documented to have returned
   to normal.
  d. As Metformin is contraindicated in the presence of
   abnormal renal function, patients who require i.v. contrast
   examinations should have their drug history reviewed by
   the appropriate physician to ensure suitability of the drug
   regime.

13. *Thyrotoxicosis.* The enormous iodine load has a statistically
 significant effect on thyroid function tests, but this is of little
 practical clinical significance.[18] Hyperthyroidism may recur
 in patients previously treated for Graves' disease.

14. *Pregnancy.* A possible teratogenic risk has not been excluded.

Contraindications to other contrast media, e.g. barium, water-soluble contrast media for the gastrointestinal tract and biliary contrast media are given in the relevant sections.

 For further discussion of contrast media see Chapter 2.

Due to the technique

Skin sepsis at the needle puncture site.

 Specific contraindications to individual techniques are discussed with each procedure.

Contrast medium

Volumes given are for a 70 kg man.

Equipment

For many procedures this will also include a trolley with a sterile upper shelf and a non-sterile lower shelf. Emergency drugs and resuscitation equipment should be readily available (see Appendix II).

 See Chapter 9 for introductory notes on angiography catheters.

 If only a simple radiography table and overcouch tube are required, then this information has been omitted from the text.

Patient preparation

1. Will admission to hospital be necessary?
2. If the patient is a woman of child-bearing age, the examination
 should be performed at a time when the risks to a possible
 fetus are minimal (see above). Any female presenting for
 radiography or a nuclear medicine examination at a time when
 her period is known to be overdue should be considered to be

pregnant unless there is information indicating the absence of pregnancy. If her cycle is so irregular that it is difficult to know whether a period has been missed and it is not practicable to defer the examination until menstruation occurs, then a pregnancy test or pelvic ultrasound (US) examination may help to determine whether she is pregnant.

The risk to a fetus irradiated during the first 4 weeks following the onset of the last menstruation is likely to be so small that there need be no special limitation on radiological exposures within these 4 weeks. The 'ten-day rule' should still apply for hysterosalpingography, so that the risks of mechanical trauma to an early pregnancy are reduced.[12]

3. The procedure should be explained to the patient and consent obtained when necessary.[19] The UK General Medical Council has published advice to medical practitioners on the issue of consent[20] and The Royal College of Radiologists has published advice on the radiological aspects of intimate examinations.[21]

The radiologist must assess a child's capacity to decide whether to consent or refuse an investigation. At age 16 years a young person can be treated as an adult and can be presumed to have the capacity to understand the nature, purpose and possible consequences of the proposed investigation, as well as the consequences of non-investigation. Following recent case law in the United Kingdom (Gillick v. West Norfolk and Wisbech Area Health Authority) and the introduction of The Children Act 1989, in which the capacity of children to consent has been linked with the concept of individual ability to understand the implications of medical treatment, there has come into existence a standard known as 'Gillick competence'. Under age 16 years children may have the capacity to decide depending on their ability to understand. Nevertheless, where there is more than one person or body who could give consent, investigation/treatment would be vetoed only where *all those who could consent had refused to do so*, i.e. a person with parental responsibility or the court may authorize investigation/treatment which is in the child's best interests. A parent has a right to consent to the treatment of a minor, and this right lasts as long as minority does (i.e. until the age of 18 years).[22]

4. If the procedure has a risk of bleeding and a bleeding disorder is suspected, e.g. liver disease or concurrent administration of warfarin, then that disorder must be investigated and appropriate steps taken to normalize blood clotting.[23,24]

5. Bowel preparation is used:
   a. prior to investigation of the gastrointestinal tract
   b. when considerable faecal loading obscures other intra-abdominal organs
   c. when opacification of an organ is likely to be poor, e.g. the gall bladder in oral cholecystography.

   For other radiological investigations of abdominal organs bowel preparation is not always necessary and when given may result in excessive bowel gas. Bowel gas may be reduced if the patient is kept ambulant prior to the examination and those who routinely take laxatives should continue to do so.[25]
6. Previous films and notes should be obtained.
7. Premedication will be necessary for painful procedures or where the patient is unlikely to cooperate for any other reason. Suggested premedication for *adults* includes:

Benzodiazepines

a. diazepam, 10 mg orally 2 h prior to the procedure, or up to 0.3 mg kg^{-1} i.v., or
b. midazolam (which has a shorter duration of action than diazepam), up to 0.1 mg kg^{-1} i.v., or intramuscularly (i.m.), or
c. temazepam (which also has a shorter action than diazepam and has a more rapid onset), 20–40 mg (elderly 10–20 mg) 1 h before the procedure, or
d. lorazepam (which produces more prolonged sedation than temazepam and has greater amnesic properties), 1–5 mg orally 2–6 h before the procedure.

(Droperidol, 5–10 mg orally, is usefully combined with a benzodiazepine to produce a quieter patient. It should not be used alone.)

Opioid analgesics

a. morphine, 10 mg i.m., or ⎫
b. papaveretum, 20 mg i.m., or ⎬ 1 h prior to the procedure
c. pethidine, 50–100 mg i.m., or ⎭
d. fentanyl, 50–200 μg i.v. or
e. alfentanil, up to 500 μg i.v. over 30 s.

Sedation of children

Sedation may be defined as the use of a drug or drugs to produce a state of depression of the central nervous system that enables treatment to be carried out but during which verbal contact with the patient is maintained throughout the period of sedation. However, most radiological procedures on children requiring sedation cannot be performed as defined above and children may require sedation of a degree which borders on rendering them unconscious.

Sedation in departments of clinical radiology should be carried out under the responsibility of a named consultant radiologist and under the supervision of a suitably trained radiologist. Ideally, when drugs are used which are likely to result in loss of consciousness the primary care of the patient should be under the direct supervision of an anaesthetist. More commonly, sedation will be undertaken by a radiologist trained in resuscitative techniques supported by the rapid availability of anaesthetic and resuscitative help. A nurse, experienced in the care of sedated children, should be present.

Each child should be individually assessed. In most circumstances parents should be encouraged to stay with the child and with patience and encouragement the need for sedation may be avoided in some cases.

EMLA cream to a suitable vein (preferably chosen by the radiologist) at the time of administration of the sedation or prior insertion of a venous cannula if venous access will be necessary during the procedure, e.g. for the administration of contrast medium.

The following categories of patients are at high risk from sedation:

1. Infants, because of variable pharmacokinetics
2. Children with airway obstruction
3. Children with respiratory failure, mitochondrial cytopathies or brain stem tumours
4. Children with raised intracranial pressure
5. Children with severe renal or hepatic failure.

Clinicians should use drugs that they are familiar with. Some patient groups are difficult to sedate, e.g. mentally retarded children and those receiving antiepileptic drugs. The following sedation regimes are in use in the UK.

Chloral hydrate

For many years chloral hydrate has been the mainstay for sedation of young children for a variety of procedures. However, the commonly recommended dose (50 mg kg^{-1}) is unpredictable in terms of the time to onset of action and the depth and duration of sedation. This is particularly important where failure to adequately sedate a patient may result in postponement of the investigation.

MRI scanning creates a particular problem due to the noise of the scanner, which creates a clear stimulus to the child to wake up. The following recommendations are made as being suitable for the majority of patients, in respect of both safety and efficacy. It is recognized that, for certain patients, deviation from these guidelines will be appropriate on clinical or weight grounds and some situations where this may be appropriate are highlighted below. Some children of 4 or 5 years of age will be cooperative and not require sedation or anaesthesia. All children will require individual assessment.

Age/Weight	Sedation	
< 1 month old	Feed only	
> 1 month old but < 5 kg	Chloral hydrate:	50–70 mg kg^{-1}
5–10 kg	Chloral hydrate:	75 mg kg^{-1} with a further 25 mg kg^{-1} if not asleep in 30 min
> 10 kg–4 years	Chloral hydrate:	100 mg kg^{-1} **(max. 2 g)**
	+ Droperidol:	10–20 kg: 2.5 mg > 20 kg: 5mg
	+ procyclidine:	10–20 kg: 2.5 mg > 20 kg: 5 mg

Chloral hydrate should be administered as 1 g in 5 ml syrup in order to reduce the dose volume to a minimum. Droperidol is available as 5 mg in 5 ml solution (or 10 mg tablets).

Vomiting. Chloral hydrate is a mucosal irritant and vomiting is not uncommon. It should be used with caution in patients with gastritis. If the child vomits the dose of chloral hydrate (or Droperidol or procyclidine) within 15 min of administration the dose may be repeated.

URTI. Chloral hydrate may make rhinitis and catarrhal symptoms worse. Consideration should be given to postponing the scan if the child presents with a cold or URTI.

Liver disease. Chloral hydrate is metabolized by alcohol dehydrogenase, a hepatic enzyme which reaches full adult activity at 5 years of age. It is also metabolized by enzymes present on erythrocytes. On the basis that its metabolism would be impaired, it should be avoided in patients with end-stage liver failure, although there is little evidence to support this advice. The majority of the drug is excreted in bile as glucuronides of chloral and the active metabolite, trichloroethanol. It should therefore also be used with caution in cholestasis, although it is likely that renal excretion would increase if biliary excretion is impaired. Cholestatic children, i.e. visible jaundice or bilirubin >70 μmol l^{-1} should receive 50–75 mg kg^{-1}, whatever the age of the patient.

Children who are not jaundiced, or after liver transplant, would be expected to metabolize chloral hydrate normally and can receive the recommended dose of 100 mg kg^{-1}. Some children, especially after liver transplantation, are very difficult to sedate and may require intravenous midazolam.

Patients receiving hepatic enzyme inducers, e.g. phenobarbitone or phenytoin. These may be expected to reduce the effectiveness of chloral and dose escalation may be considered.

Neurological impairment. Lower doses *may* be considered in such patients.

Renal impairment. Dose reduction should be considered due to the risk of accumulation of renally-excreted, active metabolites.

Warfarin. Patients anticoagulated with warfarin are at risk of haemorrhage due to displacement of warfarin from plasma protein binding sites.

Temazepam + Droperidol
Temazepam 1 mg kg^{-1} (maximum dose 30 mg) + Droperidol 0.2 mg kg^{-1} (maximum 2.5 mg) orally 1 h before the procedure.

Quinalbarbitone
Quinalbarbitone 7.5–10 mg kg^{-1} orally 30–45 min before the procedure (maximum dose 200 mg).

Advice to parents prior to MRI scanning
Try to keep the child awake for as long as possible in the time leading up to the scan. Late to bed and wake up early on the day of the scan. No 'naps' are allowed on the journey to the hospital. This will ensure that the child is already tired prior to administration of the sedation.

Children need not be starved prior to sedation/scanning but should take a light diet only on the day of the scan and nothing in the hour preceding the scan. For example, cereal, milk or toast and drink for a morning scan or a 'snack' lunch for an afternoon appointment. Babies may receive milk feeds up to 2 h prior to the scan and clear fluids up to 1 h. Avoid crisps and fizzy drinks.

Recovery

The child is considered to have recovered from the sedation when they have been able to take a drink and/or have returned to their state prior to sedation.

Complex procedures on children or very uncooperative patients will be performed under general anaesthesia.

The patient should micturate prior to the procedure so that it will not be disrupted. Some procedures are of lengthy duration.

Preliminary film

The purpose of these films is:

1. To make any final adjustments in exposure factors, centring, collimation and patient's position for which the film should always be taken using the same equipment as will be used for the remainder of the procedure.
2. To exclude prohibitive factors such as residual barium from a previous examination or excessive faecal loading.
3. To demonstrate, identify and localize opacities which may be obscured by contrast medium.
4. To elicit radiological physical signs.

Films should have on them the patient's name, registration number, date and a side marker. The examination can only proceed if satisfactory preliminary films have been obtained.

Technique

1. For aseptic technique the skin is cleaned with chlorhexidine 0.5% in 70% industrial spirit or its equivalent.
2. Local anaesthetic used is lignocaine 1% without adrenaline.
3. Gonad protection is used whenever possible, unless it obscures the region of interest.

Films

When films are taken during the procedure rather than at the end of it, they have, for convenience, been described under 'Technique':

Additional techniques *or* Modifications of technique

Aftercare

May be considered as:

1. Instructions to the patient.
2. Instructions to the ward.

Complications

Complications may be considered under three headings.

Due to the anaesthetic

1. General anaesthesia
2. Local anaesthesia:
   a. allergic – unusual
   b. toxic.

The maximum adult dose of lignocaine is 200 mg (0.3 mg kg^{-1}; 20 ml of a 1% solution). Anaesthetic lozenges contribute to the total dose.

Symptoms are of paraesthesia and muscle twitching which may progress to convulsions, cardiac arrhythmias, respiratory depression and death due to cardiac arrest.

Treatment is symptomatic and includes adequate oxygenation

Due to the contrast medium

Water-soluble contrast media See Chapter 2
Barium See Chapter 3
Biliary contrast media See Chapter 4

Due to the technique

Specific details are given with the individual procedures and may be conveniently classified as:

1. Local
2. Distant or generalized.

References

1. Russell, J.G.B. (1984) How dangerous are diagnostic X-rays? *Clin. Radiol.* **35**, 347–351.
2. MacMahon, B. (1962) Prenatal X-ray exposure and childhood cancer. *J. Natl. Cancer Inst.* **28**, 1173–1191.
3. Boice, J.D., Rosenstein, M. & Trout, E.D. (1978) Estimation of breast doses and breast cancer risk associated with repeated fluoroscopic chest examinations of women with tuberculosis. *Radiat. Res.* **73**, 373–390.
4. Kendall, G.M., Muirhead, C.R., MacGibbon, B.T., et al. (1992) Mortality and occupational exposure to radiation: first analysis of the National Registry of Radiation Workers. *Br. Med. J.* **304**, 220–225.
5. Field, S. (1992) Just how harmful are diagnostic X-rays? – the college response. *Clin. Radiol.* **46**, 295.
6. International Commission on Radiological Protection (1982) *Protection Against Ionising Radiation from External Sources used in Medicine.* ICRP Publication 33. Oxford: Pergamon Press.
7. International Commission on Radiological Protection (1973) *Implication of Commission Recommendation that Doses be Kept as Low as Readily Achievable.* ICRP Publication 22. Oxford: Pergamon Press.

8. United Nations Scientific Committee on the Effects of Atomic Radiation (1972) *Ionising Radiation: Levels and Effects.* New York: United Nations.
9. Otake, M. & Schull, V.J. (1984) In utero exposure to A bomb radiation and mental retardation: a reassessment. *Br. J. Radiol.* **57**, 409–414.
10. International Commission on Radiological Protection (1970) *Protection of the Patient in X-Ray Diagnosis.* Oxford: Pergamon Press.
11. Department of Health and Social Security (1972) *Code of Practice for the Protection of Persons Against Ionising Radiations Arising from Medical and Dental Use.* London: HMSO.
12. Russell, J.G.B. (1986) The rise and fall of the ten-day rule. *Br. J. Radiol.* **59**, 3–6.
13. Mole, R.H. (1979) Radiation effects on pre-natal development and their radiological significance. *Br. J. Radiol.* **52**, 89–101.
14. National Radiological Protection Board (1985) *Exposure to Ionising Radiation of Pregnant Women: Advice on the Diagnostic Exposure of Women who are, or who may be, Pregnant ASP8.* London: HMSO.
15. International Commission on Radiological Protection (1984) *Statement from the Washington Meeting of the ICRP.* Oxford: Pergamon Press.
16. Fischer, H. (1991) Personal communication. In: McClennan B.L. & Stolberg H.O. (eds) Intravascular contrast media. Ionic versus non-ionic: current status. *Radiol. Clin. N. Am.* **29**, 437–454.
17. *Royal College of Radiologists' Guidelines with Regard to Metformin-Induced Lactic Acidosis and X-Ray Contrast Medium Agents* (1999) London: The Royal College of Radiologists.
18. Jaffiol, C., Baldet, L., Bada, M. & Vierne, Y. (1982) The influence on thyroid function of two iodine containing radiological contrast media. *Br. J. Radiol.* **55**, 263–265.
19. Craig, J.O.M.C. (1988) Editorial. Consent in diagnostic radiology. *Clin. Radiol.* **39**, 1.
20. *Seeking Patients' Consent: The Ethical Considerations.* London: General Medical Council.
21. *Intimate Examinations* (1998) London: The Royal College of Radiologists.
22. Smith, A.McC. (1992) Consent to treatment in childhood. *Arch. Dis. Child.* **67**, 1247–1248.
23. Silverman, S.G., Mueller, P.R. & Pfister, R.C. (1990) Hemostatic evaluation before abdominal interventions: an overview and proposal. *Am. J. Roentgenol.* **154**, 233–238.
24. Rapaport, S.I. (1990) Assessing hemostatic function before abdominal interventions. *Am. J. Roentgenol.* **154**, 239–240.
25. Payne-Jeremiah, W.D. (1977) Pre-radiographic bowel preparation: a comprehensive reappraisal of factors. *Radiography* **43**, 3–14.

Further reading

Craig, O. (1985) The radiologist and the courts. *Clin. Radiol.* **36**, 475–478.

RADIONUCLIDE IMAGING RN

RADIOPHARMACEUTICALS

Radionuclides are shown in symbolic notation, the most frequently used in nuclear medicine being ^{99m}Tc, a 140-keV gamma-emitting radioisotope of the element technetium with $T_{1/2} = 6.0$ h.

Radioactive injections

In the UK, the Administration of Radioactive Substances Advisory Committee (ARSAC) advises the health ministers on the Medicines (Administration of Radioactive Substances) Regulations 1978 (MARS). These require that radioactive materials may only be administered to humans by a doctor or dentist holding a current ARSAC certificate or by a person acting under their direction. Administration of radioactive substances can only be carried out by an individual who has received appropriate theoretical and practical training, as specified in the Ionising Radiation (Medical Exposure) Regulations 2000[1] (see Appendix V). These will place responsibilities on the referrer to provide medical data to justify the exposure, the practitioner (ARSAC licence holder) to justify individual exposure, and operators (persons who carry out practical aspects relating to the exposure).

Activity administered

The maximum activity values quoted in the text are those currently recommended as diagnostic reference levels in the ARSAC Guidance Notes.[2] The unit used is the SI unit, the Megabecquerel (MBq). Millicuries (mCi) are still used in some countries, notably the US; 1 mCi = 37 MBq.

Radiation doses are quoted as the adult effective dose (ED) in millisieverts (mSv) from the ARSAC Guidance Notes.

The regulations require that doses to patients are kept as low as reasonably practicable (the ALARP principle) and that exposure follows accepted practice. Centres will frequently be able to administer activities below the maximum, depending upon the capabilities of their equipment and local protocols. Typical figures are given in the text where they differ from the diagnostic reference levels. In certain circumstances, the person clinically directing (ARSAC licence holder) may use activity higher than the recommended maximum for a named patient, for example for an obese patient where attenuation would otherwise degrade image quality.

ARSAC recommends that activities administered for paediatric investigations should be reduced according to body weight, but no longer in a linear relationship. The guidance notes include a table of suggested scaling factors based on producing comparable quality images to those expected for adults, with a minimum activity of 10% of the adult value for most purposes. However, organs develop at different rates (e.g. the brain achieves 95% of its adult size by age 5 years) and some radiopharmaceuticals behave differently in children, so the administered activity may need to be adjusted accordingly. It should be noted that when scaling activity according to the suggested factors, the radiation dose to a child may be higher than that to an adult.

Equipment

Gamma cameras usually have one or two imaging heads. Double-headed systems have the advantage of being able to image two sites simultaneously, which in many cases can roughly halve the imaging time. This can be a great advantage for SPECT (single-photon emission computed tomography) scans where minimizing patient movement can be critical.

Recent developments on double-headed systems include transmission line sources for measured attenuation correction, and coincidence imaging systems for PET (positron emission tomography).

All gamma cameras are now supplied with imaging computer systems, and the text assumes that all images are acquired to computer for appropriate processing.

Technique

Patient positioning

The resolution of gamma camera images is critically dependent on the distance of the collimator surface from the patient, falling off approximately linearly with distance. Every effort should therefore be made to position the camera as close to the patient as possible. For example, in posterior imaging with the patient supine, the thickness of the bed separates the patient from the camera, as well as interposing an attenuating medium. In this case, imaging with the patient sitting or standing directly against the camera is preferable.

Patient immobilization for the duration of image acquisition is very important. If a patient is uncomfortable or awkwardly positioned, they will have a tendency to move gradually and perhaps imperceptibly, which will have a blurring effect on the image. Point marker sources attached to the patient away from areas being examined can help to monitor and possibly permit correction for movement artefact.

'Oldendorf ' bolus injection[3]

For some investigations the Oldendorf technique is recommended to provide an abrupt bolus:

1. Place a butterfly needle (20 G or larger) in the antecubital vein.
2. Attach to a three-way tap connected to two syringes, one containing 10 ml saline and the other the radiopharmaceutical in a small volume (< 1 ml).
3. Place a blood pressure cuff on the arm and inflate to below diastolic pressure for about 1 min to suffuse veins.
4. Inflate above systolic pressure for 1–2 min to provoke reactive hyperaemia when cuff is released.
5. Inject radionuclide.
6. Release cuff and flush with saline.

Images

The image acquisition times quoted in the text should only be considered an approximate guide, since the appropriate time will depend upon such factors as the sensitivity of the available equipment, the amount of activity injected and the size of the patient. An acceptable time will usually be a compromise between the time available, the counts required for a diagnostic image and the ability of the patient to remain motionless.

Aftercare

Radiation safety

Special instructions should be given to patients who are breast feeding regarding expression of milk and interruption of feeding.[2] Precautions may have to be taken with patients leaving hospital or returning to wards, depending upon the radionuclide and activity administered. These precautions are under review following the introduction of the new Ionising Radiation Regulations 1999 and the adoption of lower dose limits to members of the public, and new guidance has been published.[4]

Complications

With few exceptions (noted in the text), the amount of biologically active substance injected with radionuclide investigations is at trace levels and very rarely causes any systemic reactions. Those that may occasionally cause problems are labelled blood products, antibodies and substances of a particulate nature.

References

1. *The Ionising Radiation (Medical Exposure) Regulations* (2000) London: HMSO.
2. Administration of Radioactive Substances Advisory Committee (1998) *Notes for Guidance on the Clinical Administration of Radiopharmaceuticals and use of Sealed Radioactive Sources.* Didcot: NRPB.
3. Oldendorf, W.H., Kitano, M. & Shimizy, F. (1965) Evaluation of a simple technique for abrupt intravenous injection of radionuclide. *J. Nucl. Med.* **6**, 205–209.
4. Working Party of the Radiation Protection Committee of the British Institute of Radiology (1999) Patients leaving hospital after administration of radioactive substances. *Br. J. Radiol.* **72**, 121–125.

COMPUTERIZED TOMOGRAPHY   CT

Patient preparation

Many CT examinations require little physical preparation. An explanation of the procedure, the time it is likely to take, the necessity for immobility and the necessity for breath-holding whilst scanning chest and abdomen should be given. Waiting times should be kept to a minimum, as this tends to increase anxiety. The patient should be as pain-free as is practical but too heavy sedation or analgesia may be counter-productive – patient cooperation is often required. Children under the age of 4 years will usually need sedation; a suitable regime is given on p. 7. Children should also have an i.v. cannula inserted at the time sedation is administered or local anaesthetic cream applied to two sites if i.v. contrast medium is needed. If these simple steps are taken the number of aborted scans will be reduced and the resultant image quality be improved.

Intravenous contrast medium

Many CT examinations will require i.v. contrast medium. Allergy and atopy should be excluded. If present, follow the relevant guidelines regarding the use of steroid prophylaxis and use LOCM. An explanation of the need for contrast enhancement should be given to the patient.

The dose will depend on the area examined: head – 50 ml; abdomen – 100 ml, given initially as a bolus of 20 ml followed by 2 ml s^{-1} during scanning. In children a maximum dose of 2 ml kg^{-1} body weight (300 mg I ml^{-1}) should be observed.

Oral contrast medium

For examinations of the abdomen, opacifying the bowel

Table 1.1   Timing and volume for oral contrast medium in CT

	Volume (ml)	Time before scan (min)
Adult		
Full abdomen and pelvis	1000	Gradually over 1 h before scanning
Upper abdomen, e.g. pancreas	500	Gradually over 0.5 h before scanning
Child		
Newborn	60–90	Full dose 1 h before scanning and a further half dose immediately prior to the scan
1 month–1 year	120–240	
1–5 years	240–360	
5–10 years	360–480	
Over 10 years	As for adult	
		If the large bowel needs to be opacified then give the contrast medium the night before or 3–4 h before scanning

satisfactorily can be problematic. Water-soluble contrast medium (2–3% Urografin flavoured to disguise the taste [15–20 ml Urografin 150 diluted in 1 l of orange squash]) or low-density barium suspensions (2% w/v) can be used. Timing of administration is given in Table 1.1. Doses of contrast media in children depend on age.

Pelvic scanning

Rarely it may be necessary to opacify the rectum using direct instillation of contrast medium or air via catheter. The concentration of contrast medium should be the same as for oral administration; 150 ml is adequate. Vaginal tampons may also be used. The air trapped by the tampon produces good negative contrast.

SAFETY IN MRI   MR

Potential hazards associated with magnetic resonance imaging which may affect patients and staff are due to:

1. Magnetic fields
   a. static field
   b. gradient field
   c. radiofrequency field
2. Auditory effects of noise
3. Inert gas quench
4. Claustrophobia
5. Intravenous contrast agents (see Chapter 2).

Table 1.2 Guidelines on exposure in MRI

	USA FDA guidelines	UK NRPB guidelines
Max. static field (Tesla)	2.0	Whole body: 2.5
		Part body: 4.0
Whole-body-specific absorption rate (W kg^{-1}); (see text)	0.4	$t^* > 30$ min: 1
		$15 < t < 30$:30/t
		$t < 15$ min: 2
Temperature rise		
Whole body (°C)	1	0.5
Skull	38	38
Trunk	39	39
Limb	40	40

t^* = time of exposure.

Effects due to magnetic fields

The effects due to magnetic fields are largely dependent on the field strengths used, and as a result guidelines have been issued by the various regulatory authorities that advise on the maximum to be used (Table 1.2).

Static field

Biological effects

Despite extensive research, no deleterious physiological effects have been found. There have been reports of minor changes, such as alteration in electrocardiogram (T wave elevation) presumed to be due to eddy currents induced in circulating electrolytes. This change is purely temporary and disappears on removal from the field. Alterations in length of cardiac cycle, changes in red cell morphology, alterations in haemostasis, increased nerve cell excitability, alterations in growth patterns and activity, alteration in behaviour in rats, changes in blood–brain barrier permeability have all been reported but do not appear to be significant in vivo. Reports of chromosomal aberrations in lymphocyte culture, and also increased malformations in chick and frog embryo development, have been made but are not considered to be a significant danger in mammalian development, and teratogenesis in humans is thought unlikely at the field strengths used in clinical MRI.

Non-biological effects

There are two main areas of concern.

1. Ferromagnetic materials may undergo rotational or translational movement as a result of the field.

Rotational movement occurs as a result of an elongated object trying to align with the field. This may result in displacement of the object, and this applies to certain types of surgical clip. Not all materials implanted are ferromagnetic and many are only weakly so. Each type should be checked individually for any such risk. In many cases, post-operative fibrosis (greater than 6 weeks) is strong enough to anchor the material so that no danger of displacement exists.

Translational movement occurs when loose ferromagnetic objects are attracted to the field. Objects such as paperclips or hairgrips may reach considerable speeds and could potentially cause severe damage to patient or equipment. This is the so-called missile effect.

2. Electrical devices such as cardiac pacemakers may be affected by the static field strengths as low as 5 Gauss. Most modern pacemakers have a sensing mechanism that can be bypassed by a magnetically operated relay and this relay can be triggered by fields as low as 5 Gauss. Relay closure can be expected in virtually all pacemakers placed in the bore of the magnet.

Gradient field

Biological effects

Sudden changes in field strength during acquisition may induce voltages in the body. The strength of these is dependent on the rate of change of the field, the cross-sectional area and the conductivity of the tissue. Possible effects include direct stimulation of nerve or muscle. Magnetophosphenes are visual flashes perceived by the subject. They are produced by direct stimulation of the optic pathways and are the most likely effects to occur since the threshold is much lower than for other direct nerve or muscle depolarization.

Non-biological effects

Rapidly varying fields can induce currents in conductors. Metal objects may heat up rapidly and cause tissue damage. Instances of partial and full thickness burns, arising when conducting loops (e.g. ECG electrodes or surface imaging coils) have come into contact with skin, are well recorded.

Radiofrequency fields

Energy is absorbed by the stimulation of protons and is largely dissipated as heat. Radiofrequency (RF) energy also induces voltages similar to the time-varying field. These voltages are oscillating, and currents thus produced are not capable of inducing depolarization but are capable of producing heat through resistive losses. Energy deposited in this way is calculated in terms of the specific absorption rate (SAR) measured in Watts per kilogram (W kg^{-1}). Total body temperature rises do occur but are insignificant (0.3°C). Of more concern are the temperature rises in tissue close to surface coils. Temperature rises of several degrees Celsius have been measured in the skin of the scrotum and the cornea. No adverse effects on spermatogenesis have yet been found within the defined power limits used.

Noise

During imaging, noise arises from vibration in the gradient coils and other parts of the scanner due to the varying magnetic fields. The amplitude of this noise does depend on such physical characteristics as the strength of the magnetic fields, pulse sequence and the design.

Noise levels may reach as much as 95 dB for long periods of time. This level is greater than agreed noise limits in industry. Temporary or even permanent hearing loss has been reported.

Where noise levels are excessive the use of earplugs or headphones is advised.

Inert gas quench

Where superconducting magnets are used the coolant gases, liquid helium or nitrogen, can vaporize should the temperature inadvertently rise. This could potentially lead to asphyxiation or exposure to extreme cold and result in frostbite. To prevent this, a well-ventilated room with some form of oxygen monitor to raise alarm should be installed.

Psychological effects

Some patients find the interior of the scanner a very disconcerting environment and report claustrophobic and even acute anxiety symptoms. This may occur in as many as 10% of patients. Approximately 1% of investigations may have to be curtailed as a result.

To decrease the number of scans aborted, the counselling, explanation to and reassurance of patients by well-trained staff should be routine.

Intravenous contrast media

See Chapter 2.

RECOMMENDATIONS FOR SAFETY

Controlled and restricted access

Access to the scanning suite should be limited. Areas should be designated as controlled (10 Gauss line) and restricted (5 Gauss line). No patient with a pacemaker should be allowed to enter the restricted area. Any person who enters this area should be made aware of the hazards of, in particular, the 'missile effect'. Any person entering the controlled area should remove all loose ferromagnetic materials such as paperclips and pens, and it is advisable that any magnetic tape or credit cards do not come near the magnet. Other considerations include the use of specially adapted cleaning equipment such as long extensions to vacuum cleaners. Fire extinguishers must be constructed from non-ferromagnetic materials. Anaesthetic equipment must be specially adapted in the same way.

Implants

As mentioned above, persons with pacemakers must not enter the controlled area. All other persons must be screened to ensure there is no danger from implanted ferromagnetic objects such as aneurysm clips. Where an object is not known to be 'magnet safe', then the person should not be scanned. Lists of safe and unsafe implants are available and some common examples are included in Table 1.3.

Occupational screening is also advisable to assess the risk of shrapnel; intraocular foreign bodies in metal workers have been known to migrate and cause further damage.

Pregnancy

Although no conclusive evidence of teratogenesis exists in humans, scanning should be avoided, particularly during the first trimester, unless alternative diagnostic procedures would involve the exposure of the fetus to ionizing radiation. Pregnant staff are advised to remain outside the controlled area (10 Gauss line) and to avoid exposure to gradient or RF fields.

References

1. Kanal, E., Shellock, F.G. & Talagala, L. (1990) Safety considerations in MR imaging. *Radiology* **176**, 593–606.

Table 1.3   Some common metallic implants

Type	Deflection*	Max. field strength tested (Tesla)
Aneurysm and haemostatic clips		
Drake DR20	Yes	1.5
Downs multipositional	Yes	1.44
Autosuture GIA	No	1.5
Hemoclip tantalum	No	1.5
Heart valves†		
Starr Edwards 1260	Yes	2.35
Bjork-Shiley	No	1.5
Intravascular devices		
Gianturco coil	Yes	1.5
Greenfield filter		
Steel	Yes	1.5
Titanium	No	1.5
Orthopaedic implants‡		
Charnley THR	No	
AO plates	No	
Dental materials		
Amalgam	No	
Wire	Yes (probably safe)	
Miscellaneous		
CSF shunt	No	
Bullet	Yes	
AMS 800 artificial sphincter	No	
IUD, copper 7	No	
Copper T	No	

*Deflection refers to rotational movement as a result of the primary field.
†Many heart valves are safe because the deflection force is insignificant when compared with the mechanical forces already present. The exception are some valves pre-1964 in origin.
‡Most orthopaedic implants are safe.

2. Jehenson, P., Duboc, D., Lavergne, T., et al. (1988) Change in human cardiac rhythm induced by a 2T static imaging field. *Radiology* **166**, 227–230.
3. Brummett, R.E., Talbot, J.M. & Charuhas, P. (1988) Potential hearing loss resulting from MR imaging. *Radiology* **169**, 539–540.
4. Quirk, M.E., Letendre, A.J., Ciottone, R.A., et al. (1989) Anxiety in patients undergoing MR imaging. *Radiology* **170**, 463–466.
5. Carrington, B.M. (1991) Biosafety. In: Hricak, H. & Carrington, B.M. (eds) *MRI of the Pelvis*, pp. 37–42. London: Martin Dunitz.

ULTRASONOGRAPHY   US

Patient preparation

For many US examinations no preparation is required. This includes examination of tissue such as thyroid, breast, testes, musculoskeletal, vascular and cardiac. In certain situations simple preparatory measures are required.

Abdomen

For optimal examination of the gallbladder it should be dilated. This requires fasting for 6–8 h before scanning.

Pelvis

To optimally visualize the pelvic contents, bowel gas must be displaced. This is easily accomplished by filling the urinary bladder to capacity. This then acts as a transonic 'window'. The patient should be instructed to drink 1–2 pints of water during the hour prior to scanning and not to empty their bladder.

In practice, both abdominal and pelvic scanning are often performed at the same attendance. Oral intake of clear fluids will not provoke gallbladder emptying and so the two preparations can be combined.

Endoscopic

Endoscopic examination of rectum or vagina requires no physical preparation but an explanation of the procedure in a sympathetic manner is needed.

Examination of the oesophagus or transoesophageal echo-cardiography require preparation similar to upper gastrointestinal endoscopy. The patient should be starved for 4 h prior to the procedure to minimize the risk of vomiting, reflux and aspiration. Anaesthesia and sedation are partly a matter of personal preference of the operator. Local anaesthesia of the pharynx can be obtained using 10% lignocaine spray. Care to avoid overdose is essential as lignocaine is rapidly absorbed via this route. The maximum dose of lignocaine should not exceed 200 mg; the xylocaine spray metered dose applicator delivers 10 mg per dose. Intravenous sedation using benzodiazepines such as Diazemuls 10 mg or midazolam 2–5 mg may also be necessary. If local anaesthetic has been used then the patient must be instructed to avoid hot food or drink until the effect has worn off (1–2 h).

Children

Ultrasound examination in children can, in most cases, be performed with no preparation apart from explanation and reassurance to both child and parent. In some cases where the child is excessively frightened or where immobility is required then sedation may be necessary. With echocardiography in infants, sedation is essential to obtain optimal recordings. The sedation regimes described on p. 7 may be used.

2 Intravascular contrast media

HISTORICAL DEVELOPMENT OF RADIOGRAPHIC AGENTS

The first report of opacification of the urinary tract by renal excretion rather than by retrograde introduction of a contrast agent appeared in 1923 when Osborne et al. took advantage of the fact that i.v. injected 10% sodium iodide solution, which was used in the treatment of syphilis, was excreted in the urine.[1] In an effort to detoxify the iodine, Binz and Rath in Berlin synthesized a number of pyridine rings containing iodine. One of these, Selectan Neutral, was excreted in the urine but the images were poor and there was anxiety about the side-effects. Swick suggested some modifications to the molecule and in 1928 and 1929 the first i.v. urograms with the compound Uroselectan were performed.[2–4] This mono-iodinated compound was developed further into the di-iodinated compounds, Uroselectan-B (Neo-ipax) and diodone (Diodrast) and in 1952 the first tri-iodinated compound, sodium acetrizoate (Urokon), was introduced into clinical radiology. Sodium acetrizoate was based on a 6-carbon ring structure, tri-iodo benzoic acid, and was the precursor of all modern water-soluble contrast media.

In 1955 a much safer derivative became available – diatrizoate (Urografin, Hypaque). This was a fully substituted benzoic acid derivative with an acetamido group at the previously unsubstituted position 5. Isomerization of diatrizoate and substitution at position 5 of N-methyl carbamyl produced the iothalamate ion (Conray) in 1962. Modern HOCM are distinguished by differences at position 5 of the anion and by the cations sodium and/or meglumine.

All conventional ionic water-soluble contrast media or high-osmolar contrast media (HOCM) are hypertonic with osmolalities of 1200–2000 mosmol kg^{-1} water, 4–7 × the osmolarity of blood. Almén first postulated that many of the adverse effects of contrast media were the result of high osmolality and that by eliminating the cation, which does not contribute to diagnostic information but is responsible for up to 50% of the osmotic effect, it would be possible to reduce the toxicity of contrast media.[5,6]

In order to decrease the osmolality without changing the iodine concentration, the ratio between the number of iodine atoms and the number of dissolved particles must be increased. Conventional ionic contrast media have a ratio of three iodine atoms per molecule to two particles in solution, i.e. a ratio of 3:2 or 1.5 (Table 2.1). In 1972, a new agent was introduced for radiculo-

Table 2.1   Schematic illustration of the development of contrast media

Name	Chemical structure	No. of iodine atoms/ions (A)	No. of particles in solution (B)	Ratio of A/B	Osmolality of a 280 mg I ml^{-1} solution
Sodium iodide	Na$^+$I$^-$	1	2	0.5	
Diodone		2	2	1	
Diatrizoate Iothalamate Metrizoate Iodamide	monomeric–monoacidic	3	2	1.5	1500
Iocarmate	dimeric–diacidic	6	3	2	1040
Ioxaglate	dimeric–monoacidic	6	2	3	490
Iopamidol Iohexol Iopramide Iopentol Ioversol	monomeric–non-ionic	3	1	3	470
Iotrolan	dimeric–non-ionic	6	1	6	

Meg = meglumine; R = an unspecified side-chain.

graphy. This was produced by linking two iothalamate molecules to form a dimer – iocarmate (Dimer X). This has since been withdrawn for toxicological reasons, but the iodine/particle ratio was increased to two and the osmolality decreased (Table 2.1).

Further development has proceeded along two separate paths. The first was, again, to combine two tri-iodinated benzene rings to produce an anion with six iodine atoms. Replacement of one of the carboxylic acid groups with a non-ionizing radical means that only one cation is necessary for each molecule. This anion, ioxaglate, is marketed as a mixed sodium and meglumine salt (Hexabrix). The alternative approach was to produce a compound that does not ionize in solution and so does not provide radiologically useless cations. Contrast media of this type include metrizamide (Amipaque), iopamidol (Niopam, Iopamiro, Iopamiron, Isovue, Solutrast), iohexol (Omnipaque), iopromide (Ultravist), iomeprol (Iomeron) and ioversol (Optiray).

For both types of contrast media the ratio of iodine atoms in the molecule to the number of particles in solution is 3:1. Compared with conventional HOCM, the new LOCM show a theoretical halving of osmolality for equi-iodine solutions. However, because of aggregation of molecules in solution the measured reduction is approximately one-third[7] (Fig. 2.1).

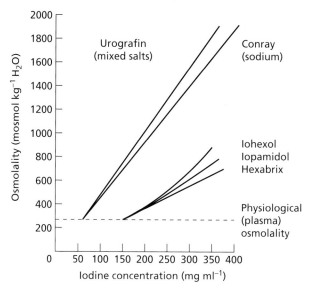

Figure 2.1   A plot of osmolality against iodine concentration for new and conventional contrast media. From Dawson et al.[8] (Reproduced by courtesy of the editor of *Clinical Radiology*.)

A further development of LOCM has been non-ionic dimers – iotrolan (Isovist) and iodixanol (Visipaque). These have a ratio of six iodine atoms for each molecule in solution, and satisfactory iodine concentrations can now be obtained at iso-osmolality. In addition to the increased financial cost these compounds also have the problem of high viscosity at room temperature.[9] With development having reached the stage of iso-osmolality, further development has been targeted on decreasing the chemotoxicity of the molecule. Increased hydrophilicity due to an increased number of hydroxyl groups provides a high affinity for water and shelters the toxic iodine atoms from the human body.

It should be noted that the terms 'low-osmolar' and 'non-ionic' are not synonymous. Iopamidol, iohexol, iotrolan, iopramide, ioversol, iopentol, iomeprol and ioxaglate are all low-osmolar, but the latter is not non-ionic. The major clinical difference between the two groups is that ionic contrast media cannot be used in the subarachnoid space.

ADVERSE EFFECTS OF INTRAVENOUS WATER-SOLUBLE CONTRAST MEDIA

When large doses of contrast medium are administered i.v. to animals to determine the LD_{50}, they show apprehension, vomiting, urination, defecation, muscle twitching and convulsions. Capillary breakdown in the lungs causes pulmonary haemorrhage and right heart failure. LOCM have lower LD_{50} values than HOCM, by a factor of approximately three (Table 2.2). Deaths in humans due to overdosage have mostly occurred in infants and children and have mostly been the result of hyperosmolar effects.

Intrinsic toxicity of contrast media is a function of osmolarity, chemical structure (chemotoxicity) or lipophilicity.

Table 2.2 LD_{50} data for some commonly used contrast media (Data from manufacturers' references)

	LD_{50} (mouse i.v. g I kg^{-1})
Urografin	7.6
Conray	8.0
Hexabrix	12.5
Niopam	21.8
Omnipaque	24.2

TOXIC EFFECTS ON SPECIFIC ORGANS

Vascular toxicity

Venous

1. Pain at the injection site – usually the result of a perivenous injection.
2. Pain extending up the arm – due to stasis of contrast medium in the vein. May be relieved by abducting the arm.
3. Delayed limb pain – due to thrombophlebitis as a result of the toxic effect on endothelium.

Immediate and delayed pain is more common with sodium-containing ionic contrast media than those containing meglumine. LOCM are less toxic to endothelium. Contrast medium-induced thrombophlebitis and venous thrombosis are particular complications of lower limb venography with a four-fold increase with HOCM compared to LOCM.

Arterial

Arterial endothelial damage and vasodilatation are mostly related to hyperosmolality. Contrast medium injected during peripheral arteriography causes a sensation of heat or pain. These symptoms are considerably reduced when LOCM are used and particularly so when non-ionic dimers are used.

Soft tissue toxicity

Pain, swelling, erythema and even sloughing of skin may occur from extravasated contrast medium. The risk is increased when pumps are used to inject large volumes of contrast medium during CT examinations. Treatment should consist of the application of cold packs and elevation of the limb should be considered. Systemic steroids, non-steroidal anti-inflammatory drugs and antibiotics have all been shown to be useful.

Cardiovascular toxicity

1. Intracoronary injection of contrast media may cause ventricular fibrillation, ventricular tachycardia, asystole, sinus bradycardia, heart block, increased QT interval, QRS prolongation, ST depression and increased T wave amplitude. HOCM are weak binders of ionic calcium.[10] Significant reductions in ionic calcium are caused by diatrizoate compounds because of the addition of the chelating agent sodium citrate as a stabilizing agent. The mechanism is in part due to calcium binding by sodium edetate. Non-ionic cause considerably less physiological cardiac disturbance.

2. Increased vagal activity may result in depression of the sino-atrial and atrio-ventricular nodes, resulting in bradycardia or asystole.
3. The injection of a hypertonic contrast medium causes significant fluid and ion shifts. Immediately after injection there is a significant increase in serum osmolality. This causes an influx of water from the interstitial space into the vascular compartment, an increase in blood volume, an increase in cardiac output and a brief increase of systemic blood pressure. Peripheral dilatation causes a more prolonged fall of blood pressure. Injection into the right heart or pulmonary artery causes transitory pulmonary hypertension and systemic hypotension; injection into the left ventricle or aorta causes brief systemic hypertension followed by a more prolonged fall.

Haematological changes

1. In the presence of a high concentration of contrast medium, such as withdrawal of blood into a syringe of contrast medium, damage to red cell walls occurs and haemolysis follows. Haemolysis and haemoglobinuria have been reported following angiocardiography with diatrizoate and acute renal failure may supervene. It is advisable not to re-inject blood that has been mixed with contrast medium.
2. Red cell aggregation and coagulation may occur in the presence of a high concentration of contrast medium, e.g. 350 mg I ml^{-1}. However, disaggregation occurs easily and this is not likely to be of any clinical significance.[11]
3. Contrast media impair blood clotting and platelet aggregation. LOCM have a minimal effect compared to HOCM.[12]
4. Contrast media have a potentiating effect on the action of heparin.
5. Thrombus formation also occurs and is more common when blood is mixed with LOCM. However, the role of the syringe is also significant and thrombus formation is maximal when blood is slowly withdrawn into a syringe so that it layers on top of the contrast medium, against the wall of the syringe. Activation of coagulation by the tube material (worse with glass syringes and those made from styrene acrylonitrile) probably plays a significant role.
6. Sickle cell crisis has been provoked by contrast medium and diatrizoate > 35% concentration causes HbSS blood to sickle

in vitro. LOCM have a lesser effect and their use is indicated in this disease.[13]

7. When red blood cells are placed in a hypertonic contrast medium, water leaves the interior of the cells by osmosis and they become more rigid. Red cell rigidity or deformability is, thus, dependent on osmolality. However, isosmolar solutions may also have an effect on red cell deformability, indicating that there may also be a chemical effect. Red cells that deform less easily are less able to pass through capillaries and may occlude them. This is the explanation for the transient rise in pulmonary arterial pressure during pulmonary arteriography[14] and the reason why LOCM should be used when there is any likelihood of pre-existing pulmonary hypertension. It may also be a factor in the deterioration of renal function that is occasionally encountered after contrast administration.[15]

8. Transient eosinophilia may occur 24–72 h after administration of contrast medium.

Nephrotoxicity

Recent reviews on the incidence of contrast-induced nephrotoxicity suggest an incidence of approximately 5%.[16–18] For the majority, the renal impairment is temporary. There are a number of predisposing factors:

1. Pre-existing impairment of renal function. This is present in 90% of reported cases of contrast medium nephrotoxicity.
2. Diabetes mellitus, which is present in 50% of cases of contrast medium nephrotoxicity. Approximately 75% of patients with juvenile onset diabetes mellitus and renal insufficiency will show deterioration of renal function after HOCM. In as many as 50% of these patients the renal function will not return to baseline levels.
3. Dehydration.
4. Age – because of the greater incidence of cardiovascular disease in the elderly.
5. Very large doses of contrast medium.
6. Multiple myeloma.
7. Other nephrotoxic drugs.

The mechanisms of contrast medium-induced nephrotoxicity have been reviewed by Dawson and are summarized below:[19]

1. Impaired renal perfusion
   a. Adverse cardiotoxic effects

   b. Increased peripheral vasodilatation
   c. Renal vascular bed changes (increased blood flow followed by a more prolonged decrease)
   d. Increased rigidity of red cells
   e. Pre-dehydration
   f. Osmotic diuresis.
2. Glomerular injury
   a. Impaired perfusion
   b. Hyperosmolar effects
   c. Chemotoxic effects.
3. Tubular injury
   a. Impaired perfusion ⎤ manifest histologically
   b. Hyperosmolar effects ⎬ as cytoplasmic
   c. Chemotoxic effects. ⎦ vacuolation.
4. Obstructive nephropathy
   a. Cytoplasmic vacuolation in tubules
   b. Precipitation of Tamm-Horsfall protein
   c. Precipitation of Bence Jones protein in multiple myeloma.

Experimental work and theoretical considerations suggest that LOCM are less nephrotoxic. However, the available evidence,[20] including a review of 43 clinical trials comparing LOCM and HOCM, concluded that there was no difference.[21]

Neurotoxicity

1. Contrast medium delivered to the brain via the arterial route may cross the blood–brain barrier. Sodium-containing HOCM are more neurotoxic than meglumine-containing HOCM. Neurotoxicity is reduced with the use of LOCM, but they do show some chemotoxic effect unrelated to osmolality.
2. Intravenous contrast medium may provoke convulsions in patients with epilepsy or cerebral tumours.[22,23] LOCM are less neurotoxic.
3. Convulsions may also occur secondary to the cerebral hypoxia caused by hypotension ± cardiac arrest.

Thyroid function

1. Thyrotoxicosis may occur in patients with non-toxic goitres, or be exacerbated in those with pre-existing thyrotoxic symptoms.
2. Contrast media may interfere with thyroid function tests.

IDIOSYNCRATIC REACTIONS

Excluding death, adverse reactions can be classified in terms of severity as:

1. Major reactions, i.e. those that interfere with the examination and require treatment.
2. Intermediate reactions, i.e. those that interfere with the examination but do not require treatment.
3. Minor reactions, i.e. those that do not interfere with the examination and require only firm assurance.

Minor and intermediate reactions are not uncommon; major adverse reactions are rare (Table 2.3).

Table 2.3   Adverse reaction rates for intravenous ionic* and non-ionic# contrast media (From Ansell et al. See Further reading)

Study	Number of examinations	Minor	Intermediate	Severe	Fatal
Shehadi [N America][24]	146 904*	1:29	1:60	1:2800	1:15000
Toniolo [Italy][14]	67 129*	1:31	1:130	1:1200	1:34000
Ansell et al. [UK][25]	164 475*	1:15	1:76	1:4200	1:45000
Hartman et al. [N America][26]	300 000*				1:75000
Palmer [Australasia][27]	79 000*	1:30	1:284	1:1117	1:40000
	30 000#	1:96	1:1010	1:6056	
Katayama et al. [Japan][28]	169 284*			1:394	1:169000
	168 363#			1:2215	1:168000
Wolf et al. [USA][29]	6006*	1:35	1:86	1:316	
	8857#	1:227	1:738	1:8857	

The incidence of severe reactions is reduced (by approximately 80%) when LOCM are used.

Fatal reactions

The number of deaths due to contrast media is small and makes comparison of ionic and non-ionic contrast media difficult. However, it is widely believed that there is no difference in the mortality rate between the two types of contrast media. Almost all fatal reactions occur in the minutes following injection and patients must be under close observation during this time. The fatal event may be preceded by trivial events, such as nausea and vomiting, or may occur without warning. The majority of deaths occur in those over 50 years of age. Causes of death include cardiac arrest, pulmonary oedema, respiratory arrest, consumption coagulopathy, bronchospasm, laryngeal oedema and angioneurotic oedema.[30]

Non-fatal reactions

1. *Flushing, metallic taste in the mouth, nausea, sneezing, cough* and *tingling* are common and related to dose and speed of injection. Ioxaglate is associated with a higher incidence of vomiting and anaphylactoid reactions, whereas LOCM in general are associated with a lower incidence.

2. *Perineal burning, a desire to empty the bladder or rectum* and *a spurious feeling of having been incontinent of urine* are more common in women.

3. *Urticaria.*

4. *Angioneurotic oedema.* Most commonly affects the face. May persist for up to 3 days and its onset may be delayed.

5. *Rigors.*

6. *Necrotizing skin lesions.* Rare and mostly in patients with pre-existing renal failure (particularly those with systemic lupus erythematosus).

7. *Bronchospasm.* Predisposed to by a history of asthma and concurrent therapy with β-blockers.[25] In most patients the bronchospasm is subclinical. Bronchospasm is much less pronounced with LOCM than with HOCM.[31] LOCM are preferable in patients with asthma and these patients should also receive steroid prophylaxis. Mechanisms for contrast medium-induced bronchospasm include:
   a. Direct histamine release from mast cells and platelets
   b. Cholinesterase inhibition
   c. Vagal overtone
   d. Complement activation
   e. Direct effect of contrast media on bronchi.

8. *Non-cardiogenic pulmonary oedema.* During acute anaphylaxis or hypotensive collapse and possibly due to increased capillary permeability.

9. *Arrhythmias.*

10. *Hypotension.* Usually accompanied by tachycardia but in some patients there is vagal over-reaction with bradycardia.[32,33] The latter is rapidly reversed by atropine 0.6–2 mg i.v. Hypotension is usually mild and is treatable by a change of posture. Rarely, it is severe and may be accompanied by pulmonary oedema.[34]

11. *Abdominal pain.* May be a symptom in anaphylactic reactions or vagal overactivity. Should be differentiated from the loin pain that may be precipitated in patients with upper urinary tract obstruction.

12. *Delayed-onset reactions – rashes, headaches, itching and parotid gland swelling.*

MECHANISMS OF IDIOSYNCRATIC CONTRAST MEDIUM REACTIONS

Histamine release

Contrast media cause the release of histamine from mast cells and basophils and this could provide a mechanism for the phenomena of flushing, urticaria, metallic taste, hypotension, collapse and angioneurotic oedema. While hyperosmolality is a factor, isosmolar concentrations of contrast media will also stimulate histamine release. The basophils of allergic individuals do release more histamine than those of normal individuals.[35] The histamine-releasing properties of contrast media differ, with LOCM causing less histamine release than HOCM. Meglumine salts have a greater effect than sodium salts and this is reflected in the four-fold increase in the incidence of bronchospasm when the former is compared with the latter. Bronchospasm may be due to the effect of contrast medium on pulmonary-bed mast cells and dysrrhythmias from the effect on cardiac mast cells.

Complement activation

Lasser et al.[36] have hypothesized that damage to vascular endothelium stimulates a complex of activation systems resulting in the formation of kinins, thrombus, fibrinogen degradation products, histamine release and haemolysis. A number of inhibitors limit the extent to which these systems function. One such inhibitor, C1-inhibitor, has been shown to be lower in those exhibiting contrast medium-induced reactions than in non-reactors and the variability of severity of reactions, both between patients and in any individual on different occasions, may be related to variable inhibitor levels. As LOCM cause less endothelial damage than HOCM it is to be expected that activation systems will be less important with the new contrast media.

Protein binding and enzyme inhibition

Contrast media are weakly protein bound and the degree of protein binding correlates well with their ability to inhibit the enzyme acetylcholinesterase.[37] Contrast medium side-effects such as vasodilatation, bradycardia, hypotension, bronchospasm and urticaria are all recognized cholinergic effects and it was postulated that they may be related more to cholinesterase inhibition than osmolality. LOCM are less effective enzyme inhibitors as well as having lower osmolality, whilst the biliary contrast agent, meglumine ioglycamide, is the most strongly protein-bound contrast agent and the most toxic. However, in vitro inhibition of acetylcholinesterase by contrast media is reversed by the addition of 1% albumen, suggesting that under physiological conditions protein binding and acetylcholinesterase inhibition do not have a significant role in contrast medium reactions.[38]

Chemotoxicity

In addition to the toxicity of the contrast medium because of its intrinsic structure, the electrical charge on the particles of the HOCM and of Hexabrix (sodium/meglumine ioxaglate) is of particular importance in intracoronary and intrathecal use. The cations are clinically more toxic than the anions and sodium is more toxic than meglumine to brain (increased incidence of convulsions in patients with altered blood–brain barrier) and myocardium (increased incidence of arrhythmias). The toxicity of intracoronary ionic agents is partly related to their greater propensity to bind calcium.[39] The high incidence of adverse reactions when LOCM or sodium/meglumine ioxaglate is introduced into the subarachnoid space is almost certainly related to the electrical charge on the particles.

Although the major adverse effect on erythrocytes is due to hyperosmolality, even contrast medium which is iso-osmolar with plasma produces changes in red blood cell morphology which reveal the intrinsic chemotoxicity of contrast medium molecules.[40]

Anxiety

Lalli[41] has postulated that most, if not all, contrast medium reactions are the result of the patient's fear and apprehension. The high autonomic nervous system activity in an anxious patient will be stimulated further when the patient experiences the administration of contrast medium. Furthermore, contrast medium crossing the blood–brain barrier can stimulate the limbic area and hypothalamus to produce further autonomic activity. This autonomic activity is responsible for contrast medium reactions by the sequence of events illustrated in Figure 2.2.

Support for Lalli's hypothesis is found in the work of Heron et al.[42] who showed a significant correlation between ECG changes and more subjective side-effects experienced after contrast injection. When compared with HOCM, LOCM resulted in less frequent ECG abnormalities and subjective side-effects.

PROPHYLAXIS FOR ADVERSE CONTRAST MEDIUM REACTIONS

1. *Pre-testing*. Involves applying contrast medium to the cornea or injecting a 1 ml test dose intravenously a few minutes prior

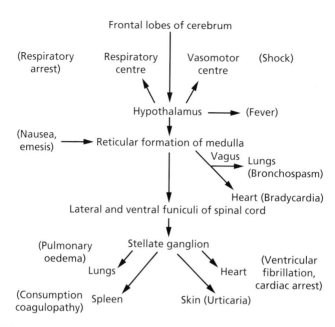

Figure 2.2 Central nervous system and contrast media reactions. From Lalli.[41] (Reproduced by courtesy of the editor of *Radiology*.)

to the full intravenous injection. However, a negative result does not preclude a major reaction when the full dose is given and a severe reaction may result from the test dose itself. The technique has, therefore, fallen into disfavour.

2. *Pre-treatment with steroids*. Those who have had a previous severe adverse reaction or who are 'at risk' may benefit from pre-treatment with steroids.[43] A suggested regime is methyl prednisolone 32 mg orally 12 and 2 h prior to injection of contrast medium.[44] However, the reduction in the incidence of adverse reactions using oral steroids is not as great as that achieved by the use of LOCM.[45] High-risk patients should be given a LOCM and steroid premedication. For the emergency administration of contrast medium to high-risk patients, when oral premedication is not possible, Greenberger et al. recommend 200 mg hydrocortisone i.v. immediately and every 4 h until the procedure is completed, and 50 mg diphenhydramine i.v. 1 h before the procedure.[46]

3. *Pre-treatment with antihistamines*. Prophylactic chlorpheniramine (Piriton) is of no benefit and, when given, is associated with a threefold increase in the incidence of flushing.[47]

4. *Change of contrast medium to a LOCM*. This is the most important factor in the reduction of contrast medium adverse reactions.
5. *Reduction of patient anxiety and apprehension*.[30] Lalli described nine patients who had previously suffered severe hypotension resulting in loss of consciousness during urography. Repeat urography after reassurance only was not accompanied by a further adverse event.[48]

INDICATIONS FOR THE USE OF LOCM

The advantages of LOCM are:

1. More comfortable arteriograms and i.v. injections.
2. Less tissue toxicity.
3. Reduction in adverse reactions.

If it were not for their expense, there would have been a complete switch to LOCM many years ago.[49] The financial implications of using LOCM for all patients and all procedures are so great that a selection process to identify those at risk must be instituted. The following should receive LOCM in preference to HOCM:[50,51]

1. Those at high risk from the hyperosmolar effects:
   a. Infants and small children and the elderly
   b. Those with renal and/or cardiac failure
   c. Poorly hydrated patients
   d. Patients with diabetes, myelomatosis or sickle cell anaemia
   e. Patients who have had a previous severe contrast medium reaction with LOCM or those with a strong allergic history
   f. High-dose procedures.
2. Those who would suffer unnecessarily from the hyperosmolar effects of HOCM, e.g. arteriography under local anaesthesia.

References

1. Osborne, E.D., Sutherland, C.G., Scholl, A.J., et al. (1923) Roentgenography of the urinary tract during excretion of sodium iodide. *JAMA* **80**, 368–373.
2. Swick, M. (1929) Darstellung der niere und harnwege in roentgenbild durch intravenose einbringung eines neuen kontraststoffes: des uroselectans. *Klin. Wochenschr.* **8**, 2087–2089.
3. Von Lichtenberg, A. & Swick, M. (1929) Klinische prüfung des uroselectans. *Klin. Wochenschr.* **8**, 2089–2091.
4. Swick, M. (1978) Radiographic media in urology. The discovery of excretion urography: historical and developmental aspects of the organically bound urographic media and their role in the varied diagnostic angiographic areas. *Surg. Clin. N. Am.* **58**, 977–994.

5. Almén, T. (1969) Contrast agent design. Some aspects of synthesis of water-soluble contrast agents of low osmolality. *J. Theor. Biol.* **24**, 216–226.
6. Almén, T. (1985) Development of nonionic contrast media. *Invest. Radiol.* **20 (suppl)**, S2–S9.
7. Grainger, R.G. (1980) Osmolality of intravascular radiological contrast media. *Br. J. Radiol.* **53**, 739–746.
8. Dawson, P., Grainger, R.G. & Pitfield, J. (1983) The new low-osmolar contrast media: a simple guide. *Clin. Radiol.* **34**, 221–226.
9. Dawson, P. & Howel, M. (1986) The non-ionic dimers: a new class of contrast agents. *Br. J. Radiol.* **59**, 987–991.
10. Morris, T.W., Sahler, L.G. & Fisher, H.W. (1982) Calcium binding in radiographic media. *Invest. Radiol.* **17**, 501–505.
11. Dawson, P., McCarthy, P., Allison, D.J., et al. (1988) Non-ionic contrast agents, red cell aggregation and coagulation. *Br. J. Radiol.* **61**, 963–965.
12. Dawson, P., Hewitt, M.R., Mackie, I.J., et al. (1986) Contrast, coagulation and fibrinolysis. *Invest. Radiol.* **21**, 248–252.
13. Rao, V.M., Rao, A.K., Steiner, R.M., Burka, E.R., Grainger, R.G. & Ballas, S.K. (1982) The effect of ionic and nonionic contrast media on the sickling phenomenon. *Radiology* **144**, 291–293.
14. Effros, R.M. (1972) Impairment of red cell transit through the canine lungs following injections of hypertonic fluids. *Circ. Res.* **31**, 590–601.
15. Golman, K. & Holtas, S. (1980) Proteinuria produced by urographic contrast media. *Invest. Radiol.* **15**, S61–S66.
16. Gomes, A.S., Lois, J.F., Baker, J.D., McGlade, C.T., Bunnell, D.H. & Hartzman, S. (1989) Acute renal dysfunction in high risk patients after angiography: Comparison of ionic and nonionic contrast media. *Radiology* **170**, 65-68.
17. Parfrey, P.S., Griffiths, S.M., Barrett, B.J., et al. (1989) Contrast material induced renal failure in patients with diabetes mellitus, renal insufficiency or both: a prospective controlled study. *N. Engl. J. Med.* **320**, 143–149.
18. Schwab, S.J., Hlatky, M.A., Pieper, K.S., et al. (1989) Contrast nephrotoxicity: a randomized control trial of nonionic and ionic radiographic contrast agent. *N. Engl. J. Med.* **320**, 149–153.
19. Dawson, P. (1985) Contrast agent nephrotoxicity. *Br. J. Radiol.* **58**, 121–124.
20. Schwab, S.J., Hlatky, M.A., Piepers, K.S., et al. (1989) Contrast nephrotoxicity. A randomised controlled trial of a non-ionic (iopamidol) and an ionic radiographic contrast agent (diatrizoate). *N. Engl. J. Med.* **320**, 149–153.
21. Kinnison, M.L., Powe, N.R. & Steinberg, E.P. (1989) Results of radiologic controlled trials of low vs high osmolality contrast media. *Radiology* **170**, 381–389.
22. Scott, W.R. (1980) Seizures, a reaction to contrast media for computed tomography of the brain. *Radiology* **137**, 359–361.
23. Fischer, H.W. (1980) Occurrence of seizures during cranial computed tomography. *Radiology* **137**, 563–564.
24. Shehadi, W.H. & Toniolo, G. (1980) Adverse reactions to contrast media. A report from the Committee on Safety of Contrast Media of the International Society of Radiology. *Radiology* **137**, 299–302.
25. Ansell, G., Tweedie, M.C.K., West, C.R., et al. (1980) The current status of reactions to intravenous contrast media. *Invest. Radiol.* **15 (Suppl)**, S32–S39.
26. Hartman, G.W., Hattery, R.R., Witten, D.M. et al. (1982) Mortality during excretory urography: Mayo Clinic experience. *Am. J. Roentgenol.* **139**, 919–922.
27. Palmer, F.G. (1988) The R.A.C.R. survey of intravenous contrast media reactions: final report. *Australas. Radiol.* **32**, 426–428.

28. Katayama, H., Yamaguchi, K., Kozuka, T., et al. (1990) Adverse reactions to ionic and non-ionic media. A report from the Japanese Committee on the Safety of Contrast Media. *Radiology* **175**, 621–628.
29. Wolf, G.L., Mishkin, M.M., Roux S.G., et al. (1991) Ionic contrast agents, ionic agents combined with steroids and nonionic agents. *Invest. Radiol.* **26**, 404–410.
30. Lalli, A.F. (1980) Contrast media reactions: data analysis and hypothesis. *Radiology* **134**, 1–12.
31. Dawson, P., Pitfield, J. & Britton, J. (1983) Contrast media and bronchospasm: a study with iopamidol. *Clin. Radiol.* **34**, 227–230.
32. Andrews, E.J. (1976) The vagus reaction as a possible cause of severe complications of radiological procedures. *Radiology* **34**, 227–230.
33. Stanley, R.J. & Pfister, R.C. (1976) Bradycardia and hypotension following use of intravenous contrast media. *Radiology* **121**, 5–7.
34. Chamberlin, W.H., Stockman, G.D. & Wray, N.P. (1979) Shock and noncardiogneic pulmonary edema following meglumine diatrizoate for intravenous pyelography. *Am. J. Med.* **67**, 684–686.
35. Arroyave, C.M. (1980) An in vitro assay for radiographic contrast media idiosyncracy. *Invest. Radiol.* **15**, S21–S25.
36. Lasser, E.C., Lang, J.H., Hamblin, A.E., Lyon, S.G. & Howard, M. (1980) Activation systems in contrast idiosyncracy. *Invest. Radiol.* **15**, S2–S5.
37. Dawson, P. & Edgerton, D. (1983) Contrast media and enzyme inhibition. 1. Cholinesterase. *Br. J. Radiol.* **56**, 653–656.
38. Tamura, A., Suzuki, T., Yamasaki, T., et al. (1991) Effect of radiological iodinated contrast media on acetylcholinesterase activity. *Br. J. Radiol.* **64**, 768–770.
39. Haywood, R. & Dawson, P. (1984) Contrast agents in angiocardiography. *Br. Heart. J.* **52**, 361–368.
40. Dawson, P., Harrison, M.J.G. & Weisblatt, E. (1983) Effect of contrast media on red cell filtrability and morphology. *Br. J. Radiol.* **56**, 707–710.
41. Lalli, A.F. (1974) Urographic contrast media reactions and anxiety. *Radiology* **112**, 267–271.
42. Heron, C.W., Underwood, S.R. & Dawson, P. (1984) Electrocardiographic changes during intravenous urography: a study with sodium iothalamate and iohexol. *Clin. Radiol.* **35**, 137–141.
43. Lasser, E.C., Lang, J., Sovak, M., Kollo, W., Lyon, S. & Hamlin, A.E. (1977) Steroids: theoretical and experimental basis for utilization in prevention of contrast media reactions. *Radiology* **125**, 1–9.
44. Lasser, E.C., Berry, C.C., Talner, L.B., et al. (1987) Pretreatment with corticosteroids to alleviate reactions to intravenous contrast material. *N. Engl. J. Med.* **317**, 845–849.
45. Wolf, G.L., Mishkin, M.M., Roux, S.G., et al. (1991) Comparison of the rates of adverse drug reactions: ionic contrast agents, ionic agents combined with steroids, and nonionic agents. *Invest. Radiol.* **26**, 404–410.
46. Greenberger, P.A., Halwig, M., Patterson, R., et al. (1986) *J. Allergy Clin. Immunol.* **77**, 630–634.
47. Davies, P., Roberts, M.B. & Roylance, J. (1975) Acute reactions to urographic contrast media. *Br. Med. J.* **ii**, 434–437.
48. Lalli, A.F. (1975) Editorial. Urography, shock reaction and repeated urography. *Am. J. Roentgenol.* **125**, 264–268.
49. Grainger, R.G. (1987) Annotation: radiological contrast media. *Clin. Radiol.* **38**, 3–5.
50. Grainger, R.G. (1984) The clinical and financial implications of the low-osmolar contrast media. *Clin. Radiol.* **35**, 251–252.
51. Granger, R. & Dawson, P. (1991) Guidelines for use of low osmolar intravascular contrast media. *Fac. Clin. Radiol. Roy. Coll. Radiol.* London.

Further reading

Ansell, G., Bettmann, M.A., Kaufman, J.A. & Wilkins, R.A. (1996) *Complications in Diagnostic Imaging and Interventional Radiology.* Oxford: Blackwell Science.

Dawson, P., Cosgrove, D.O. & Grainger, R.G. (1999) *Textbook of Contrast Media.* Oxford: Isis Medical Media.

Grainger, R.G. (1982) Intravascular contrast media – the past, the present and the future. *Br. J. Radiol.* **55**, 1–18.

CONTRAST AGENTS IN MRI

MRI

MECHANISM OF ACTION

To enhance the inherent contrast between tissues, MRI contrast agents must alter the rate of relaxation of the protons within the tissues. The changes in relaxation must vary for different tissues in order to produce differential enhancement of the signal (see Figs 2.3 and 2.4). These show that, for a given time t, if the T1 relaxation is more rapid then a larger signal is obtained (brighter images), but the opposite is true for T2 relaxation where more rapid relaxation produces reduced signal intensity (darker images).

MRI contrast agents must exert a large magnetic field density (a property imparted by their unpaired electrons) to interact with the magnetic moments of the protons in the tissues and so shorten their T1 relaxation time which will produce an increase in signal intensity (see Fig. 2.3). The electron magnetic moments also cause local changes in the magnetic field, which promotes more rapid

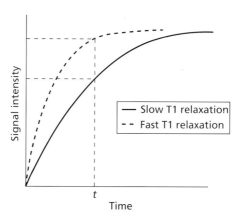

Figure 2.3 Signal intensity and T1 relaxation time.

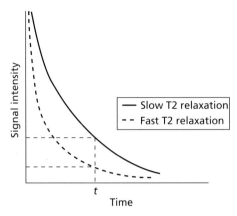

Figure 2.4   Signal intensity and T2 relaxation time.

proton dephasing and so shortens the T2 relaxation time. Agents with unpaired electron spins are therefore potential contrast agents in MRI. These may be classified into three groups:

1. *Ferromagnetic.* These have magnetic moments which align with the scanner's applied field. They will maintain their alignment even when the applied field is removed. This retained magnetism may cause particle aggregation and interfere with cell function, making them unsafe as MR contrast agents.
2. *Paramagnetic* – e.g. gadolinium (see below). These agents have magnetic moments which align to the applied field, but once the gradient field is turned off, thermal energy within the tissue is enough to overcome the alignment. They may be made soluble by chelation and can therefore be injected intravenously. Their maximum effect is on protons in the water molecule, shortening the T1 relaxation time and hence producing increased signal intensity (white) on T1 images (Fig. 2.3).
3. *Superparamagnetic* – e.g. ferrite. These are aggregates of paramagnetic ions in a crystalline lattice. They cause abrupt changes in the local magnetic field which results in rapid proton dephasing and reduction in the T2 relaxation time, and hence producing decreased signal intensity (black) on T2 images (Fig. 2.4). They are less soluble than paramagnetic agents, due to their chemical structure and so are available only as a colloidal suspension.

Both paramagnetic and superparamagnetic substances can be used as gastrointestinal contrast agents (see below).

GADOLINIUM (GD)

Chemistry

There are a number of gadolinium chelates:

1. Gd-diethylenetriaminepenta-acetic acid (DTPA), dimeglumine gadopentetate (Magnevist, Schering)
2. Gd-tetraazacyclododecanetetra-acetic acid (DOTA), meglumine gadoterate (Dotarem)
3. Gadodiamide (Gd-DTPA-bismethylamide) (Omniscan, Nycomed Amersham)
4. Gadoversetamide (Optimark)
5. Gd-DO3A, Gadoteridol (ProHance, Bracco, Merck, Squibb)
6. Gd-butrol, Gadobutrol (Gadovist)

Indications

1. CNS tumours – particularly small acoustic neuromas and spinal seedlings from posterior fossa tumours.
2. Demyelinating diseases – for differentiating acute from chronic plaques.
3. More accurate delineation of tumour margins from oedema.
4. Discrimination of tumour recurrence from post-therapy fibrosis (although fibrosis may enhance even several years after therapy, particularly if due to radiation).
5. Discrimination of recurrent intervertebral disc prolapse from postoperative fibrosis. Images must be obtained within 30 min of the injection as fibrosis enhances immediately but disc material may enhance approximately 20 min after injection.
6. Cardiac/aortic imaging.

Contraindications

No absolute contraindications are known, but roughly they are contraindicated in similar situations to iodinated contrast media. There is limited experience with any form of MRI during pregnancy and even less with the use of contrast agents, particularly in the first trimester.

Dose

Usually, 0.1 mmol kg^{-1} body weight (e.g. 0.2 ml of Magnevist kg^{-1}); up to 0.2 mmol kg^{-1} when used in low-field magnets.

Administration should be by relatively slow intravenous injection (60 s for a 40 kg individual, up to 120 s for a 100 kg person) to reduce side-effects.

Side-effects

Few are described and include:
1. Warmth
2. Pain at injection site
3. Seizure
4. Strange taste
5. Nausea
6. Headache
7. Dizziness
8. Anaphylactoid reactions may occur (at the present time seven episodes have been reported to Schering worldwide) and so medical cover should be readily available, as should resuscitation equipment.

Of these the first two are the most common, but in all they add up to only about 3% of injections (Schering Technical Brochure).

GASTROINTESTINAL CONTRAST AGENTS

These are used to distinguish bowel from adjacent soft tissue masses. As with CT, all bowel contrast agents need to mix readily with the bowel contents to ensure even distribution. They must also be palatable. They can be divided into two groups:

Positive agents

e.g. fatty oils and gadolinium.

Act by T1-shortening effects.

Appear white on T1 images.

Disadvantages

1. The high signal increases the effect of bowel motion artefact.
2. The effect varies with the pulse sequence and the contrast concentration within the bowel. This can produce non-uniformity in the signal which may cause confusion.
3. Expensive.

Negative agents

e.g. ferrite and barium sulphate (60–70% w/w).

Act by T2-shortening.

Appear black on T2 images.

Disadvantages

1. High concentrations result in image distortion and blurring of adjacent structures.
2. The required dose of ferrite is a potentially lethal dose and so enteric preparations need to be chelated to reduce the absorption of iron.
3. Rather unpalatable.

Other aids to abdominal MRI

1. Prone position of the patient results in reduced respiratory artefact
2. Smooth muscle relaxants help reduce motion artefact due to bowel peristalsis
3. Saturation pulses reduce motion artefact due to diaphragmatic movement
4. Breath holding
5. Fast pulse sequences
6. Corsets.

CONTRAST AGENTS IN ULTRASONOGRAPHY   US

Although gas microbubbles are an effective US contrast agent, bubbles smaller than 7 μm must be used to pass the pulmonary filter and bubbles of this size only remain intact for a few seconds in the blood. All US contrast media depend on the interaction between encapsulated microbubbles and the US beam. US contrast agents allow imaging of vascular structures which cannot be evaluated even with sophisticated Doppler techniques.

Levovist (Schering)

The most widely used microbubble contrast agent. Microbubbles of air enclosed by a thin layer of palmitic acid in a galactose solution. Stable in blood for 1–4 min.

Echovist (Schering)

The precursor of Levovist. Bubbles in a galactose solution but lacking the palmitic acid coating. These microbubbles cannot pass the pulmonary filter and are mostly employed to assess tubal patency.

Albunex (Molecular Biosystems Inc.)

Sonicated air microbubbles coated with human serum albumen. Used in echocardiography. Survives only a short time in the left ventricle. Little enhancement of the arterial tree.

EchoGen (Abbott)

An emulsion of dodecafluoropentane which changes its phase converting to echogenic gas microbubbles by hypobaric activation prior to i.v. injection.

SonoVue (Bracco)

An aqueous suspension of stabilized sulphur hexafluoride microbubbles. After reconstitution of the lyophilisate with saline, the suspension is stable and can be used for up to 4 h.

Further reading

Calliada, F., Campani, R., Bottinelli, O., et al. (1998) Ultrasound contrast agents. Basic principles. *Eur. J. Radiol.* **27**, S157–S160.

Dalla-Palma, L. (ed) (2000) Ultrasonography today and tomorrow: new developments and contrast media. *Eur. Radiol.* **9 (suppl 3)**.

3 Gastrointestinal tract

Methods of imaging the gastrointestinal tract

1. Plain film
2. Barium swallow
3. Barium meal
4. Barium follow-through
5. Small bowel enema
6. Barium enema
7. Ultrasound
   - Transcutaneous
   - Endosonography
8. CT
9. MRI
10. Angiography
11. Radionuclide imaging
    - Inflammatory bowel disease
    - Gastro-oesophageal reflux
    - Gastric emptying
    - Bile reflux study
    - Meckel's scan
    - Gastrointestinal bleeding.

Further reading

Kelvin, F.M. (ed.) (1992) Radiology of the alimentary tract. *Radiol. Clin. N. Am.* **20(4)**.

Nolan, D.J. (1998) Imaging of the small intestine. *Schweiz. Med. Wochenschr.* **128**, 109–114.

Ott, D.J. & Gelfand, D.W. (1997) The future of barium radiology. *Br. J. Radiol.* **5**, 171–176.

Sivit, C.J. (1997) Gastrointestinal emergencies in older infants and children. *Radiol. Clin. N. Am.* **35**, 865–877.

INTRODUCTION TO CONTRAST MEDIA

BARIUM

Barium suspension is made up from pure barium sulphate.

(Barium carbonate is poisonous.) The particles of barium must be small (0.1–3 μm), since this makes them more stable in suspension. A non-ionic suspension medium is used, for otherwise the barium particles would aggregate into clumps. The resulting solution has a pH of 5.3, which makes it stable in gastric acid.

There are many varieties of barium suspensions in use. Exact formulations are secret. In most situations the preparation may be diluted with water to give a lower density.

Proprietary name	Density (w/v)
Baritop 100	100%
EPI-C	150%
E-Z-Cat	1–2%
E-Z HD	250%
E-Z Paque	100%
Micropaque DC	100%
Micropaque liquid	100%
Micropaque powder	76%
Polibar	115%
Polibar Rapid	100%

Examinations of different parts of the gastrointestinal tract require barium preparations with differing properties.

1. *Barium swallow*, e.g. E-Z HD 250% 100 ml (or more, as required).
2. *Barium meal*, e.g. E-Z HD 250% w/v 135 ml. A high-density, low-viscosity barium is required for a double-contrast barium meal to give a good thin coating that is still sufficiently dense to give satisfactory opacification. E-Z HD fulfils these requirements. It also contains simethicone (an anti-foaming and coating agent) and sorbitol (a coating agent).[1]
3. *Barium follow-through*, e.g. E-Z Paque 60–100% w/v 300 ml (150 ml if performed after a barium meal). This preparation is partially resistant to flocculation.
4. *Small bowel enema*, e.g. two tubs of E-Z Paque made up to 1500 ml (60% w/v). N.B. As the transit time through the small bowel is relatively short in this investigation, there is a reduced chance of flocculation. This enables the use of barium preparations which are not flocculation-resistant. Some advocate the addition of Gastrografin to the mixture as this may help reduce the transit time still further.
5. *Barium enema*, e.g. Polibar 115% w/v 500 ml (or more, as required).

Advantages

1. The main advantage when compared to water soluble contrast agents is the excellent coating which can be achieved with barium, allowing the demonstration of normal and abnormal mucosal patterns.
2. Cost.

Disadvantages

1. High morbidity associated with barium in the peritoneal cavity.
2. Subsequent abdominal CT and US are rendered difficult (if not impossible) to interpret. Patients may be asked to wait for up to 2 weeks to allow satisfactory clearance of the barium. If also required, it is advised that the CT and/or US be performed before the barium study.

Complications

1. *Perforation.* The escape of barium into the peritoneal cavity is extremely serious, and will produce pain and severe hypovolaemic shock. Despite treatment, which should consist of i.v. fluids, steroids and antibiotics, there is still a 50% mortality rate. Of those that survive, 30% will develop peritoneal adhesions and granulomata. Intramediastinal barium also has a significant mortality rate. It is therefore imperative that a water-soluble contrast medium is used for any investigation in which there is a risk of perforation, or in which perforation is already suspected.
2. *Aspiration.* Barium if aspirated is relatively harmless. Sequelae include pneumonitis and granuloma formation. Physiotherapy is the only treatment required (for both aspirated barium and LOCM), and should be arranged before the patient leaves hospital.
3. *Intravasation.* This may result in a barium pulmonary embolus, which carries a mortality of 80%.

For further complications (e.g. constipation and impaction), see the specific procedure involved.

Further reading

Karanikas, I.D., Kakoulidis, D.D., Gouvas, Z.T., et al. (1997) Barium peritonitis: a rare complication of upper gastrointestinal contrast investigation. *Postgrad. Med J.* **73**, 297–298.

Lintott, D.J., Simpkins, K.C., de Dombal, F.T., et al. (1978) Assessment of double contrast barium meal: method and application. *Clin. Radiol.* **29**, 313–321.

WATER-SOLUBLE CONTRAST MEDIA e.g. Gastromiro, Gastrografin

Proprietary name	Chemical name	Iodine concentration (mg ml^{-1})
Gastromiro	iopamidol 61% w/v	300
Gastrografin	{meglumine diatrizoate 66% w/v} {sodium diatrizoate 10% w/v}	370

Indications

1. Suspected perforation.
2. Meconium ileus.
3. To distinguish bowel from other structures on CT. A dilute solution of water-soluble contrast medium (e.g. 15 ml of Gastrografin in 1 l of flavoured drink) is used so that minimal artefact 'shadow' is produced.
4. LOCM is used if aspiration is a possibility.

Complications

1. Pulmonary oedema if aspirated (not LOCM).
2. Hypovolaemia in children – due to the hyperosmolality of the contrast media drawing fluid into the bowel (not with LOCM).
3. Allergic reactions – due to absorbed contrast media.
4. May precipitate in hyperchlorhydric gastric acid (i.e. 0.1 N HCl) – not non-ionics.
5. Ileus – may occur in 4% of patients examined in the postoperative phase.

GASES

Carbon dioxide and, less often, air are used in conjunction with barium to achieve a 'double contrast' effect.

For the upper gastrointestinal tract, CO_2 is administered orally in the form of gas producing granules/powder.

The requirements of these agents are as follows:[1]

a. production of an adequate volume of gas – 200–400 ml
b. non-interference with barium coating
c. no bubble production
d. rapid dissolution, leaving no residue
e. easily swallowed
f. low cost.

Carbex granules and fluid satisfy most of these requirements, but have the disadvantage of being relatively costly.

For the large bowel, room air is administered per rectum via a hand pump attached to the enema tube. Carbon dioxide is said to cause less abdominal pain, but inferior bowel distension when compared to air.[2]

References

1. de Lacey, G.J., Wignall, B.K. & Bray, C. (1979) Effervescent granules for the barium meal. *Br. J. Radiol.* **52**, 405–408.
2. Holemans, J.A., Matson, M.B. Hughes, J.A., et al. (1998) A comparison of air, carbon dioxide and air/carbon dioxide mixture as insufflation agents for double contrast barium enema. *Eur. Radiol.* **8**, 274–276.

Further reading

Gellett, L.R., Farrow, R., Bloor, C., et al. (1999) Pain after small bowel meal and pneumocolon: a randomized controlled trial of carbon dioxide versus air insufflation. *Clin. Radiol.* **54**, 381–383.

PHARMACOLOGICAL AGENTS

Hyoscine-N-butyl bromide (Buscopan)

This is an antimuscarinic agent and therefore inhibits both intestinal motility and gastric secretion.

Adult dose

20 mg i.v.

Advantages

1. Immediate onset of action
2. Short duration of action (approx. 15 min)
3. Cost.

Disadvantages

Antimuscarinic side-effects:

1. Blurring of vision
2. Dry mouth
3. Tachycardia
4. Urinary retention
5. Acute gastric dilatation.

Contraindications[1]

1. Closed angle glaucoma
2. Myasthenia gravis

3. Paralytic ileus
4. Pyloric stenosis
5. Prostatic enlargement.

Glucagon may be used in these circumstances.

Glucagon

This polypeptide hormone produced by the alpha cells of the islets of Langerhans in the pancreas, has a predominantly hyper-glycaemic effect but also causes smooth muscle relaxation.

Adult dose

0.3 mg i.v. for barium meal.
1.0 mg i.v. for barium enema.

Paediatric dose

0.5–1.0 μg kg⁻¹ for barium meal.
0.8–1.25 μg kg⁻¹ for barium enema.[2]
(NB: a smooth muscle relaxant is rarely required in paediatric practice.)

NB: Glucagon is available in vials which contain either 1 unit or 10 units. Both sizes are supplied with a diluent, but if the 10-unit vials are reconstituted they contain a bactericide which enables them to be stored in a refrigerator for up to 1 week provided the temperature of the refrigerator is 4°C.

Advantages

1. It is a more potent smooth muscle relaxant than Buscopan.
2. Short duration of action (approx. 15 min).
3. It does not interfere with the small bowel transit time.

Disadvantages

1. Hypersensitivity reactions are possible, as it is a protein molecule.
2. Relatively long onset of action (1 min).
3. Cost.

Contraindications

1. Phaeochromocytoma. Glucagon can cause the tumour to release catecholamines, resulting in sudden and marked hypertension. 5–10 mg phentolamine mesylate may be administered i.v. in an attempt to control the blood pressure.
2. Caution is advised in the following conditions:[1]
   a. insulinoma: an initial increase in blood glucose may be followed by severe hypoglycaemia
   b. glucagonoma.

Metoclopramide (Maxolon)

This dopamine antagonist stimulates gastric emptying and small intestinal transit.

Adult dose

20 mg oral or i.v.

Advantages

1. Enhanced transit of barium during a follow-through examination.
2. Anti-emetic.

Disadvantages

Extrapyramidal side-effects may occur if the dose exceeds 0.5 mg kg^{-1}. This is more likely to occur in children/young adults.

References

1. *British National Formulary*, 37 March 1999
2. Ratcliffe, J.F. (1980) Glucagon in barium examinations in infants and children: special reference to dosage. *Br. J. Radiol.* **53**, 860–862.

General Points

Although digital systems are increasingly being used, a tilting table and fluoroscopic unit with a spot film device (and tube angulation facilities) are standard equipment for all barium investigations. The need for these will not be mentioned further in the text.

In all barium work a high-kV technique is used (90–110 kV).

As in all radiological procedures, the ALARP (*As Low As Reasonably Practicable*) principle should be adhered to.

As regards women of child bearing age, the 'ten-day rule' is generally applied for both upper and lower gastrointestinal investigations.

For the radiation doses associated with various procedures, see Appendix III.

CONTRAST SWALLOW

Barium has superior contrast qualities and unless there are specific contraindications, its use (rather than water-soluble agents) is preferred. The barium swallow is virtually always done in conjunction with a barium meal.

Indications

1. Dysphagia
2. Anaemia

3. Pain
4. Assessment of tracheo-oesophageal fistulae
5. Assessment of the site of perforation.

Contraindications

None.

Contrast medium

1. E-Z HD 250% 100 ml (or more, as required)
2. Gastrografin
3. LOCM (approx. 350 mg I ml^{-1}).

N.B.

1. Gastrografin should NOT be used for the investigation of a tracheo-oesophageal fistula or when aspiration is a possibility.
2. Barium should NOT be used if perforation is suspected.

Equipment

Rapid serial radiography (2 frames per s) or video recording may be required for assessment of the laryngopharynx and upper oesophagus during deglutition.

Patient preparation

None (but as for barium meal if the stomach is also to be examined – see p. 57)

Preliminary film

A control film is advised prior to a water-soluble study if perforation is suspected.

Technique

1. The patient is in the erect RAO position to throw the oesophagus clear of the spine. An ample mouthful of barium is swallowed, and spot films of the upper and lower oesophagus are taken. Oesophageal varices are better seen in the prone RPO position, as they will be more distended.
2. If rapid serial radiography is required, it may be performed in the right lateral, RAO and PA positions.

Modification of technique

To demonstrate a tracheo-oesophageal fistula in infants, a nasogastric tube is introduced to the level of the mid-oesophagus, and the contrast agent (barium or LOCM) is syringed in to distend the oesophagus. This will force the contrast medium through any small fistula which may be present. It is important to take radiographs in the lateral projection during simultaneous injection of the contrast medium and withdrawal of the tube. Although some authors recommend that the infant be examined in the prone position whilst lying on the footstep of a vertical tilting table, satisfactory results are possible with children on their side on a horizontal table.

When this technique is used as part of a conventional upper gastrointestinal examination with the infant being fed from a bottle, it is important that it be performed first, before there is any possibility of aspiration into the airway from overspill. Overspill may lead to the incorrect diagnosis of tracheo-oesophageal fistula if it is not possible to determine whether contrast medium in the bronchi is due to a small fistula, which is difficult to see, or due to aspiration.

Aftercare

None.

Complications

1. Leakage of barium from an unsuspected perforation
2. Aspiration.

BARIUM MEAL

Methods

1. *Double contrast* – the method of choice to demonstrate mucosal pattern.
2. *Single contrast* – uses:
   a. children – since it usually is not necessary to demonstrate mucosal pattern
   b. very ill adults – to demonstrate gross pathology only.

Indications

1. Dyspepsia
2. Weight loss
3. Upper abdominal mass
4. Gastrointestinal haemorrhage (or unexplained iron-deficiency anaemia)
5. Partial obstruction
6. Assessment of site of perforation – it is essential that a water-soluble contrast medium, e.g. Gastrografin or LOCM, is used.

Contraindications

Complete large bowel obstruction.

Contrast medium

1. E-Z HD 250% w/v 135 ml
2. Carbex granules (double contrast technique).

Patient preparation

1. Nil orally for 6 h prior to the examination.
2. The patient is advised not to smoke on the day of the examination, as it increases gastric motility.
3. It should be ensured that there are no contraindications to the pharmacological agents used.

Preliminary film

None.

Technique

The double contrast method (Fig. 3.1)

1. A gas-producing agent is swallowed.
2. The patient then drinks the barium while lying on the left side, supported by the elbow. This position prevents the barium from reaching the duodenum too quickly and so obscuring the greater curve of the stomach.
3. The patient then lies supine and slightly on the right side, to bring the barium up against the gastro-oesophageal junction. This manoeuvre is screened to check for reflux, which may be revealed by asking the patient to cough or to swallow water while in this position. The significance of reflux produced by tipping the patient's head down is debatable, as this is an unphysiological position. If reflux is observed, spot films are taken to record the level to which it ascends.
4. An i.v. injection of a smooth muscle relaxant (Buscopan 20 mg or glucagon 0.3 mg) is given. The administration of Buscopan has been shown not to effect the detection of gastro-oesophageal reflux or hiatus hernia.[1]
5. The patient is asked to roll onto the right side and then quickly over in a complete circle, to finish in an RAO position. This roll is performed to coat the gastric mucosa with barium. Good coating has been achieved if the areae gastricae in the antrum are visible.

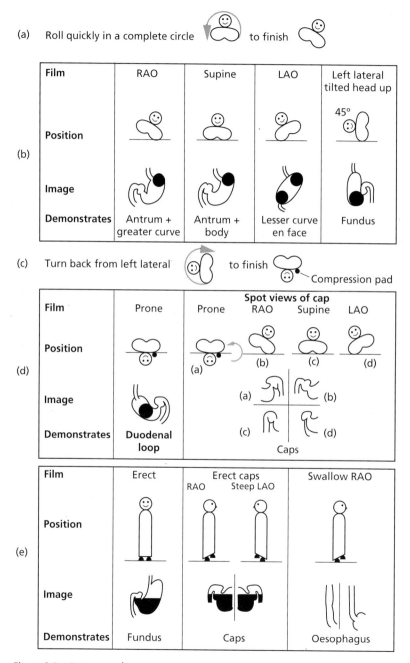

Figure 3.1   Barium meal sequence.

Films

There is a great variation in views recommended, and the following is only the scheme used in our departments. In some departments fewer films are taken to reduce the cost and radiation dose.

1. Spot films of the stomach (lying):
   a. RAO – to demonstrate the antrum and greater curve
   b. supine – to demonstrate the antrum and body
   c. LAO – to demonstrate the lesser curve *en face*
   d. left lateral tilted, head up 45° – to demonstrate the fundus. From the left lateral position the patient returns to a supine position and then rolls onto the left side and over into a prone position. This sequence of movement is required to avoid barium flooding into the duodenal loop, which would occur if the patient were to roll onto the right side to achieve a prone position.
2. Spot film of the duodenal loop (lying):
   a. prone – the patient lies on a compression pad to prevent barium from flooding into the duodenum.
   An additional view to demonstrate the anterior wall of the duodenal loop may be taken in an RAO position.
3. Spot films of the duodenal cap (lying):
   a. prone
   b. RAO – the patient attains this position from the prone position by rolling first onto the left side, for the reasons mentioned above
   c. supine
   d. LAO.
4. Additional views of the fundus in an erect position may be taken at this stage, if there is suspicion of a fundal lesion.
5. Spot films of the oesophagus are taken, while barium is being swallowed, to complete the examination.

Modification of technique for young children

The main indication will be to identify a cause for vomiting. The examination is modified to identify the three major causes of vomiting – gastro-oesophageal reflux, pyloric obstruction and malrotation, and it is essential that the position of the duodeno-jejunal flexure is demonstrated.

1. Single contrast technique using 30% w/v barium sulphate and no paralytic agent.

2. A relatively small volume of barium – enough to just fill the fundus – is given to the infant in the supine position. A film of the distended oesophagus is exposed.
3. The child is turned semi-prone into a LPO or RAO position. A film is exposed as barium passes through the pylorus. The pylorus is shown to even better advantage if 20–40° caudocranial angulation can be employed with an overhead screening unit. Gastric emptying is prolonged if the child is upset. A dummy coated with glycerine is a useful pacifier.
4. Once barium enters the duodenum, the infant is returned to the supine position, and with the child perfectly straight a second film is exposed as barium passes around the duodenojejunal flexure.
5. Once malrotation has been diagnosed or excluded, a further volume of barium is administered until the stomach is reasonably full and barium lies against the gastro-oesophageal junction. The child is gently rotated through 180° in an attempt to elicit gastro-oesophageal reflux.

In newborn infants with upper intestinal obstruction, e.g. duodenal atresia, the diagnosis may be confirmed if 20 ml air are injected down the nasogastric tube (which will almost certainly have already been introduced by the medical staff). If the diagnosis remains in doubt, it can be replaced by a positive contrast agent (dilute barium or LOCM if the risk of aspiration is high).

Aftercare

1. The patient should be warned that his bowel motions will be white for a few days after the examination and may be difficult to flush away.
2. The patient should be advised to drink adequate volumes of water to avoid barium impaction. Laxatives may be taken if required.
3. The patient must not leave the department until any blurring of vision produced by the Buscopan has resolved.

Complications

1. Leakage of barium from an unsuspected perforation.
2. Aspiration of stomach contents due to the Buscopan.
3. Conversion of a partial large bowel obstruction into a complete obstruction by the impaction of barium.
4. Barium appendicitis, if barium impacts in the appendix.
5. Side-effects of the pharmacological agents used.

N.B. It must be emphasized that there are many variations in technique, according to individual preference, and that the best way of becoming familiar with the sequence of positioning is actually to perform the procedure oneself.

Further reading

Dzik-Jurasz, A.S. & Mumcuoglu, E.A. (1997) Does 100 mm photofluorography always have a dose advantage over conventional film-screen radiography in barium meals? *Br. J. Radiol.* **70**, 168–171.

Rajah, R.R. (1990) Effects of Buscopan on gastro-oesophageal reflux and hiatus hernia. *Clin. Radiol.* **41**, 250–252.

BARIUM FOLLOW-THROUGH

Methods

1. Single contrast
2. With the addition of an effervescent agent
3. With the addition of a pneumocolon technique.

Indications

1. Pain
2. Diarrhoea
3. Anaemia/gastrointestinal bleeding
4. Partial obstruction
5. Malabsorption
6. Abdominal mass
7. Failed small bowel enema.

Contraindications

1. Complete obstruction
2. Suspected perforation (unless a water-soluble contrast medium is used).

Contrast medium

E-Z Paque 100% w/v 300 ml (150 ml if performed immediately after a barium meal). The transit time through the small bowel has been shown to be reduced by the addition of 10 ml of Gastrografin to the barium. In children, 3–4 ml kg^{-1} is a suitable volume.

In situations where barium is contraindicated, non-ionic water-soluble solutions have been shown to be a satisfactory alternative.[1]

Patient preparation

Metoclopramide 20 mg orally may be given 20 min before the examination.

Preliminary film

Plain abdominal film.

Technique

The aim is to deliver a single column of barium into the small bowel. This is achieved by lying the patient on the right side after the barium has been ingested. Metoclopramide enhances the rate of gastric emptying. If the transit time through the small bowel is found to be slow, a dry meal may help to speed it up. If a follow-through examination is combined with a barium meal, glucagon is used for the duodenal cap views rather than Buscopan because it has a short length of action and does not interfere with the small-bowel transit time.

Films

1. Prone PA films of the abdomen are taken every 20 min during the first hour, and subsequently every 30 min until the colon is reached. The prone position is used because the pressure on the abdomen helps to separate the loops of small bowel.
2. Spot films of the terminal ileum are taken supine. A compression pad is used to displace any overlying loops of small bowel that are obscuring the terminal ileum.

Additional films

1. To separate loops of small bowel:
   a. obliques
   b. with X-ray tube angled into the pelvis
   c. with the patient tilted head down.
2. To demonstrate diverticula:
   a. erect – this position will reveal any fluid levels caused by contrast medium retained within the diverticula.

Aftercare

As for barium meal.

Complications

As for barium meal.

References

1. Jobling, C., Halligan, S. & Bartram, C. (1999) The use of water-soluble contrast agents for small bowel follow-through examinations. *Eur. Radiol.* **9**, 706–710.

Further reading

Ha, H.K., Shin, J.H., Rha, S.E., et al. (1999) Modified small bowel follow through: use of methylcellulose to improve bowel transradiance and prepare barium suspension. *Radiology* **211**, 197–201.
Maglinte, D.D.T., Kelvin, F.M., O'Connor, K., et al. (1996) Current status of small bowel radiography. *Abdom. Imaging* **21**, 247–257.

SMALL BOWEL ENEMA

Advantage

This procedure gives better visualization of the small bowel than that achieved by a barium follow-through because rapid infusion of a large, continuous column of contrast medium directly into the jejunum avoids segmentation of the barium column and does not allow time for flocculation to occur.

Disadvantages

1. Intubation may be unpleasant for the patient, and may occasionally prove difficult.
2. It is more time-consuming for the radiologist.
3. There is a higher radiation dose to the patient (screening the tube into position).

Indications
Contraindications

The same as for a barium follow-through. In some departments it is only performed in the case of an equivocal follow-through.

Contrast medium

E-Z Paque 70% w/v.

This is diluted with tap water to give a 20% solution (total volume 1500 ml). The reduced viscosity produces better mucosal coating, and the reduced density permits the visualization of bowel loops which may otherwise have been obscured by a denser contrast medium in an overlying loop.

An alternative way to gain a double contrast effect is to use 600 ml of 0.5% methylcellulose after 500 ml of 70% w/v barium.[1]

Even with these modifications, it may still be difficult to obtain good distension and double contrast effect of the distal small bowel and terminal ileum.

Equipment

A choice of tubes is available.

1. Bilbao-Dotter tube with a guide-wire (the tube is longer than the wire so that there is reduced risk of perforation when introducing the wire).
2. Silk tube (E. Merck Ltd). This is a 10-F, 140-cm long tube with a tungsten-filled guide-tip. It is made of polyurethane and the stylet and the internal lumen of the tube are coated with a water-activated lubricant to facilitate the smooth removal of the stylet after insertion.

Patient preparation

1. A low-residue diet for 2 days prior to the examination.
2. If the patient is taking any antispasmodic drugs, they must be stopped 1 day prior to the examination.
3. Amethocaine lozenge 30 mg, 30 min before the examination.

Immediately before the examination the pharynx is anaesthetized with lignocaine spray.

Preliminary film

Plain abdominal film if a small bowel obstruction is suspected.

Technique

1. The patient sits on the edge of the X-ray table. The pharynx is thoroughly anaesthetized with lignocaine spray. If a per nasal approach is planned the patency of the nasal passages is checked by asking the patient to sniff with one nostril occluded. The Silk tube should be passed with the guide-wire pre-lubricated and fully within the tube, whereas for the Bilbao-Dotter tube it may be more comfortable to introduce the guide-wire after the tube tip is in the stomach.
2. The tube is then passed through the nose or the mouth, and brief lateral screening of the neck may be helpful in negotiating the epiglottic region. The patient is asked to swallow as the tube is passed through the pharynx. The tube is then advanced into the gastric antrum.
3. The patient then lies down and the tube is passed into the duodenum. Various manoeuvres may be used alone or in

combination, to help this part of the procedure, which may be difficult.

   a. Lie the patient on the left side so that the gastric air bubble rises to the antrum, thus straightening out the stomach.
   b. Advance the tube whilst applying clockwise rotational motion (as viewed from the head of the patient looking towards the feet).
   c. In the case of the Bilbao-Dotter tube, introduce the guide-wire.
   d. In the case of the Silk tube, lie the patient on the right side, as the tube has a tungsten-weighted guide-tip which will then tend to fall towards the antrum.
   e. Get the patient to sit up, to try to overcome the tendency of the tube to coil in the fundus of the stomach.
   f. Metoclopramide (20 mg i.v.) may help.

4. When the tip of the tube has been passed through the pylorus, the guide-wire tip is maintained at the pylorus as the tube is passed over it along the duodenum to the level of the ligament of Treitz. Clockwise torque applied to the tube may again help in getting past the junction of the first and second parts of the duodenum. The tube is passed as far as the duodenojejunal flexure to diminish the risk of aspiration due to reflux of barium into the stomach.

5. Barium is then run in quickly, and spot films are taken of the barium column and its leading edge at the regions of interest, until the colon is reached. If methylcellulose is used, it is infused continuously, after an initial bolus of 500 ml of barium, until the barium has reached the colon.

6. The tube is then withdrawn, aspirating any residual fluid in the stomach. Again, this is to decrease the risk of aspiration.

7. Finally, prone and supine abdominal films are taken.

Modification of technique

In patients with malabsorption, especially if an excess of fluid has been shown on the preliminary film, the volume of barium should be increased (240–260 ml). Compression views of bowel loops should be obtained before obtaining double contrast. Flocculation is likely to occur early. It is important to obtain images of the duodenum and the catheter tip should be sited proximal to the ligament of Trietz.[2]

Aftercare

1. Nil orally for 5 h after the procedure.

2. The patient should be warned that diarrhoea may occur as a result of the large volume of fluid given.

Complications

1. Aspiration
2. Perforation of the bowel owing to manipulation of the guide-wire.

Reference

1. Ha, H.K., Paik, K.B., Kim, P.N., et al. (1998) Use of methylcellulose in the small bowel follow through examination: comparison with conventional series in normal subjects. *Abdom. Imaging* **23**, 281–285.
2. Herlinger, H. (1992) Editorial. Radiology in malabsorption. *Clin. Radiol.* **45**, 73–78.

Further reading

Nolan, D.J. (1997) The true yield of the small intestinal barium study. *Endoscopy* **29**, 447–453.

BARIUM ENEMA

In females, the ten-day rule should apply.

Methods

1. *Double contrast* – the method of choice to demonstrate mucosal pattern.
2. *Single contrast* – uses:
    a. children – since it is usually not necessary to demonstrate mucosal pattern
    b. reduction of an intussusception (see p. 75).

Indications

1. Change in bowel habit
2. Pain
3. Mass
4. Melaena/anaemia
5. Obstruction.

N.B. If a tight stricture is demonstrated, only run a small volume of barium proximally to define the upper margin, for otherwise the barium may impact.

Contraindications

Absolute

1. Toxic megacolon (double contrast barium enema is said to be no better than clinical judgement in this situation, and is clearly more dangerous[1])
2. Pseudomembranous colitis
3. Rectal biopsy via:
   a. rigid endoscope within previous 5 days[2]
   b. flexible endoscope within previous 24 h.[2]

Relative

1. Incomplete bowel preparation
2. Recent barium meal – it is advised to wait for 7–10 days
3. Patient frailty.

Contrast medium

1. Polibar 115% w/v 500 ml (or more, as required)
2. Air.

Equipment

Miller disposable enema tube. If the patient is incontinent, it is permissible to use a tube with an inflatable cuff. However, its use should be confined to such cases, owing to the increased risk of perforation (see 'complications' p. 72).

Patient preparation

Many regimes for bowel preparation exist. A suggested regime is as follows:

For 3 days prior to examination

Low residue diet.

On the day prior to examination

1. Fluids only
2. Picolax – at 08.00 h and 18:00 h.

On the day of the examination

Patients with prosthetic heart valves, a previous history of endocarditis or a surgically constructed systemic pulmonary shunt or conduit require antibiotic prophylaxis. Suitable regimes as recommended by The Royal College of Radiologists are:[3]

Adults
Not allergic to penicillins
Amoxycillin 1 g + gentamicin 120 mg i.v. 15 min prior to the procedure
Followed by amoxicillin 500 mg orally 6 h later

Allergic to penicillins or who have had a penicillin more than once in the previous month

Vancomycin 1 g by slow i.v. infusion over 100 min + gentamicin 120 mg i.v. immediately prior to the start of the procedure
OR
Teicoplanin 400 mg i.v. + gentamicin 120 mg immediately prior to the start of the procedure

Children (< 10 years)
Not allergic to penicillins

Amoxycillin 500 mg + gentamicin 2 mg kg^{-1} i.v. 15 min prior to the procedure
Followed by amoxicillin (0–4 years 125 mg; 5–9 years 250 mg) orally 6 h later

Allergic to penicillins

Vancomycin 20 mg kg^{-1} by slow i.v. infusion over 100 min + gentamicin 2 mg kg^{-1} i.v. immediately prior to the start of the procedure
OR
Teicoplanin 6 mg kg^{-1} i.v. + gentamicin 2 mg kg^{-1} i.v. immediately prior to the start of the procedure

NB:
1. Consider admitting the elderly and those with social problems.
2. It is advisable to place diabetics first on the list.

Preliminary film

A preliminary plain abdominal film is not necessary unless:
1. severe constipation renders the effectiveness of bowel preparation doubtful
2. toxic megacolon is suspected.

Technique

The double contrast method (Fig. 3.2)

1. The patient lies on one side on an incontinence sheet, and the catheter is inserted gently into the rectum. It is taped firmly in position. Connections are made to the barium reservoir and the hand pump for injecting air.
2. An i.v. injection of Buscopan (20 mg) or glucagon (1 mg) is given. Some radiologists choose to give the muscle relaxant half way through the procedure.
3. The infusion of barium is commenced. Intermittent screening is required to check the progress of the barium. The infusion is terminated when the barium reaches the hepatic flexure. The

column of barium within the sigmoid colon is run back out by either lowering the infusion bag to the floor or tilting the table erect.

4. Air is gently pumped into the bowel, forcing the column of barium round towards the caecum, and producing the double contrast effect. Some centres use CO_2 as the negative contrast agent as it has been shown to reduce the incidence of severe post-double contrast enema pain.[4]

5. From the prone position, the patient rolls onto the left side and over into an RAO position so that the barium coats the bowel mucosa.

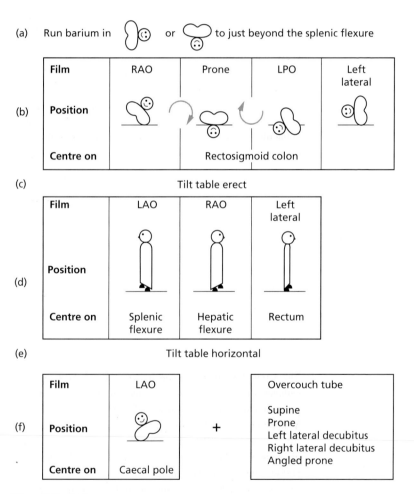

Figure 3.2   Barium enema sequence.

Films

There is a great variation in views recommended, and the following is only the scheme used in this department. Fewer films may be taken to reduce the radiation dose and cost.

The sequence of positioning enables the barium to flow proximally to reach the caecal pole. Air is pumped in as required to distend the colon.

1. Spot films of the rectum and sigmoid colon (lying):
   a. RAO
   b. Prone
   c. LPO
   d. Left lateral of the rectum.
2. Spot films of the hepatic flexure, splenic flexure and rectum (erect):
   a. LAO to open out the splenic flexure
   b. RAO to open out the hepatic flexure
   c. Right lateral of the rectum.
3. Spot film of the caecum (lying). Positioning of the patient supine, lying slightly on the right side and with a slight head-down tilt will usually give a double contrast effect in the caecum. Some compression with a lead-gloved hand may be necessary to persuade a stubborn pool of barium out of the caecal pole.
4. Overcouch films (usually with a ceiling tube) to demonstrate all of the large bowel (lying):
   a. Supine
   b. Prone
   c. Left lateral decubitus
   d. Right lateral decubitus
   e. Prone, with the tube angled 45° caudad and centred 5 cm above the posterior superior iliac spines. This view separates overlying loops of sigmoid colon.
5. The post-evacuation film is not taken routinely, but may allow improved assessment of the caecum when the other films have failed (e.g. if the procedure has been poorly tolerated by the patient).
6. Extra spot films of any regions of abnormality are taken as required.

Aftercare

1. Patients should be warned that their bowel motions will be white for a few days after the examination, and to keep their

bowels open with laxatives to avoid barium impaction, which can be painful (see barium meal).

2. The patient must not leave the department until any blurring of vision produced by the Buscopan (in 5% of patients) has resolved.

Complications

1. Perforation of the bowel. There is an increased risk of this in:
   a. Infants and the elderly
   b. Obstructing neoplasm
   c. Ulceration of the bowel wall
   d. Inflation of a Foley catheter balloon in a colostomy, or the rectum
   e. Patients on steroid therapy
   f. Hypothyroidism.
2. Transient bacteraemia.
3. Side-effects of the pharmacological agents used (see page 53).
4. Cardiac arrhythmia due to rectal distension.
5. Intramural barium.
6. Venous intravasation. This may result in a barium pulmonary embolus, which carries 80% mortality.

References

1. Marion, J.F. & Present, D.H. (1997) The modern medical management of acute severe ulcerative colitis. *Eur. J. Gastroenterol. Hepatol.* **9**, 831.
2. Low, V.H. (1998) What is the correct waiting time for performance of a gastrointestinal barium study after endoscopic biopsy of the upper or lower gastrointestinal tract? *Am. J. Roentgenol.* **170**, 1104–1105.
3. *Antibiotic Prophylaxis Prior to Barium Enema in Patients at High Risk of Endocarditis* (1999) London: The Royal College of Radiologists.
4. Taylor, P.N. & Beckley, D.E. (1991) Use of air in double contrast barium enema: is it still acceptable? *Clin. Radiol.* **44**, 183–184.

Further reading

Cittadini, G., Sardanelli, F., De Cicco, E., et al. (1999) Bowel preparation for the double contrast barium enema: How to maintain coating with cleansing? *Clin. Radiol.* **54**, 216–220.

Foster, D.R. (1998) Audit of barium enema examinations in the diagnosis of colorectal carcinoma. *Australas. Radiol.* **42**, 197–198.

Rudman, R.H. (1998) A simple technique to perform double contrast barium enema after air distension of the colon due to previous colonoscopy or sigmoidoscopy. *Am. J. Roentgenol.* **170**, 509–510.

Smiddy, P.F., Quinn, A.D., Freyne, P.J., et al. (1996) Dose reduction in double contrast barium enema by use of low fluoroscopic current. *Br. J. Radiol.* **69**, 852–854.

THE 'INSTANT' ENEMA

Indications

1. To identify the level of suspected large bowel obstruction.
2. To show the extent and severity of mucosal lesions in active ulcerative colitis.

Contraindications

1. Toxic megacolon
2. Rectal biopsy (as for barium enema)
3. Chronic ulcerative colitis – a formal barium enema should be performed to exclude a carcinoma
4. Crohn's colitis – assessment in this situation is unreliable.

Contrast medium

Water-soluble contrast.

Preliminary film

Plain abdominal film – to exclude
a. toxic megacolon
b. perforation.

Technique

1. The contrast medium is run until it flows into
   a. an obstructing lesion
   b. dilated bowel loops
   c. the caecum.
2. Air insufflation is not required – i.e. single contrast technique.

Films

These are obtained as required, e.g.

1. Prone   2. Left lateral decubitus   3. Erect.

BALLOON DILATATION OF OESOPHAGEAL STRICTURES

Indications

1. Peptic strictures
2. Oesophageal tumours
3. Anastomotic strictures
4. Achalasia of the cardia.

Contraindications

1. Tracheo-oesophageal fistula.

Contrast medium

Because there is a risk of aspiration, LOCM 350 should always be used to outline the oesophagus and to define the stricture.

Equipment

1. Fluoroscopy unit, with a facility for spot films
2. Oesophageal dilatation balloons (15 and 22 mm diameter)
3. Long guide-wire with floppy tip (long enough to allow the wire to traverse the stricture with sufficient outside the mouth to pass and exchange balloons over)
4. Lignocaine local anaesthetic spray.

Patient preparation

1. Nil by mouth 6 h prior to the procedure.
2. An easily accessible i.v. line should be available to allow for the administration of sedative or analgesic agents, as necessary.

Technique

1. The patient is made comfortable on the screening table.
2. A contrast swallow is performed to determine the level and the degree of the stricture. The contrast also outlines the gastrointestinal tract distal to the stricture.
3. The pharynx is anaesthetized using lignocaine spray.
4. The guide-wire is passed, floppy tip first. This manoeuvre may be aided by the use of fluoroscopy and a femorovisceral catheter which allows the wire tip to be directed appropriately.
5. The guide-wire is passed through the stricture, under screening guidance. The wire is passed so that a stable position is attained; placing the tip about 30 cm distal to the stricture is usually possible.
6. The stricture is progressively dilated using the graded balloons. Very tight stenoses may require the use of angioplasty balloons initially. Hand inflation of the balloon using a syringe is performed until the 'waist' in the balloon, caused by the stricture, has been overcome. This inflation is maintained for approx. 60 s. A 22-mm balloon is usually a sufficient maximum diameter.

Aftercare

The patient should remain nil by mouth for at least 4 h after the procedure, with hourly observations of pulse and blood pressure.

Complications

1. Oesophageal rupture
2. Mediastinitis secondary to oesophageal injury.

Further reading

Sandgren, K. & Malfors, G. (1998) Balloon dilatation of oesophageal strictures in children. *Eur. J. Pediatr. Surg.* **8**, 9–11.

REDUCTION OF AN INTUSSUSCEPTION

This procedure should only be attempted in full consultation with the surgeon in charge of the case and when an anaesthetist with adequate paediatric training and experience and paediatric anaesthetic equipment is available.[1,2]

Methods

1. Using air and fluoroscopy.[3]
   Compared with barium this method has the following advantages:
   a. more rapid reduction, because the low viscosity of air permits rapid filling of the colon
   b. reduced radiation dose because of the above
   c. more effective reduction
   d. in the presence of a perforation, air in the peritoneal cavity is preferable to barium, and gut organisms are not washed into the peritoneal cavity
   e. there is more accurate control of intraluminal pressure
   f. less mess, and a dry infant will not lose heat
   g. cost
2. Using barium/water-soluble contrast agent and fluoroscopy.[4]
3. Using a water-soluble contrast medium and ultrasound.

Contraindications

1. Peritonitis or perforation.
2. Advanced intestinal obstruction (> 24 h). In these instances, successful reduction is less likely and there is a higher incidence of perforation of gangrenous bowel.

3. The pneumatic method should probably not be used in children over 4 years of age as there is a higher incidence of significant lead points which may be missed.[5]

Patient preparation

1. Sedation is of questionable value, but analgesia is important (e.g. morphine 50 µg kg^{-1} if < 1 year or 50–100 µg kg^{-1} if > 1 year).
2. Some institutions perform the examination under general anaesthesia. This has the advantages of greater muscle relaxation, which may increase the likelihood of successful reduction, and also enables the child to go to surgery quickly in the event of a failed radiological reduction.
3. Correction of fluid and electrolyte imbalance. The child has an i.v. line in-situ.
4. Antibiotic cover is not routine.

Preliminary investigations

1. Plain abdominal film – to assess bowel distension and to exclude perforation. A right-side-up decubitus film is often helpful in confirming the diagnosis by showing a failure of caecal filling with bowel gas because of the presence of the soft tissue mass of the intussusception. Normal plain films do not exclude the diagnosis and the clinical findings and/or history should be sufficient indications.
2. Ultrasound – should confirm or exclude the diagnosis. Absence of blood flow within the intussusceptum on colour-flow Doppler should lead to cautious reduction.[6,7] Ultrasound may identify a lead point; if so, even attempted reduction (to facilitate surgery) should be followed by surgery. If ultrasound identifies fluid trapped between the intussusceptum and intussuscipiens, the success rate is significantly reduced.[8]

Contrast medium

1. Air
2. Barium sulphate 100% w/v
3. Water-soluble contrast, e.g. LOCM 150 or dilute Gastrografin (1 part Gastrografin to 4 or 5 parts water).

Technique

A 16–22-F balloon catheter is inserted into the rectum and the buttocks taped tightly together to provide a seal. It may be necessary to inflate the balloon but if this is done it should be performed under fluoroscopic control so that the rectum is not overdistended.

Pneumatic reduction

1. The child is placed in the prone position so that it is easier to maintain the catheter in the rectum and the child is disturbed as little as possible during the procedure.
2. Air is instilled by a hand or mechanical pump and the intussusception is pushed back by a sustained pressure of up to 80 mmHg. If this fails, the pressure may be increased to 120 mmHg. Pressure should be monitored at all times and there should be a pressure release valve in the system to ensure that excessive pressures are not delivered.
3. Reduction is successful when there is free flow of air into the distal ileum.
4. If the intussusception does not move after 3 min of sustained pressure, the pressure is reduced and the child rested for 3 min. If, after three similar attempts, the intussusception is still immovable it is considered irreducible and arrangements are made for surgery.
5. The intussusception is only considered completely reduced when the terminal ileum is filled with air. However, it is not uncommon for there to be a persisting filling defect in the caecum at the end of the procedure, with or without reflux of air into the terminal ileum. This is often due to an oedematous ileocaecal valve. In the presence of a soft tissue caecal mass, a clinically well and stable child should be returned to the ward to await a further attempt at reduction after a period of 2–8 h rather than proceed to surgery. A second enema is often successful at complete reduction or showing resolution of the oedematous ileocaecal valve.[9]
6. When air (or barium) dissects between the two layers of the intussusception – the dissection sign - reduction is less likely.[10]

Barium reduction

1. Patient positioning is as for the pneumatic method.
2. The bag containing barium is raised 100 cm above the table top and barium run in under hydrostatic pressure. Progress of the column of barium is monitored by intermittent fluoroscopy.
3. If the intussusception does not move after 3 min of sustained pressure, the bag of barium is lowered to table-top height and the child rested for 3 min. If, after three similar attempts, the intussusception is still immovable it is considered irreducible and arrangements are made for surgery.

4. The points regarding failed or incomplete reduction discussed above also apply to hydrostatic reduction.

Ultrasound reduction

1. To facilitate scanning the child must be supine.
2. The intussusception can be identified with ultrasound. The contrast medium is run as far as the obstruction and its passage around the colon and the reducing head of the intussusception monitored by ultrasound.
3. The points regarding failed or incomplete reduction discussed above also apply to this technique.

Films

1. Spot films as required
2. Post-reduction film.

Aftercare

1. Observation in hospital for 24 h.

Complications

Perforation. For the pneumatic method, if a pump is used without a pressure-monitoring valve, perforation may result in a tension pneumoperitoneum, resulting in respiratory embarrassment. Puncture of the peritoneal cavity with a 'green' 23-G needle may be life-saving.

References

1. The Royal College of Anaesthetists. (1999) Guidelines for the Provision of Anaesthetic Services. Guidance on the Provision of Paediatric Anaesthesia, pp 24–26. London: Royal College of Anaesthetists.
2. The British Association of Paediatric Surgeons. (1994, revised 1995) A Guide for Purchasers and Providers of Paediatric Surgeons. London: British Association of Paediatric Surgeons.
3. Kirks, D.R. (1995) Air intussusception reduction: 'The winds of change'. Pediatr. Radiol. 25, 89–91.
4. Poznanski, A.K. (1995) Why I still use barium for intussusception. Pediatr. Radiol. 25, 92–93.
5. Stringer, D.A. & Ein, S.H. (1990) Pneumatic reduction: advantages, risks and indications. Pediatr. Radiol. 20, 475–477.
6. Lam, A.H. & Firman, K. (1992) Value of sonography including colour Doppler in the diagnosis and management of long-standing intussusception. Pediatr. Radiol. 22, 112–114.
7. Lim, H.K., Bae, S.H., Lee, K.H., et al. (1994) Assessment of reducibility of ileocolic intussusception in children: usefulness of color Doppler sonography. Radiology 191, 781–785.
8. Britton, I. & Wilkinson, A.G. (1999) Ultrasound features of intussusception predicting outcome of air enema. Pediatr. Radiol. 29, 705–710.

9. Gorenstein, A., Raucher, A., Serour, F., et al. (1998) Intussusception in children: reduction with repeated, delayed air enema. *Radiology* **206**, 721–724.
10. Barr, L.L., Stansberry S.D. & Swischuk, L.E. (1990) Significance of age, duration, obstruction and the dissection sign in intussusception. *Pediatr. Radiol.* **20**, 454–456.

CONTRAST ENEMA IN NEONATAL LOW INTESTINAL OBSTRUCTION

The differential diagnosis of low intestinal obstruction in the newborn consists of five conditions which comprise nearly all causes. Three involve the colon: Hirschsprung's disease, functional immaturity of the colon (small left colon syndrome, meconium plug syndrome) and colonic atresia. Two involve the distal ileum: meconium ileus and ileal atresia. All infants with low intestinal obstruction require a contrast enema.

Contraindications

1. Perforation.

Patient preparation

1. The baby should already have i.v. access and be well hydrated prior to the procedure.

Contrast medium

Dilute ionic contrast medium as is used for cystography, e.g. Urografin 150. This has the advantage of not provoking large fluid shifts and being dense enough to provide satisfactory images. Non-ionic contrast media and barium offer no advantages and the latter is contraindicated with perforation as a possibility. Infants with meconium ileus or functional immaturity will benefit from a water-soluble contrast enema and so their therapeutic enema commences with the diagnostic study. The non-operative treatment of meconium ileus was first described using the hypertonic agent Gastrografin,[1] which dislodged the sticky meconium by drawing water into the bowel lumen. However, most paediatric radiologists now believe that a hypertonic agent is not necessary for successful treatment.[2]

Technique

If the enema demonstrates that the entire colon is small (a microcolon; < 1 cm in diameter) then the diagnosis is likely to be meconium ileus or ileal atresia. (The microcolon of prematurity and total colonic Hirschsprung's disease are alternative rare diagnoses.) For the treatment of meconium ileus, the aim is to run the water-soluble contrast medium into the small bowel to surround the meconium. An attempt should be made to get the contrast medium back into dilated small bowel. If successful, meconium should be passed in the next hour. If no result is seen and the infant's condition deteriorates then surgical intervention will be necessary. If the passage of meconium is incomplete and the clinical condition remains stable, multiple enemas over the succeeding few days will be necessary to ensure complete resolution of the obstruction.

Overall success rate is approximately 50–60%, with a perforation rate of 2%.[2]

References

1. Noblett, H. (1969) Treatment of meconium ileus by Gastrografin enema. *J. Pediatr. Surg.* **4**, 190–197.
2. Kao, S.C.S. & Franken, E.A. Jr. (1995) Nonoperative treatment of simple meconium ileus: a survey of The Society for Pediatric Radiology. *Pediatr. Radiol.* **25**, 97–100.

SINOGRAM

1. A low osmolar contrast medium should be used, e.g. LOCM 150.
2. A preliminary film is taken to exclude the presence of a radio-opaque foreign body.
3. A fine catheter is then inserted into the orifice of the sinus, next to which a metal marker has been placed.
4. After a gauze pad has been firmly placed over the orifice to discourage reflux, the contrast medium is injected under fluoroscopic control.
5. Spot films are taken as required, including tangential views.

LOOPOGRAM

Bowel proximal to a colostomy

1. The tip of a Foley catheter is inserted a few centimetres into the appropriate stoma.

2. The balloon is carefully inflated within the lumen of the bowel proximal to the stoma to provide a seal.
3. Barium is run into the bowel and spot films taken as required.

Bowel distal to a colostomy

1. The bowel distal to a colostomy may be investigated by running barium per rectum in the usual manner, as this is easier and safer.
2. If there is any suspicion of an anastomotic break-down, a water-soluble contrast medium must be used.

HERNIOGRAM

Indications

1. History suggestive of a hernia with a normal/inconclusive physical examination.
2. Undiagnosed groin pain.

Contraindications

1. Infancy
2. Pregnancy
3. Intestinal obstruction
4. Allergy to contrast medium.

Patient preparation

1. The patient is asked to empty their bladder just prior to the examination.

Technique

1. The patient lies supine on the X-ray table.
2. An aseptic technique is employed.
3. 5–10 ml of 1% lignocaine is injected into the skin, subcutaneous tissues and peritoneum. The injection site varies between operators; the midpoint of the left lateral rectus muscle is one variation.
4. A 19-G spinal needle is introduced into the peritoneal cavity.

Contrast medium

50–100 ml water-soluble medium (e.g. Omnipaque 300)

Films

1. Supine
2. Prone
3. Erect films: frontal, obliques, lateral.

The patient is asked to cough and perform the Valsalva manoeuvre while these are taken. The tube may be angled 25° caudally.

Complications

These are uncommon, and patient admission for observation is all that is usually required.

1. Pain
2. Visceral puncture
3. Vascular puncture
4. Injection into the abdominal wall
5. Haematoma at the injection site
6. Allergy to contrast medium.

Further reading

Baomddoja, M., Bush, I.M., Angres, G., et al. (2000) The role of herniography in undiagnosed groin pain. In: *Inguinal Hernia Advances or Controversies?*, pp. 323–331. London: Radcliffe Medical Press.

Ekberg, O. (1981) Inguinal herniography in adults: technique, normal anatomy, and diagnostic criteria for hernias. *Radiology* **138**, 31–36.

Ekberg, O. (1983) Complications after herniography in adults. *Am. J. Roentgenol.* **140**, 490–495.

Jones, R.L. & Wingate J.P. (1998) Herniography in the investigation of groin pain in adults. *Clin. Radiol.* **53**, 805–808.

DEFECATING PROCTOGRAM

Indications

1. Anorectal incontinence
2. Constipation
3. Suspected pelvic floor weakness
   a. anterior (cystocoele/urinary stress incontinence)
   b. middle (uterus/vaginal vault)
   c. posterior (rectocoele/enterocoele/rectal intussuception).

NB: Opacification of other pelvic viscera may aid diagnosis.

Contraindications

None.

Methods[1]

1. Evacuation proctography
2. Dynamic magnetic resonance imaging.

EVACUATION PROCTOGRAPHY

Contrast medium

Thick barium paste (although commercial pastes are available, this may be satisfactorily prepared with barium powder and ultrasound coupling gel).

Technique

1. A Foley's catheter (balloon deflated) is inserted just beyond the anal margin with the patient in the left lateral position.
2. Approximately 120 ml of barium paste (or enough to fill the rectosigmoid colon) are instilled via a bladder syringe.

Films

1. These are taken in a lateral projection with the patient sitting on a commode
2. Spot films at rest and during the Valsalva manoeuvre
3. Single spot films during defecation (rather than rapid sequence) to minimize patient dose.

Reference

1. Healey, J.C., Halligan, S., Reznek, R.H., et al. (1997) Dynamic MR imaging compared with evacuation proctography when evaluating anorectal configuration and pelvic floor movement. *Am. J. Roentgenol.* **169**, 775–779.

Further reading

Hamlin, J.A. & Kahn, A.M. (1998) Herniography: a review of 333 herniograms. *Am. Surg.* **64**, 965–969.

Kelvin, F.M., Maglinte, D.D.T., Hornback, J.A. et al. (1992) Pelvic prolapse: assessment with evacuation proctography (defecography). *Radiology* **184**, 547–551.

COELIAC AXIS, SUPERIOR MESENTERIC AND INFERIOR MESENTERIC ARTERIOGRAPHY

Indications

1. Gastrointestinal haemorrhage
2. Staging tumours prior to intervention (surgical or radiological)
3. Gastrointestinal ischaemia
4. Portal venography.

Contrast medium

LOCM 370.

Equipment

1. Digital fluoroscopy with angiography facility
2. Pump injector
4. Catheter – selective femorovisceral or cobra catheter (Figs 3.3 and 3.4).

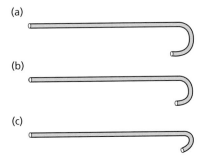

(a)

(b)

(c)

Figure 3.3 Selective femorovisceral catheters. (a) For coeliac and superior mesenteric arteries in larger patients. (b) For coeliac and superior mesenteric arteries in smaller patients. (c) For inferior mesenteric artery.

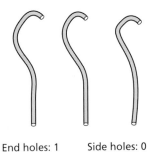

End holes: 1   Side holes: 0

Figure 3.4 Cobra catheters.

Technique

1. Femoral artery puncture – Seldinger technique.
2. Bowel movement causing subtraction artefact can be reduced by using a smooth muscle relaxant (e.g. Buscopan 10–20 mg) and abdominal compression.
3. When performed for gastrointestinal bleeding, provided that the patient is bleeding at the time, a blood loss of 0.5–0.6 ml min^{-1} can be demonstrated. The site of active bleeding is

revealed by extravasated contrast medium remaining in the bowel on the late films, when intravascular contrast has cleared. Vascular malformations, tumours and varices may be demonstrated.

Coeliac axis

Patient supine; 36 ml contrast medium at 6 ml s^{-1}.
(Angiography of the pancreas is best achieved by selective injection into the splenic, dorsal pancreatic and gastroduodenal arteries.)

Superior mesenteric artery

Patient supine; 42 ml contrast medium at 7 ml s^{-1}.

Late phase visceral arteriography

Patient slightly RPO.

When selective catheterization of the coeliac or SMA has been achieved, delayed venous phase films will show the portal vein.

NB: If splenic vein opacification is required, then a late phase coeliac arteriogram is necessary.

Inferior mesenteric artery

If the inferior mesenteric artery is to be examined as part of a procedure which will examine the superior mesenteric artery or coeliac axis as well, e.g. to find the source of gastrointestinal bleeding, then the inferior mesenteric artery should be examined first so that contrast medium in the bladder will not obscure its terminal branches.

Patient 30° LPO (to open the sigmoid loop). Hand injection of 10 ml of contrast medium.

ULTRASOUND OF THE GASTROINTESTINAL TRACT

US

ENDOLUMINAL EXAMINATION OF THE OESOPHAGUS AND STOMACH

Indications

1. Staging of primary malignant disease
2. Ultrasound-guided biopsy of primary tumours or suspected nodal disease.

Equipment

Echoendoscope with 7.5–10-MHz 360° rotary transducer.

Patient preparation

Slight sedation may be required.

Technique

Monitoring with a pulse oximeter is recommended. If the stomach is to be examined, this is filled with de-aerated water through the working channel before the patient is examined in a left lateral decubitus position. The US transducer is passed during endoscopy, either combined with direct vision or blind by an experienced endoscopist. A 360° rotary transducer will provide transverse scans with respect to the long axis of the tube.

Aftercare

The patient should be observed by experienced nursing staff until the effects of any sedation have worn off.

Further reading

Botet, J.F. & Lightdale, C. (1991) Endoscopic sonography of the upper gastrointestinal tract. *Am. J. Roentgenol.* **156**, 63–68.

Botet, J.F. & Lightdale, C. (1992) Endoscopic ultrasonography of the upper gastrointestinal tract. *Radiol. Clin. N. Am.* **30**, 1067–1083.

Shorvon, P.J. (1990) Endoscopic ultrasound in oesophageal cancer: the way forward? *Clin. Radiol.* **42**, 149–151.

TRANSABDOMINAL EXAMINATION OF THE LOWER OESOPHAGUS AND STOMACH

Indications

1. Oesophageal and fundal varices
2. Gastro-oesophageal reflux
3. Staging of malignant disease from adjacent organs (endoluminal ultrasound is more accurate).

Equipment

3.5–5-MHz transducer.

Patient preparation

None.

Technique

1. A transcutaneous epigastric approach is used, scanning either transversely or longitudinally. The oesophagus can be identified posterior to the liver as it passes through the diaphragmatic hiatus. It can be readily recognized by the presence of high reflectivity air within its lumen.

2. Oesophageal varices are seen as hypo-echoic channels within a thickened oesophageal wall and can be interrogated by colour and duplex Doppler.

3. The normal gastric wall has five recognizable sonographic layers and should not measure more than 6–7 mm.

HYPERTROPHIC PYLORIC STENOSIS

The typical patient is a 6-week-old male infant with non-bilious projectile vomiting.

Equipment

5–7.5-MHz linear or sector transducer.

Technique

1. The right upper quadrant is scanned with the patient supine. If the stomach is very distended, the pylorus will be displaced posteriorly and the stomach should be decompressed with a nasogastric tube. If the stomach is collapsed, the introduction of some dextrose, by mouth or via a nasogastric tube, will distend the antrum and differentiate it from the pylorus.

2. The pylorus is scanned in its longitudinal and transverse planes and images will resemble an olive and a doughnut, respectively. The poorly echogenic muscle is easily differentiated from the bright mucosa. Antral peristalsis can be seen and the volume of fluid passing through the pylorus with each antral wave can be assessed.

3. A number of measurements can be made. These include muscle thickness, canal length, pyloric volume and muscle thickness/wall diameter ratio, but there is no universal agreement as to which is the most discriminating parameter.

Further reading

King, S.J. (1997) Ultrasound of the hollow gastrointestinal tract in children. *Eur. Radiol.* **7**, 559–565.

Misra, D., Akhter, A., Potts, S.R., et al. (1997) Pyloric stenosis. Is over reliance on ultrasound scans leading to negative explorations? *Eur. J. Ped. Surg.* **7**, 328–330.

SMALL BOWEL

Indications

1. It is infrequent that US is used as a primary investigation for patients with suspected small-bowel disease, but the small bowel can be included in an examination of the abdomen,

especially if the patient has right iliac fossa pain, inflammatory bowel disease or suspected small-bowel obstruction.
2. Midgut malrotation.[1]

Technique

1. Dilated small-bowel loops and bowel wall thickening may be readily recognized. Doppler examination of the mesenteric vessels may be included to assess activity of inflammatory bowel disease.
2. Malrotation of the small bowel may be diagnosed by alteration of the normal relationship between the superior mesenteric artery and vein. The vein should lie anterior and to the right of the artery.

Reference

1. Gaines, P.A., Saunders, A.J.S. & Drake, D. (1987) Midgut malrotation diagnosed by ultrasound. *Clin. Radiol.* **38**, 51–53.

APPENDIX

Indications

Diagnosis of appendicitis and its complications.

Equipment

5–7.5-MHz linear array transducer.

Patient preparation

None.

Technique

The US transducer is used to apply graded compression to the right lower quadrant of the abdomen. This displaces bowel loops and compresses the caecum. The normal appendix should be compressible and have a maximum diameter of 6 mm. It should also exhibit peristalsis.

Further reading

Brown, G.J. (1991) Acute appendicitis – the radiologist's role. *Radiology* **180**, 13–14.
Šimonovský, V. (1999) Sonographic detection of normal and abnormal appendix. *Clin. Radiol.* **54**, 533–539.

LARGE BOWEL

Indications

At present, colonoscopy or barium examinations are first line imaging investigations but large-bowel masses can be visualized by US or CT during a routine abdominal scan.

RECTUM AND ANUS

Indications

1. Staging of primary rectal carcinoma or suspected local recurrence
2. Incontinence and suspected anal sphincter defects
3. Intersphincteric fistula.

Patient preparation

Simple bowel preparation using a small self-administered disposable enema.

Equipment

5–7-MHz radially scanning transducer. A linear transducer can be used but is less satisfactory.

Technique

1. The patient is placed in the left lateral position.
2. A careful digital rectal examination is carried out.
3. The probe is covered with a latex sheath containing contact jelly, and all air bubbles are expelled.
4. More jelly is placed over the latex sheath and the probe is introduced into the rectum.

Aftercare

None.

Further reading

Beynon, J., Feifel, G., Hildebrandt, U., et al. (1991) *An Atlas of Rectal Endosonography*. Berlin: Springer-Verlag.

CT OF THE GASTROINTESTINAL TRACT   CT

Indications

1. Abdominal mass
2. Tumour staging
3. Appendicitis – focused appendiceal CT (FACT)
4. Bowel tumours.

Oral and i.v. contrast media are usually employed.

NB: CT gives a high radiation dose (see Appendix IV).

Further reading

Domjan, J., Blaquiere, R. & Odurny, A. (1998) Is minimal preparation CT comparable with barium enema in elderly patients with colonic symptoms? *Clin. Radiol.* **53**, 894–898.

Herts, B.R., Einstein, D.M. & Paushter, D.M. (1993) Spiral CT of the abdomen: artefacts and potential pitfalls. *Am. J. Roentgenol.* **161**, 1185–1190.

Peck, J.J., Milleson, T. & Phelan, J. (1999) The role of computed tomography with contrast and small bowel follow-through in the management of small bowel obstruction. *Am. J. Surg.* **177**, 375–378.

Rao, P.M. & Boland, G.W. (1998) Imaging of acute right lower abdominal quadrant pain (1998). *Clin. Radiol.* **53**, 639–649.

Zeman, R.K., Fox, S.H., Silverman, P.M., et al. (1993) Helical (spiral) CT of the abdomen. *Am. J. Roentgenol.* **160**, 719–725.

MRI OF THE GASTROINTESTINAL TRACT

Contrast agents

Contrast agents that can be used to alter the signal intensity within the bowel can be classified as positive contrast agents (high signal on T1-weighting) or negative agents (low signal on T2-weighting). Further information about these can be found in Chapter 2. However, air itself (within bowel) is a natural contrast agent and the addition of expensive contrast agents is not often necessary. One area where negative contrast agents have a role is in magnetic resonance cholangiopancreatography (MRCP) where fluid in the stomach and duodenum can obscure the biliary tree and pancreatic duct, and the introduction of a negative contrast agent can remove signal due to this fluid.

Motion artefacts

The time taken to obtain a scan can be in the order of several minutes if spin echo sequences are used. Consequently it is important to minimize peristalsis and respiration artefacts. Glucagon may be used to try and minimize peristalsis. A prone position or a compression band can be used to help reduce respiratory motion of the anterior abdominal wall. The artefact, which is propagated from the anterior abdominal wall during respiration, is also due to the high signal from fat. Consequently, fat suppression sequences can help to minimize this.

Pulse sequences

The sequences used for imaging the abdomen and gastrointestinal tract will depend on the nature of the clinical problem. Very fast sequences such as breath-hold gradient echo and single-shot fast-spin echo sequences may be used to minimize any movement artefact. However, they do suffer from relatively poor contrast resolution. Standard fast-spin echo T1-weighted and T2-weighted sequences (with gadolinium and fat suppression added as necessary) are often used as baseline sequences, but on occasion suffer from movement artefact. The plane of the sequences will depend on the clinical problem but axial scans are frequently used in the first instance in an orthogonal plane (coronal or sagittal) as required.

Further reading

1. Ferrucci, J.T. (1998) Advances in abdominal MR imaging. *Radiographics* **18**, 1569–1586.
2. Paley, M.R. & Ros, P.R. (1997) MRI of the gastrointestinal tract. *Eur. Radiol.* **7**, 1387–1397.

RADIONUCLIDE GASTRO-OESOPHAGEAL REFLUX STUDY

RN

Indications

1. Diagnosis and quantification of suspected gastro-oesophageal reflux.

Contraindications

None.

Radiopharmaceuticals

^{99m}Tc-colloid or ^{99m}Tc-DTPA mixed with:

1. *Adults and older children*: 150–300 ml orange juice acidified with an equal volume of 0.1 M hydrochloric acid.
2. *Infants and young children*: normal milk feed.

Typical adult dose is 10–20 MBq, max. 40 MBq (0.9 mSv ED).

Equipment

1. Gamma-camera
2. Low-energy general purpose collimator
3. Abdominal binder for compression test.

Patient preparation

Nil by mouth for 4–6 h. Infants may be studied at normal feed times.

Technique

Physiological test[1,2] – adults and older children

1. The liquid containing the tracer is given and washed down with unlabelled liquid to clear residual activity from the oesophagus.
2. The patient lies semi-recumbent with the camera centred over the stomach and lower oesophagus.
3. Dynamic imaging is commenced with 5-s 64×64 frames for 30–60 min.

Milk scan[1,2] – infants and younger children

1. The milk feed is divided into two parts and one mixed with the tracer.
2. The radiolabelled milk is given and washed down with the remaining unlabelled milk.
3. After eructation, the child is placed either supine or prone, according to natural behaviour (although reflux appears to occur more readily in the supine position), with the camera anterior over stomach and oesophagus.
4. Dynamic imaging is commenced with 5-s 64×64 frames for 30–60 min.
5. If pulmonary aspiration of feed is suspected, later imaging at 4 h may be performed. The test is specific but not very sensitive for this purpose.

Provocation with abdominal compression[1,3] – adults and older children

1. The abdominal binder is placed around the upper abdomen.
2. The radiolabelled liquid is given as above.
3. The patient lies supine with the camera centred over the stomach and lower oesophagus.
4. A 30-s image is taken.
5. The pressure in the binder is increased in steps of 20 mmHg up to 100 mmHg, being maintained at each step for 30 s while an image is taken.
6. The test is terminated as soon as significant reflux is seen.

Analysis

1. For dynamic studies, regions are drawn round the stomach and lower, middle and upper oesophagus.
2. Time–activity curves of these regions are produced, from which may be calculated the size, extent, frequency and duration of any reflux episodes.

Additional techniques

Oesophageal transit[1]

The reflux study may be combined with a bolus transport investigation by fast-frame (0.2–0.5 s) dynamic imaging during swallowing and generation of a functional compressed image incorporating information from each frame.[4]

Aftercare

None.

Complications

None.

References

1. Harding, L.K. & Robinson, P.J.A. (1990) The oesophagus. In: *Clinician's Guide to Nuclear Medicine: Gastroenterology*, pp. 6–21. London: Churchill Livingstone.
2. Guillet, J., Basse-Cathalinat, B., Christophe, E., et al. (1984) Routine studies of swallowed radionuclide transit in paediatrics: experience with 400 patients. *Eur. J. Nucl. Med.* **9**, 86–90.
3. Martins, J.C.R., Isaacs, P.E.T., Sladen, G.E., et al. (1984) Gastro-oesophageal reflux scintigraphy compared with pH probe monitoring. *Nucl. Med. Commun.* **5**, 201–204.
4. Klein, H.A. & Wald, A. (1984) Computer analysis of radionuclide esophageal transit studies. *J. Nucl. Med.* **25**, 957–964.

Further reading

Heyman S (1994) Gastroesophageal reflux, esophageal transit, gastric emptying, and pulmonary aspiration. In: Treves S. (ed) *Pediatric Nuclear Medicine*, 2nd edn, pp. 430–452. New York: Springer-Verlag.

Heyman S (1995) Paediatric gastrointestinal motility studies. *Semin. Nucl. Med.* **25**, 339–347.

Kjellen, G., Brudin, L. & Hakansson, H.O. (1991) Is scintigraphy of value in the diagnosis of gastro-oesophageal reflux disease? *Scand. J. Gastroenterol.* **26**, 425–430.

RADIONUCLIDE GASTRIC EMPTYING STUDY   RN

Indications

1. Investigation of symptoms suggestive of gastroparesis
2. Before or after gastric surgery
3. Investigation of the effects of gastric motility-altering drugs.

Contraindications

High probability of vomiting.

Radiopharmaceuticals

Many radiolabelled meals have been designed for gastric emptying studies, but as yet no standard has emerged. Emptying rate measured by radiolabelling is influenced by many factors, for example meal bulk, fat content, calorie content, patient position during imaging and labelling stability in vivo. For this reason, so-called 'normal' emptying times need to be taken in the context of the particular meal and protocol used to generate them. It is important that the meal used is physiological and reproducible. For centres new to the technique, it is better to use a meal for which published data exists than to create yet another formulation with inherently different behaviour.

Both liquid and solid studies may be performed, separately or simultaneously as a dual isotope study. Liquids have generally shorter emptying times than solids, and tend to follow an exponential emptying pattern. Solids tend to empty linearly after a lag phase. Prolonged solid emptying is highly correlated with prolonged liquid emptying, and there is debate therefore as to whether both studies are routinely necessary.[1] Examples of meals used are:

1. *Liquid meal*: Max. 12 MBq ^{99m}Tc-tin colloid (0.3 mSv ED) mixed with 200 ml orange juice, or with milk or formula feed for infants.
2. *Solid meal*: Scrambled egg prepared with max. 12 MBq ^{99m}Tc-colloid[2] (0.3 mSv ED) or ^{99m}Tc-DTPA.[3] Bulk is made up with other non-labelled foods such as bread and milk.
3. *Dual isotope combined liquid and solid meal:*[4]
   a. *Liquid*: 12 MBq ^{99m}Tc-colloid (0.3 mSv ED) mixed with 200 ml orange juice.
   b. *Solid*: 2 MBq ^{111}In-labelled resin beads (0.7 mSv ED) incorporated into a pancake containing 27 g fat, 18 g protein, 625 calories. Bulk is made up with other non-labelled foods. Only 2 MBq of ^{111}In is suggested (ARSAC max. is 12 MBq, 4 mSv ED) in order to minimize the downscatter into the ^{99m}Tc energy window.[5]

Equipment

1. Gamma-camera, preferably dual-headed
2. Low-energy general purpose collimator for ^{99m}Tc, medium energy for ^{111}In/^{99m}Tc.

Patient preparation

1. Nil by mouth for 8 h.
2. No smoking or alcohol from midnight before test.

3. Where practical, stop medications affecting gastric motility such as dopaminergic agonists (e.g. metoclopramide, domperidone), cholinergic agonists (e.g. bethanechol), tricyclic antidepressants and anticholinergics for 24 h or more prior to the study, depending upon their biological half-life.

Technique

Imaging from a single projection can cause significant errors due to movement of the meal anteriorly as it transfers to the antrum, thereby altering the amount of tissue attenuation of gamma-photons. The problem is likely to be exacerbated in obese patients. This can largely be overcome by taking pairs of opposing views (simultaneously for dual-head systems, consecutively for single heads) and calculating the geometric mean stomach activity in each pair.

1. The patient ingests the meal as quickly as they comfortably can. (If dumping syndrome is suspected, the meal should be eaten in front of the camera with a fast-frame dynamic acquisition running, or the dumping episode may be missed.)
2. The patient is positioned standing in front of the camera.
3. Every 5 min, a pair of 1-min anterior and posterior 128×128 images are obtained. Care should be taken to accurately reposition the patient for successive images.
4. The patient sits and relaxes between images.
5. A liquid study should be continued for up to 60 min and a solid study for up to 90 min. If it can be seen that the majority of the meal has emptied inside this time, the study may be terminated.
6. If emptying is very slow, later pairs of images may be acquired at intervals of 30–60 min.

If this protocol is impractical and an error of up to 20% can be tolerated in the calculated half-emptying time, then a single dynamic study in the anterior position (128×128 acquisition with 1-min frame time) may be performed with the patient sitting or semi-recumbent, or, for an infant, lying prone directly on the surface of a horizontal gamma camera.

Analysis

1. Stomach region of interest is drawn. Depending upon analysis software, this may be facilitated by aligning frames first.
2. Stomach time-activity curve is produced, using geometric mean if anterior and posterior imaging performed.

3. Half-emptying time is calculated, either from direct observation or by curve-fitting.
4. Other parameters may be calculated, e.g. lag phase duration for solid studies, or percentage left in the stomach at various time points.

Additional techniques

1. The small bowel transit time (SBTT) can be ascertained by continuing imaging at intervals until the caecum is seen. Since the position of the caecum is often not obvious and may be overlain by small bowel, a 12–24 h image can be useful to determine the position of the large bowel. This is convenient to perform if a two-stage solid and liquid test is being undertaken on consecutive days. Anatomical marking of the anterior superior iliac spine may help to locate the caecum. However, it must be recognized that there will still be a significant minority of cases where the SBTT can not be obtained with any certainty.
2. Frequency analysis of fast dynamic scans (1-s frame time) can be used to characterize antral contraction patterns.[6,7]

Aftercare

None.

Complications

None.

References

1. Siegel, J.A., Krevsky, B., Maurer, A.H., et al. (1989) Scintigraphic evaluation of gastric emptying: are radiolabeled solids necessary? *Clin. Nucl. Med.* **14**, 40–46.
2. Malmud, L.S., Fisher, R.S., Knight, L.C., et al. (1982) Scintigraphic evaluation of gastric emptying. *Semin. Nucl. Med.* **12**, 116–125.
3. Jonderko, K. (1987) Radionuclide studies on gastric evacuatory function in health and in the duodenal ulcer disease. I. Types of solid meal distribution within the stomach and their relation to gastric emptying. *Nucl. Med. Commun.* **8**, 671–680.
4. Mather, S.J., Ellison, D., Nightingale, J., et al. (1991) The design of a two-phase radiolabelled meal for gastric emptying studies. *Nucl. Med. Commun.* **12**, 409–416.
5. Heyman, S. (1988) Gastric emptying, gastroesophageal reflux, and esophageal motility. In: Gelfand, M.J. & Thomas, S.R. (eds) *Effective Use of Computers in Nuclear Medicine*, pp. 412–437. New York: McGraw-Hill.
6. Urbain, J.-L., Vekemans, M.C., Bouillon, R., et al. (1993) Characterisation of gastric antral motility disturbances in diabetes using the scintigraphic technique. *J. Nucl. Med.* **34**, 576–581.
7. Urbain J-L, & Charkes, N.D. (1995) Recent advances in gastric emptying. *Semin. Nucl. Med.* **25**, 318–325.

Further reading

Malmud, L.S. (1990) Gastric emptying. *J. Nucl. Med.* **31**, 1499–1500.
Maughan, R.J. & Leiper, J.B. (1996) Methods for the assessment of gastric emptying in humans: an overview. *Diabet Med.* **13(suppl 5)**, S6–10.

RADIONUCLIDE BILE REFLUX STUDY   RN

Indications[1]

1. Persistent symptoms after peptic ulcer surgery or gastrectomy.
2. Persistent flatulent dyspepsia after cholecystectomy after other causes have been ruled out.

Contraindications

None.

Radiopharmaceuticals

^{99m}Tc-trimethylbromoiminodiacetic acid (TBIDA) or other iminodiacetic acid (IDA) derivative, 80 MBq typical (1 mSv ED), 150 MBq max (2 mSv ED). ^{99m}Tc-pertechnetate 10 MBq (0.13 mSv ED) to demonstrate stomach outline.

IDA compounds are rapidly cleared from the circulation by the hepatocytes and secreted into bile in a similar way to bilirubin.

Equipment

1. Gamma-camera
2. Low-energy general purpose collimator.

Patient preparation

Nil by mouth for 6 h.

Technique

1. ^{99m}Tc-TBIDA is administered i.v.
2. 20–30 min post-injection, the patient lies supine with the camera anterior. Marker sources may be placed on the iliac crests to monitor patient movement.
3. Imaging is commenced at 1 min per frame for 60–70 min.
4. 30–45 min post-injection when the gallbladder is well visualized, either 70 units of cholecystokinin (CCK) are administered i.v. over 2 min, or a liquid fatty meal (e.g. 300 ml

full cream milk) is given through a straw to stimulate gallbladder contraction. CCK is more effective at provoking reflux.

5. If images are suggestive of reflux, 100–200 ml of water is given through a straw to diffuse any activity in the stomach and thereby differentiate it from nearby bowel activity.

6. 4 min before the end of imaging, 100 ml of water containing 10 MBq ^{99m}Tc-pertechnetate is given to delineate the stomach.

Additional techniques

1. A standard series of manoeuvres such as Valsalva (forced exhalation against a closed glottis) and coughing may be performed to provoke further reflux into the oesophagus.[2]

2. Functional evaluation of the complete oesophagogastroduodenal tract may be performed with a combined ^{99m}Tc-HIDA and radiolabelled swallow study.[3]

4. Region of interest analysis has been used to attempt to quantify reflux.[3]

Aftercare

None.

Complications

Possibility of severe colic or hypotension following CCK injection.

References

1. Harding, L.K. & Robinson, P.J.A. (1990) Hepatobiliary studies: bile reflux, jaundice and acute cholecystitis. In: *Clinician's Guide to Nuclear Medicine: Gastroenterology*, pp. 31–48. London: Churchill Livingstone.

2. Bortolotti, M., Abbati, A., Turba, E., et al. (1985) ^{99m}Tc-HIDA dynamic scintigraphy for the diagnosis of gastroesophageal reflux of bile. *Eur. J. Nucl. Med.* **10**, 549–550.

3. Borsato, N., Bonavina, L., Zanco, P. et al. (1991) Proposal of a modified scintigraphic method to evaluate duodenogastroesophageal reflux. *J. Nucl. Med.* **32**, 436–440.

Further reading

Drane, W.E., Karvelis, K., Johnson, D.A., et al. (1987) Scintigraphic evaluation of duodenogastric reflux: problems, pitfalls, and technical review. *Clin. Nucl. Med.* **12**, 377–384.

Mittal, B.R., Ibrarullah, M., Agarwal, D.K., et al. (1994) Comparative evaluation of scintigraphy and upper gastrointestinal tract endoscopy for detection of duodenogastric reflux. *Ann. Nucl. Med.* **8**, 183–186.

Szarszewski, A., Korzon, M., Kaminska, B., et al. (1999) Duodenogastric reflux: clinical and therapeutic aspects. *Arch. Dis. Child.* **81**, 16–20.

RADIONUCLIDE MECKEL'S DIVERTICULUM SCAN RN

Indications

Detection of a Meckel's diverticulum as a cause for gastro-intestinal bleeding, obstruction or abdominal pain.

Contraindications

1. Barium study in previous 2–3 days (barium causes significant attenuation of gamma photons and may mask a bleeding site).
2. *In vivo* labelled red blood cell study in previous few days (due to likelihood of pertechnetate adhering to red cells).
3. Precautions and contraindications to any pre-administered drugs should be observed.

Radiopharmaceuticals

^{99m}Tc-pertechnetate, 200 MBq typical (2.5 mSv ED), 400 MBq max (5 mSv ED). Injected ^{99m}Tc-pertechnetate localizes in ectopic gastric mucosa within a diverticulum.

Equipment

1. Gamma-camera
2. Low-energy general purpose collimator.

Patient preparation

1. Nil by mouth for 6 h, unless emergency.
2. It may be possible to enhance detection by prior administration of drugs aimed at increasing the uptake of ^{99m}Tc-pertechnetate into gastric mucosa and inhibiting its release into the lumen of the stomach and progression into the bowel. The following regimes have been suggested:[1]
   a. pentagastrin (6 µg kg^{-1} subcutaneously 15 min before imaging)
   b. pentagastrin as above in combination with glucagon (0.25–2 mg i.v.)
   c. cimetidine (300 mg orally 4 times daily for 48 h before test, or 300 mg in 100 ml 5% glucose infused i.v. over 20 min, 1 h before imaging)
   d. ranitidine (1 mg kg^{-1}, up to a maximum of 50 mg, in sodium chloride 0.9%, infused i.v. over 20 min, 1 h before imaging).

Technique

1. The bladder is emptied – a full bladder may obscure the diverticulum.

2. The patient lies supine with the camera over the abdomen and pelvis. The stomach must be included in the field of view because diagnosis is dependent on demonstrating uptake of radionuclide in the diverticulum concurrent with uptake by gastric mucosa.
3. Pertechnetate is administered i.v.
4. A 128×128 dynamic acquisition is begun immediately with 2-s images for 1 min to demonstrate vascular blood pool anatomy, followed by 1 min images up to 45 min.
5. Posterior and lateral images as required.

Aftercare

None.

Complications

Pre-administered drug sensitivity and side-effects.

Reference

1. Datz, F.L., Christian, P.E., Hutson, W.R., et al. (1991) Physiological and pharmacological interventions in radionuclide imaging of tubular gastrointestinal tract. *Semin. Nucl. Med.* **21**, 140–152.

Further reading

Ford, P.V., Bartold, S.P., Fink-Bennett, D.M., et al. (1999) Procedure guidelines for gastrointestinal bleeding and Meckel's diverticulum scintigraphy. *J. Nucl. Med.* **40**, 1226–1232.

Harding, L.K. & Notghi, A. (1998) Gastrointestinal tract and liver. In: Sharp, P.F., Gemmell, H.G. & Smith, F.W. (eds) *Practical Nuclear Medicine*, pp. 193–209. Oxford: Oxford University Press.

Rossi, P., Gourtsoyiannis, N., Bezzi, M., et al. (1996) Meckel's diverticulum: imaging diagnosis. *Am. J. Roentgenol.* **166**, 567–573.

RADIONUCLIDE IMAGING OF GASTROINTESTINAL BLEEDING   RN

Indications

Gastrointestinal bleeding of unknown origin.

Contraindications

1. No active bleeding at time scheduled for study.
2. Slow bleeding of less than approx. 0.5 ml min^{-1}.

3. Barium study in previous 2–3 days (barium causes significant attenuation of gamma photons and may mask a bleeding site).

Radiopharmaceuticals

1. *^{99m}Tc-labelled red blood cells*, 400 MBq max (4 mSv ED). Red cells are pre-treated with a stannous agent. ^{99m}Tc-pertechnetate is added and is reduced by the stannous ions, causing it to be retained intracellularly. Labelling efficiency is important, as false positive scans can result from accumulations of free pertechnetate. In vitro preparation gives the best labelling efficiency, but is most complex and time-consuming.[1] However, commercial kits are available which can reduce the preparation time to around 30 min (e.g. 'Ultratag', Mallinckrodt Medical). In vivo labelling is least efficient, and there is also a compromise in vivo/vitro method where the labelling occurs in the syringe as blood is withdrawn from the patient.[2,3]

2. *^{99m}Tc-colloid*, 400 MBq max (4 mSv ED). This used to be a commonly used alternative to labelled red cells (for a protocol see Harding & Robinson[4]), but a number of studies have shown it to be a less sensitive tracer for detecting bleeding sites,[2,5] hence it is not recommended. Colloids are rapidly extracted from the circulation, so bleeding occurring only within 10 min or so of injection can be detected. Also localizes intensely in liver and spleen, masking upper gastrointestinal bleeding sites.

Equipment

1. Gamma-camera
2. Low-energy general purpose collimator.

Patient preparation

1. In vivo or in vivo/vitro methods: 'Cold' stannous agent (15 µg kg^{-1} tin) is administered directly into a vein 20–30 min before the ^{99m}Tc-pertechnetate injection. (Injection via a plastic cannula will result in a poor label.)
2. The patient is asked to empty their bladder before each image is taken. Catheterization is ideal if appropriate.

Technique

1. The patient lies supine.
2. The camera is positioned over the anterior abdomen with the symphysis pubis at the bottom of the field of view.

3. ^{99m}Tc-pertechnetate (in vivo method) or ^{99m}Tc-labelled red cells (in vitro or in vivo/vitro methods) are injected i.v.

4. A 128×128 dynamic acquisition is begun immediately with 2-s images for 1 min to help to demonstrate vascular blood pool anatomy, followed by 1-min images up to 45 min. Dynamic imaging permits cinematic viewing of images to detect bleed sites and movement through bowel.[6]

5. Further 15×1-min dynamic image sets are acquired at 1, 2, 4, 6, 8 and 24 h or until bleeding site is detected (imaging much beyond 24 h is limited by radioactive decay).

6. Oblique and lateral views may help to localize any abnormal collections of activity.

Aftercare

None.

Complications

None.

References

1. Jones, J. & Mollison, P.L. (1978) A simple and efficient method of labelling red cells with ^{99m}Tc for the determination of red cell volume. *Br. J. Haematol.* **38**, 141–148.
2. Chaudhuri, T.K. (1991) Radionuclide methods of detecting acute gastrointestinal bleeding. *Nucl. Med. Biol. Int. J. Radiat. Appl. Instrum. Part B* **18**, 655–661.
3. Callahan, R.J., Froelich, J.W., McKusick, K.A., et al. (1982) A modified method for the in vivo labeling of red blood cells with Tc-99m: concise communication. *J. Nucl. Med.* **23**, 315–318.
4. Harding, L.K. & Robinson P.J.A. (1990) Hepatobiliary studies: Localisation of gastrointestinal bleeding. In: *Clinician's Guide to Nuclear Medicine: Gastroenterology*, pp 116–128. London: Churchill Livingstone.
5. Bunker, S.R., Lull, R.J., Tanasescu, D.E., et al. (1984) Scintigraphy of gastrointestinal hemorrhage: superiority of ^{99m}Tc red blood cells over ^{99m}Tc sulfur colloid. *Am. J. Roentgenol.* **143**, 543–548.
6. Maurer, A.H. (1996) Gastrointestinal bleeding and cine-scintigraphy. *Semin. Nucl. Med.* **26**, 43–50.

Further reading

Ford, P.V., Bartold, S.P., Fink-Bennett, D.M., et al. (1999) Procedure guidelines for gastrointestinal bleeding and Meckel's diverticulum scintigraphy. *J. Nucl. Med.* **40**, 1226–1232.

Nicholson, M.L., Neoptolemos, J.P., Sharp, J.F., et al. (1989) Localization of lower gastrointestinal bleeding using in vivo technetium-99m-labelled red blood cell scintigraphy. *Br. J. Surg.* **76**, 358–361.

4 Liver, biliary tract and pancreas

Methods of imaging the hepatobiliary system

1. Plain film
2. Oral cholecystography
3. Operative cholangiography
4. Postoperative (T-tube) cholangiography
5. Endoscopic retrograde cholangiopancreatography (ERCP)
6. Percutaneous transhepatic cholangiography (PTC)
7. US
8. Radionuclide imaging
   – static, with colloid
   – dynamic, with iminodiacetic acid derivatives
9. CT
10. MRI.

Methods of imaging the pancreas

1. Chest radiography
2. Plain abdominal films
3. Hypotonic duodenography
4. ERCP
5. PTC
6. Arteriography
   – coeliac axis
   – superior mesenteric artery
7. Venography
   – percutaneous transhepatic method
   – umbilical vein catheterization
8. US
   – transcutaneous
   – intraoperative
   – endoscopic
9. CT
10. MRI.

BILIARY CONTRAST MEDIA

Like conventional urographic contrast media, biliary contrast media are also tri-iodo benzoic acid derivatives. Iopanoic acid (Telepaque) was introduced in 1951 and the later compounds were all modifications of it. Differences occur in the prosthetic group (position 1) and the amino group (position 3).

Iopanoic acid
(Telepaque)

The oral agents have a single benzene ring, whilst the only i.v. contrast medium, meglumine iotroxate (Biliscopin) is a dimer with a polymethylene chain connecting the two rings.

Meglumine iotroxate (Biliscopin)

It is the absence of a prosthetic group at position 5 in both the oral and i.v. agents that determines biliary rather than renal excretion.

METABOLIC PATHWAY

1. Absorption of oral contrast media from the gut requires that they have both hydrophilic and lipophilic properties.
2. Passive diffusion occurs across the lipid membrane of the gastrointestinal mucosa. (Iotroxate, although very water-soluble, is insoluble in lipids and is, therefore, not absorbed when given orally.)

3. After absorption they are bound to albumen and carried in the portal vein to the liver. Intravenous biliary contrast medium is also albumen-bound. Toxicity is proportional to albumen binding.
4. In the liver they are taken up by the hepatocyte, possibly via the Y and Z receptors.
5. Intravenous contrast medium is not altered in the hepatocyte and is excreted into the bile unchanged. Oral agents are conjugated with glucuronic acid to form more water-soluble glucuronides.
6. Excretion into bile is an active transport process which can become saturated and is the rate-limiting step.
7. Oral agents are concentrated in the gallbladder by the absorption of water, peak opacification of the gallbladder occurring approximately 12 h after ingestion.
8. Oral agents are finally excreted in the stool. Reabsorption is severely limited because after conjugation they are no longer lipophilic. The intravenous agent, being water-soluble, is excreted by glomerular filtration when the infusion rate is high and biliary excretion is saturated.

ORAL CHOLECYSTOGRAPHY

Indications

This is an investigation which has largely become redundant over the last decade with the widespread use of US and, to a lesser extent, of other more sophisticated imaging tools such as endoscopic retrograde cholangiography (ERCP) and magnetic resonance cholangiography (MRCP). The indication for its use now is to demonstrate suspected pathology in the gallbladder when ultrasound is not available or has failed to demonstrate the gallbladder.[1,2]

The cystic duct and common bile duct may also be seen. The examination is unlikely to be successful when the serum bilirubin is greater than 34 μmol l^{-1}.

Contraindications

1. Severe hepatic or renal disease
2. Acute cholecystitis
3. Dehydration
4. Intravenous cholangiography within the previous week (although this is now a rarely undertaken investigation)
5. Previous cholecystectomy.

Contrast medium

1. Sodium ipodate (Biloptin); 6 capsules each containing 500 mg. This is the most widely used agent.
2. Iopanoic acid (Telepaque); 6 capsules each containing 500 mg.

Patient preparation for Biloptin

1. A laxative 2 days prior to the examination.
2. Light, fat-free diet on the day before the examination.
3. No food from 18:00 h on the day before the examination until after the examination has been completed. Liquids (without milk) are allowed. The cholecystographic agent is taken with water after the last meal prior to the patient's appointment.

Preliminary film

Prone 20° LAO, centred 7.5 cm to the right of the spinous processes, 2.5 cm cephalad to the lower costal margin.

This film is taken when the patient makes an appointment. There has been controversy regarding the usefulness of this film. Some believe that 5% of calculi will be missed if it is omitted,[3] while others believe that virtually all radio-opaque gallstones are seen within the opacified gallbladder.[4] Other pathology, outside the gallbladder, may be found in 5% of patients.[5]

Films

1. Prone 20° LAO – contrast medium fills the fundus of the gallbladder.
2. Supine 20° RPO – contrast medium fills the neck and Hartmann's pouch.
3. Erect 20° LAO – may demonstrate floating gallstones.
4. Overlying bowel shadows may be removed by rotating the patient under fluoroscopic control or by tomography.
5. Prone 20° LAO, 30 min after a fatty meal (chocolate or a proprietary fat emulsion). The value of this film was assessed by Harvey et al.,[6] who found it was:
   a. essential for the cholecystographic diagnosis of adenomyomatosis[7] and cholesterolosis
   b. occasionally helpful in diagnosing small stones
   c. of little value in assessing the biliary ducts or separating the gallbladder from overlying bowel gas
   d. of no value in the diagnosis of functional biliary tract disorders.

If the gallbladder is not seen on the first film, the patient is asked the following questions:

1. What time were the tablets taken? (Sufficient time is needed for absorption and concentration in the gallbladder.)
2. How many tablets were taken?
3. Did diarrhoea or vomiting develop after the tablets were taken?

If the tablets have been taken, a 35×43-cm supine abdominal film is taken. This may demonstrate:

a. a gallbladder in an abnormal position, or
b. unabsorbed contrast medium. This has a flakey appearance and can be distinguished from esterified contrast medium that has passed through the liver and biliary tract, which causes a more uniform, fainter opacification.

If the gallbladder is only poorly seen, the patient is given a further standard dose to be taken that evening and repeat films are taken the following day.

Additional techniques

For better visualization of the ducts, manufacturers make the following recommendations:

1. Biloptin – (i) 12 capsules at the usual time or (ii) 6 capsules 10–12 h before the examination plus another 6 capsules 3 h before.
2. Telepaque – 3–6 tablets are taken 4 h after a fatty lunch on the day preceding the examination, and then a full dose of 6 tablets after a fat-free meal in the evening.

Aftercare

None.

Complications

Side-effects, even of a trivial nature, are rare with sodium ipodate. Mild gastrointestinal disturbances – nausea, with or without vomiting and diarrhoea – may occur. The incidence of diarrhoea is greatest with iopanoic acid. Skin reactions – urticaria, vasodilatation and pruritus – have been recorded. Cholecystographic agents have a uricosuric action and alteration of serum urate may precipitate an attack of gout.

References

1. Amberg, J.R. & Leopold, G.R. (1988) Is oral cholecystography still useful? *Am. J. Roentgenol.* **151**, 73–74.

2. Gelfand, D.W., Wolfman, N.T., Ott, D.J., et al. (1988) Oral cholecystography vs gallbladder sonography. A prospective, blinded reappraisal. *Am. J. Roentgenol.* **151**, 69–72.
3. Twomey, B., de Lacey, G. & Gajjar, B. (1983) The plain radiograph in oral cholecystography – should it be abandoned? *Br. J. Radiol.* **56**, 99–100.
4. Anderson, J.F. & Madsen, P.E. (1979) The value of plain radiographs prior to oral cholecystography. *Radiology* **133**, 309–310.
5. Karned, R.K. & LeVeen, R.F. (1978) Preliminary abdominal films in oral cholecystography: are they necessary? *Am. J. Roentgenol.* **130**, 477–479.
6. Harvey, I.C., Thwe, M. & Low-Beer, T.S. (1976) The value of the fatty meal in oral cholecystography. *Clin. Radiol.* **27**, 117–121.
7. Gajjar, B., Twomey, B. & de Lacey, G. (1976) The fatty meal and acalculous gallbladder disease. *Clin. Radiol.* **35**, 405–408.

INTRAVENOUS CHOLANGIOGRAPHY

This investigation is now very rarely undertaken because of improved and significantly safer imaging by US, ERCP and MRCP. Complications of meglumine iotroxate (Biliscopin 50 infusion) are similar to urographic contrast media but it is more toxic.

PREOPERATIVE CHOLANGIOGRAPHY

Indications

During cholecystectomy or bile duct surgery, to avoid surgical exploration of the common bile duct.

Contraindications

None.

Contrast medium

HOCM or LOCM 150, i.e. low iodine content so as not to obscure any calculi; 20 ml.

Equipment

1. Operating table with a film cassette tunnel.
2. Mobile X-ray machine.

Patient preparation

As for surgery.

Technique

The surgeon cannulates the cystic duct with a fine catheter. This is prefilled with contrast medium to exclude air bubbles which might simulate calculi.

Films

1. After 5 ml have been injected.
2. After 20 ml have been injected. Contrast medium should flow freely into the duodenum. Spasm of the sphincter of Oddi is a fairly frequent occurrence and may be due to anaesthetic agents or surgical manipulation. It may be relieved by glucagon, propantheline or amyl nitrite.

The criteria for a normal operative choledochogram are given by Le Quesne[1] as:

1. Common bile duct width not greater than 12 mm.
2. Free flow of contrast medium into the duodenum.
3. The terminal narrow segment of the duct is clearly seen.
4. There are no filling defects.
5. There is no excess retrograde filling of the hepatic ducts.

Reference

1. Le Quesne, L.P. (1960) Discussion on cholangiography. *Proc. R. Soc. Med.* **53**, 852–855.

Further reading

Chant, A.D.B., Dewbury, K.G., Guyer, P.B., et al. (1982) Operative cholangiography reassessed. *Clin. Radiol.* **33**, 289–291.
Faris, I., Thomson, J.P.S., Grundy, D.J., et al. (1975) Operative cholangiography: a re-appraisal based on a review of 400 cholangiograms. *Br. J. Surg.* **62**, 966–972.
Millward, S.F. (1982) Post-exploratory operative cholangiography: is it a useful technique to check clearance of the common bile duct? *Clin. Radiol.* **33**, 535–538.

POSTOPERATIVE (T-TUBE) CHOLANGIOGRAPHY

Indications

1. To exclude biliary tract calculi where (a) operative cholangiography was not performed, or (b) the results of operative cholangiography are not satisfactory or are suspect.
2. Assessment of biliary leaks following biliary surgery.

Contraindications

None.

Contrast medium

HOCM or LOCM 150; 20–30 ml.

Equipment

Fluoroscopy unit with spot film device.

Patient preparation

None.

Preliminary film

Coned supine PA of the right side of the abdomen.

Technique

1. The examination is performed on or about the tenth postoperative day, prior to pulling out the T-tube.
2. The patient lies supine on the X-ray table. The drainage tube is clamped off near to the patient and cleaned thoroughly with antiseptic.
3. A 23-G needle, extension tubing and 20 ml syringe are assembled and filled with contrast medium. After all air bubbles have been expelled the needle is inserted into the tubing between the patient and the clamp. The injection is made under fluoroscopic control, the total volume depending on duct filling.

Films

PA and oblique views positioned under fluoroscopic control.

Aftercare

None.

Complications

Due to the contrast medium

The biliary ducts do absorb contrast medium and cholangiovenous reflux can occur with high injection pressures. Adverse reactions are, therefore, possible but the incidence is small.

Due to the technique

Injection of contrast medium under high pressure into an obstructed biliary tract can produce septicaemia.

PERCUTANEOUS EXTRACTION OF RETAINED BILIARY CALCULI (BURHENNE TECHNIQUE)

Indications

Retained biliary calculi seen on the T-tube cholangiogram (incidence 3%).

Contraindications

1. Small T-tube (< 12F)
2. Tortuous T-tube course in soft tissues
3. Acute pancreatitis
4. Drain in situ (cross connections exist between the drain tract and the T-tube tract).

Contrast medium

HOCM or LOCM 150. (Low-density contrast medium is used to avoid obscuring the calculus.)

Equipment

1. Fluoroscopy unit with spot film device.
2. Medi-Tech steerable catheter system with wire baskets.

Patient preparation

1. T-tube should be greater than 12F.
2. T-tube should be brought out obliquely towards the right flank (to avoid irradiation of the radiologist's fingers).
3. Following discovery of the retained stone on the tenth day post-T-tube cholangiogram, the patient should be discharged with the T-tube clamped for at least 4 weeks to allow the formation of a solid fistulous tract.
4. Admission to hospital on the day prior to the procedure.
5. Prophylactic antibiotics and pre-medication 1 h prior to the procedure.
6. Analgesia during the procedure.

Technique

1. The patient lies supine on the X-ray table. A T-tube cholangiogram is performed to accurately localize the retained calculus.
2. The T-tube is slowly withdrawn from the patient.
3. The steerable catheter is advanced down the T-tube track and its tip is positioned just beyond the calculus. A basket is then inserted through the catheter and opened beyond the stone. The

opened basket and catheter are then slowly withdrawn and the stone engaged. The basket should not be closed as the stone may be disengaged or fragmented. The catheter system with the engaged stone in the basket should be slowly withdrawn to the skin surface in one movement.

4. The duct system is opacified by intermittent injections of contrast through the steerable catheter.

5. At the end of the procedure a suction catheter or similar is manipulated into the duct system and sutured to the skin.

6. Stones up to 10 mm in diameter may be extracted through a 14-F tract. Stones greater than 10 mm will require fragmentation (if soft) or endoscopic sphincterotomy/surgery. Multiple stones may require repeated procedures.

7. A completion cholangiogram should be performed via the suction catheter on the day following the procedure, when the gas bubbles have cleared.

Aftercare

1. Pulse and blood pressure half-hourly for 6 h.
2. Bed rest for 12 h.

Complications

Morbidity 4%.

Due to the contrast medium

1. 'Allergic' reactions – rare
2. Pancreatitis.

Due to the technique

1. Fever
2. Perforation of the T-tube tract.

Further reading

Burhenne, H.J. (1980) Percutaneous extraction of retained biliary stones: 661 patients. *Am. J. Roentgenol.* **134**, 888–898.

Mason, R. (1980) Percutaneous extraction of retained gallstones via the T-tube track – British experience of 131 cases. *Clin. Radiol.* **31**, 497–499.

ENDOSCOPIC RETROGRADE CHOLANGIOPANCREATOGRAPHY

Although percutaneous transhepatic cholangiography (PTC) has a higher success rate for demonstrating bile ducts, ERCP has three advantages over PTC:[1]

1. The ability to visualize and biopsy ampullary lesions.
2. The demonstration of biliary tree and pancreatic duct.
3. Greater therapeutic potential.

ERCP is usually performed by physicians or surgeons rather than radiologists.

Indications

1. Investigation of extrahepatic biliary obstruction
2. Post-cholecystectomy syndrome
3. Investigation of diffuse biliary disease, e.g. sclerosing cholangitis
4. Pancreatic disease.

Contraindications

1. Australia antigen-positive; HIV-positive
2. Oesophageal obstruction; varices; pyloric stenosis
3. Previous gastric surgery
4. Acute pancreatitis
5. Pancreatic pseudocyst
6. When glucagon or Buscopan are contraindicated
7. Severe cardio/respiratory disease.

Contrast medium

Pancreas

LOCM 240.

Bile ducts

LOCM 150; dilute contrast medium ensures that calculi will not be obscured.

Equipment

1. Side-viewing endoscope
2. Polythene catheters
3. Fluoroscopic unit with spot film facilities.

Patient preparation

1. Nil orally for 4 h prior to procedure
2. Premedication (see Chapter 1)
3. Antibiotic cover.

Preliminary film

Prone AP and LAO of the upper abdomen, to check for opaque gallstones and pancreatic calcification/calculi.

Technique

The pharynx is anaesthetized with 4% Xylocaine spray and the patient is given diazepam 5 mg min^{-1} i.v. until sedated. The patient then lies on the left side and the endoscope is introduced. The ampulla of Vater is located and the patient is turned prone. A polythene catheter prefilled with contrast medium is inserted into the ampulla, having ensured that all air bubbles are excluded. A small test injection of contrast under fluoroscopic control is made to determine the position of the cannula. It is important to avoid over-filling of the pancreas. If it is desirable to opacify both the biliary tree and pancreatic duct, then the latter should be cannulated first. A sample of bile should be sent for culture and sensitivity if there is evidence of biliary obstruction.

Films

Pancreas (using fine focal spot)

1. Prone, both posterior obliques.

Bile ducts

1. Early filling films to show calculi
   a. Prone – straight and posterior obliques
   b. Supine – straight, both obliques; Trendelenburg to fill intrahepatic ducts; semi-erect to fill lower end of common bile duct and gallbladder.
2. Films following removal of the endoscope, which may obscure the duct.
3. Delayed films to assess the gallbladder and emptying of the common bile duct.

Aftercare

1. Nil orally until sensation has returned to the pharynx (0.5–3 h).
2. Pulse, temperature and blood pressure half-hourly for 6 h.
3. Maintain antibiotics if there is biliary or pancreatic obstruction.
4. Serum/urinary amylase if pancreatitis is suspected.

Complications

Due to the contrast medium

1. 'Allergic reactions' – rare
2. Acute pancreatitis – more likely with large volumes, high-pressure injections.

Due to the technique

Local

Damage by the endoscope, e.g. rupture of the oesophagus, damage to the ampulla, proximal pancreatic duct and distal common duct.

Distant

Bacteraemia, septicaemia, aspiration pneumonitis, hyperamylasaemia (approx. 70%). Acute pancreatitis (0.7–7.4%).

Reference

1. Summerfield, J.A. (1988) Biliary obstruction is best managed by endoscopists. *Gut* **29**, 741–745.

Further reading

Freeman, A. & Martin, D. (1991) Editorial. New trends with endoscopic retrograde cholangiopancreatography. *Clin. Radiol.* **43**, 223–226.

Frost, R.A. (1996) Complications of gastrointestinal tract interventional endoscopy. In: Ansell, G., Bettmann, M.A., Kaufman, J.A., et al. (eds) *Complications in Diagnostic Imaging and Interventional Radiology*, pp. 546–562. Oxford: Blackwell Science.

PERCUTANEOUS TRANSHEPATIC CHOLANGIOGRAPHY

Indications

1. Cholestatic jaundice, to confirm or exclude extrahepatic bile duct obstruction.
2. Prior to therapeutic intervention, e.g. biliary drainage procedure.

Contraindications

1. Bleeding tendency:
   - platelets less than 100 000
   - prothrombin time 2 s greater than control
2. Biliary tract sepsis
3. Non-availability of prompt surgical facilities should they be necessary, or a patient who is unfit for surgery
4. Hydatid disease.

Contrast medium

LOCM 150; 20–60 ml.

Equipment

1. Fluoroscopy unit with spot film device and tilting table
2. Chiba needle (a fine, flexible 22-G needle, 18-cm long).

Patient preparation

1. Haemoglobin, prothrombin time and platelets are checked, and corrected if necessary.
2. Prophylactic antibiotics – ampicillin 500 mg q.d.s. – to commence 24 h before and continue for 3 days after the examination.
3. Nil by mouth for 5 h prior to the procedure.
4. Premedication (see Chapter 1).

Preliminary film

Supine PA of the right side of the abdomen.

Technique

1. The patient lies supine. Under fluoroscopic control a metal marker is placed on the skin in the right mid-axillary line such that its position overlies the liver during full inspiration and expiration. A second metal marker is placed on the xiphisternum.
2. Using aseptic technique the skin, deeper tissues and liver capsule are anaesthetized at the site of the first metal marker.
3. During suspended respiration the Chiba needle is inserted into the liver, but once it is within the liver parenchyma the patient is allowed shallow respirations. It is advanced parallel to the table top in the direction of the xiphisternum until just short of the right lateral margin of the spine.
4. The stilette is withdrawn and the needle connected to a syringe and extension tubing prefilled with contrast medium. Contrast medium is injected under fluoroscopic control while the needle is slowly withdrawn. If a duct is not entered at the first attempt, the needle tip is withdrawn to approximately 2–3 cm from the liver capsule and further passes are made, directing the needle tip more cranially, caudally, anteriorly or posteriorly until a duct is entered. If a duct has not been entered after ten attempts, the procedure is terminated and the assumption is made that the ducts are not dilated. The incidence of complications is not related to the number of passes and the likelihood of success is directly related to the degree of duct dilatation and the number of passes made.
5. Excessive parenchymal injection should be avoided and when it does occur it results in opacification of intrahepatic

lymphatics. Injection of contrast medium into a vein or artery is followed by rapid dispersion.

6. If the intrahepatic ducts are seen to be dilated, bile should be aspirated and sent for microbiological examination. (The incidence of infected bile is high in such cases.)

7. Contrast medium is injected to fill the duct system and define the lower end of an obstruction (if present). The needle is withdrawn. Care should be taken not to overfill an obstructed duct system because septic shock may be precipitated.

Films

Contrast medium is heavier than bile and the sequence of duct opacification is, therefore, gravity-dependent and determined by the site of injection and the position of the patient.

Using the undercouch tube with the patient *horizontal*:

1. PA
2. 45° RPO
3. Right lateral
4. Trendelenburg
5. Spot views of the gallbladder, if this has been opacified.

Using the undercouch tube with the patient *erect*:

1. PA
2. 45° RPO
3. Right lateral
4. Spot views of the gallbladder
5. When the above films have shown an obstruction at the level of the porta hepatis, a further film after the patient has been in the erect position for 30 min may show the level of obstruction to be lower than originally thought.

Additional films

Hypotonic duodenography

This may be performed to give additional information regarding the site of an obstruction and its position relative to the duodenum. (For method and films see p. 59.)

Delayed films

Films taken after several hours, or the next day, may show contrast medium in the gallbladder if this was not achieved during the initial part of the investigation.

Aftercare

Pulse and blood pressure half-hourly for 6 h.

Complications

Morbidity approximately 3%; mortality less than 0.1%.

Due to the contrast medium

Allergic/idiosyncratic reactions – very uncommon.

Due to the technique

Local

1. Puncture of extrahepatic structures – usually no serious sequelae
2. Intrathoracic injection
3. Cholangitis
4. Bile leakage – may lead to biliary peritonitis (incidence 0.5%). More likely if the ducts are under pressure and if there are multiple puncture attempts. Less likely if a drainage catheter is left in situ prior to surgery. (See 'Biliary drainage' below)
5. Subphrenic abscess
6. Haemorrhage
7. Shock – owing to injection into the region of the coeliac plexus.

Generalized

Bacteraemia, septicaemia and endotoxic shock. The likelihood of sepsis is greatest in the presence of choledocholithiasis because of the higher incidence of pre-existing infected bile.

Further reading

Fraser, G.M., Cruickshank, J.G., Sumerling, M.D., et al. (1978) Percutaneous transhepatic cholangiography with the Chiba needle. *Clin. Radiol.* **29**, 101–112.

Harbin, W.P., Mueller, M.D. & Ferrucci J.T. Jr. (1980) Transhepatic cholangiography: complications and use patterns of the fine needle technique. *Radiology* **135**, 15–22.

Jacques, P.F. & Bream, C.A. (1978) Barium duodenography as an adjunct to percutaneous transhepatic cholangiography. *Am. J. Roentgenol.* **130**, 693–696.

Jacques, P.F., Mauro, M.A. & Scatliff, J.H. (1980) The failed transhepatic cholangiogram. *Radiology* **134**, 33–35.

Jain, S., Long, R.G., Scott, J., et al. (1977) Percutaneous transhepatic cholangiography using the Chiba needle. *Br. J. Radiol.* **50**, 175–180.

BILIARY DRAINAGE

EXTERNAL DRAINAGE

This is achieved following transhepatic cannulation of the biliary tree. It has been used to reduce operative morbidity in jaundiced patients but this has not gained widespread acceptance.

INTERNAL DRAINAGE

This is achieved following transhepatic or endoscopic cannulation of the biliary tree. An endoprosthesis with proximal and distal side-holes or a transhepatic catheter is sited across a stricture. The endoprosthesis method is preferable because of the complications of long-term transhepatic catheterization.

Indications

1. Proven malignant biliary stricture, not amenable to surgery
2. Benign stricture following balloon dilatation.

Contraindications

As for percutaneous transhepatic cholangiography.

Contrast media

LOCM 200; 20–60 ml.

Equipment

1. Wide-channelled endoscope for introduction of endoprosthesis.
2. A biplane fluoroscope facility is useful but not essential for transhepatic puncture.
3. Set including guide-wires, dilators and endoprosthesis.

Patient preparation

1. Nil orally for 4 h before procedure.
2. Premedication including analgesia, e.g. pethidine 75 mg i.v., and pethidine 25 mg i.v. during the procedure, if necessary. An anti-emetic, e.g. Stemetil 12.5 mg, may be added.
3. Antibiotic before and for at least 3 days following, e.g. Cefuroxine 750 mg i.v. 6-hourly.
4. Intravenous line for fluids to avoid dehydration and as a route for i.v. drugs during the procedure.

Technique

Transhepatic

1. A percutaneous transhepatic cholangiogram is performed.
2. A duct in the right lobe of the liver is chosen that has a horizontal or caudal course to the porta hepatis. This duct is studied on AP and lateral fluoroscopy (if possible) to judge its depth and then an 18-G 25-cm sheathed needle is introduced following percutaneous puncture through an intercostal space

in the mid-axillary line. The chosen duct is punctured on fluoroscopy, care being taken not to push the needle tip through the medial wall of the duct. If the duct is not successfully punctured, the needle is reinserted into the sheath and a further pass is made without removing the sheath from the liver, thus minimizing the number of punctures of the capsule.

3. Upon successful puncture a J guide-wire is inserted through the sheath and manoeuvred towards or through the obstruction, if possible. The sheath is then advanced over the guide-wire as far as possible. The wire is exchanged for a more rigid Lunderquist guide-wire and over this dilators are passed to facilitate passage of the catheter/endoprosthesis. If passage through the stricture with the internal guide is not possible other wires that can be shaped may be successful. Failing this, external drainage is instituted and further attempts are made to pass the stricture a few days later.

4. An endoprosthesis is pushed through the stricture and sited with its side-holes above and below the stricture so that internal drainage is instituted. An internal/external catheter may be placed across the stricture and secured to the skin with sutures or a locking disc device.

Endoscopic

1. Cholangiography following cannulation of the biliary tree
2. Endoscopic sphincterotomy
3. A guide-wire is placed via the channel of the endoscope through the sphincter and pushed past the stricture using fluoroscopy to monitor progress
4. Following dilatation of the stricture the endoprosthesis is pushed over the guide-wire and sited with its side-holes above and below the stricture.

Aftercare

1. As for percutaneous transhepatic cholangiography.
2. Antibiotics for at least 3 days.
3. An externally draining catheter should be regularly flushed through with normal saline and exchanged at 3-monthly intervals.

Complications

1. As for PTC, ERCP and sphincterotomy.
2. Sepsis – particularly common with externally draining catheters.

3. Dislodgement of catheters, endoprostheses.
4. Blockage of catheters/endoprostheses.
5. Perforation of bile duct above the stricture on passage of guide-wires.

Further reading

Braasch, J.W. & Gray, B.N. (1977) Considerations that lower pancreatoduodenectomy mortality. *Am. J. Surg.* **129**, 480–483.

Dooley, J.S. Dick, R., Irving, D., et al. (1981) Relief of bile duct obstruction by the percutaneous transhepatic insertion of an endoprosthesis. *Clin. Radiol.* **32**, 163–172.

Ferrucci, J.T., Mueller, P.R. & Harbin, W.P. (1980) Percutaneous transhepatic biliary drainage. Technique, results and applications. *Radiology* **135**, 1–13.

Molnar, W. & Stockum, A.E. (1974) Relief of obstructive jaundice through percutaneous transhepatic catheter – a new therapeutic method. *Am. J. Roentgenol.* **122**, 356–367.

Ring, E.J., Oleaga, J.A., Freiman, D.B., et al. (1978) Therapeutic applications of catheter cholangiography. *Radiology* **128**, 333–338.

Ring, E.J., Husted, J.W., Oleaga, J.A., et al. (1979) A multihole catheter for maintaining longterm percutaneous antegrade biliary drainage. *Radiology* **132**, 752–754.

ULTRASOUND OF THE LIVER   US

Indications

1. Suspected focal or diffuse liver lesion
2. Staging known extrahepatic malignancy
3. Right upper quadrant pain or mass
4. Hepatomegaly
5. Jaundice
6. Abnormal liver function tests
7. Suspected portal hypertension
8. Pyrexia of unknown origin
9. To facilitate the placement of needles for biopsy, etc
10. Assessment of portal vein, hepatic artery or hepatic veins
11. Assessment of patients with surgical shunts or TIPS procedures
12. Follow-up after surgical resection or liver transplant.

Contraindications

None.

Patient preparation

Not imperative, but fasting or clear fluids only required if the gallbladder is also to be studied.

Equipment

3–5-MHz transducer. Small scan head may be better for an intercostal approach, e.g. phased or annular array.

Technique

1. Patient supine
2. Time-gain compensation set to give uniform reflectivity throughout the right lobe of the liver
3. Suspended inspiration
4. Longitudinal scans from epigastrium or left subcostal region across to right subcostal region. The transducer should be angled up to include the whole of the left and right lobes
5. Transverse scans, subcostally, to visualize the whole liver
6. If visualization is incomplete, due to a small or high liver, then right intercostal, longitudinal, transverse and oblique scans may be useful. Suspended respiration without deep inspiration may suffice for intercostal scanning. In patients who are unable to hold their breath, real time scanning during quiet respiration is often adequate. Upright or left lateral decubitus positions are alternatives if visualization is still incomplete
7. Doppler studies:
   a. pulsed Doppler
   b. colour Doppler
   c. power Doppler
   d. Doppler with ultrasound contrast media or 'ultrasound echo-enhancing agents'
   e. second harmonic Doppler with contrast
   f. pulse inversion Doppler with contrast.

Additional views

Hepatic veins

Best seen using a transverse intercostal or epigastric approach. During inspiration, in real time, these can be seen traversing the liver to enter the inferior vena cava (IVC). Hepatic vein walls do not have increased reflectivity in comparison to normal liver parenchyma. The normal hepatic vein waveform on Doppler is tri-phasic reflecting right atrial pressures. Power Doppler may be useful to examine flow within the hepatic segment of the IVC since it is angle-independent.

Portal vein

Longitudinal view of the portal vein is shown by an oblique subcostal or intercostal approach. Portal vein walls are of increased reflectivity in comparison to parenchyma. The normal portal vein blood flow is towards the liver. There is usually continuous flow but the velocity may vary with respiration.

Hepatic artery

May be traced from the coeliac axis, which is recognized by the 'seagull' appearance of the origins of the common hepatic artery and splenic artery. There is normally forward flow throughout systole and diastole with a sharp systolic peak.

Common bile duct

See 'Ultrasound of the Gallbladder and Biliary System', p. 124.

The spleen size should be measured in all cases of suspected liver disease or portal hypertension. 95% of normal adult spleens measure 12 cm or less in length, and less than 7×5 cm in thickness. The spleen size is commonly assessed by 'eyeballing' and measurement of the longest diameter.[1] In children, splenomegaly should be suspected if the spleen is more than 1.25 times the length of the adjacent kidney.[2]

References

1. Rumack, C.M., Wilson, S.R. & Charboneau, J.W. (1991) *Diagnostic Ultrasound*, Vol. 1, p. 92. St Louis: Mosby Year Book.
2. Loftus, W.K. & Metreweli, C. (1998) Ultrasound assessment of mild splenomegaly: spleen/kidney ratio. *Pediatr. Radiol.* **28**, 98–100.

Further reading

Abbitt, P.L. (1998) Ultrasonography. Update on liver technique. *Radiol. Clin. N. Am.* **36 (2)**, 299–307.

Ernst, H., Hahn, E.G., Balzer, T., et al. (1996) Colour Doppler ultrasound of liver lesions: signal enhancement after intravenous injection of the ultrasound contrast agent Levovist. *J. Clin. Ultrasound* **24**, 31–35

Fisher, A.J., Paulson, E.K., Kliewer, M.A., et al. (1998) Doppler sonography of the portal vein and hepatic artery: measurement of a prandial effect. I. Healthy subjects. *Radiology* **207**, 711–715.

Meire, H., Cosgrove, D., Dewbury, K. (2000) *Clinical Ultrasound: Abdominal and General Ultrasound*. Edinburgh; by Churchill Livingstone.

Shapiro, R.S., Wagreich, J., Parsons, R.B., et al. (1998) Tissue harmonic imaging sonography: evaluation of image quality compared with conventional sonography. *Am. J. Roentgenol.* **171**, 1203–1206

ULTRASOUND OF THE GALLBLADDER AND BILIARY SYSTEM

US

Indications

1. Suspected gallstones
2. Right upper quadrant pain
3. Jaundice
4. Fever of unknown origin
5. Acute pancreatitis
6. To assess gallbladder function
7. Guided percutaneous procedures.

Contraindications

None.

Patient preparation

Fasting for at least 6 h, preferably overnight. Water may be permitted.

Equipment

3–5-MHz transducer. A stand-off may be used for a very anterior gallbladder. Small scan head may be optimal.

Technique

1. Patient supine.
2. The gallbladder can be located by following the reflective main lobar fissure from the right portal vein to the gallbladder fossa.
3. Developmental anomalies are rare but the gallbladder may be intrahepatic or on a long mesentery.
4. The gallbladder is scanned slowly along its long axis and transversely from the fundus to the neck leading to the cystic duct.
5. It must be re-scanned in the left lateral decubitus or erect positions because stones may be missed if only supine scans are used.
6. Visualization of the neck and cystic ducts may be improved by head down tilt.

The normal gallbladder wall is never more than 3-mm thick.

Additional views

Assessment of gallbladder function

1. Fasting gallbladder volume may be assessed by measuring longitudinal, transverse and AP diameters.
2. Normal gallbladder contraction reduces the volume by more than 25%, 30 min after a standard fatty meal. Somatostatin, calcitonin, indomethacin and nifedipine antagonize this contraction.

Intrahepatic bile ducts

1. Left lobe: transverse epigastric scan.
2. Right lobe: subcostal or intercostal longitudinal oblique.

Normal intrahepatic ducts may be visualized with modern scanners. Intrahepatic ducts are dilated if their diameter is more than 40% of the accompanying portal vein branch. There is normally acoustic enhancement posterior to dilated ducts but not portal veins. Dilated ducts have a beaded branching appearance.

Extrahepatic bile ducts

1. Patient supine or in the right anterior oblique position.
2. The upper common duct is demonstrated on a longitudinal oblique, subcostal or intercostal scan running anterior to the portal vein. The right hepatic artery is often seen crossing transversely between the two.
3. The common duct may be followed downwards along its length through the head of the pancreas to the ampulla and, when visualized, transverse scans should also be performed to improve detection of intraduct stones.

The internal diameter of the common hepatic duct is 4 mm or less in a normal adult; 5 mm is borderline and 6 mm is considered dilated. The lower common duct (common bile duct) is normally 6 mm or less. Distinction of the common hepatic duct from the common bile duct depends on identification of the junction with the cystic duct. This is usually not possible with US. Colour flow Doppler enables quick distinction of bile duct from ectatic hepatic artery. In 17% of patients the artery lies anterior to the bile duct.[1]

Post-cholecystectomy

There is disagreement as to whether the normal common duct dilates after cholecystectomy. Symptomatic patients and those with abnormal liver function tests should have further investigation if the common duct measures more than 6 mm.

References

1. Berland, L.L., Lawson, T.L. & Foley, W.D. (1982) Porta hepatis: sonographic discrimination of bile ducts from arteries with pulsed doppler with new anatomic criteria. *Am. J. Roentgenol.* **138**, 833–840.

Further reading

Laing, F.C. (1987) Ultrasonography of the gallbladder and biliary tree. In: Sarti, D.A. (ed.) *Diagnostic Ultrasound Text and Cases*, 2nd edn, pp. 142–146. St Louis: Year Book Medical.

Meire, H., Cosgrove, D. & Dewbury, K. (2000) *Clinical Ultrasound: Abdominal and General Ultrasound.* Edinburgh: Churchill Livingstone.

Mittelstaedt, C.A. (1987) The biliary system. In: Bates, J. (ed.) *Abdominal Ultrasound*, pp. 81–89. Edinburgh: Churchill Livingstone.

Morgan, B., Rathod, A. & Crozier, A., et al. (1996) Biliary distensibility during per-operative cholangiography as compared to pre-operative ultrasound: 4-year follow-up study. *Clin. Radiol.* **51**, 338–340

ULTRASOUND OF THE PANCREAS   US

Indications

1. Suspected pancreatic tumour
2. Pancreatitis or its complications
3. Epigastric mass
4. Epigastric pain
5. Jaundice
6. To facilitate guided biopsy.

Contraindications

None.

Patient preparation

Nil by mouth, preferably overnight.

Equipment

3–5-MHz transducer. A stand-off may be required in thin patients.

Technique

1. Patient supine.
2. The body of the pancreas is located anterior to the splenic vein in a transverse epigastric scan.
3. The transducer is angled transversely and obliquely to visualize the head and tail.
4. The tail may be demonstrated from a left intercostal view using the spleen as an acoustic window.

5. Longitudinal epigastric scans may be useful.
6. The pancreatic parenchyma increases in reflectivity with age, being equal to liver reflectivity in young adults.
7. Gastric or colonic gas may prevent complete visualization. This may be overcome by left and right oblique decubitus scans or by scanning with the patient erect. Water may be drunk to improve the window through the stomach and the scans repeated in all positions. One cup is usually sufficient. Degassed water preferable.

The pancreatic duct should not measure more than 3 mm in the head or 2 mm in the body.

RADIOLABELLED COLLOID LIVER SCAN RN

Indications

This procedure has largely been succeeded by US and CT, and is now rarely performed except in combination with other specialized nuclear medicine procedures. It may occasionally be useful in cases where the liver cannot be properly visualized with US.

1. Hepatic space occupying lesions – primary and secondary tumours, abscesses and cysts
2. Diffuse liver disease.

Contraindications

None.

Radiopharmaceuticals

^{99m}Tc-colloid, 80 MBq max (0.8 mSv ED), 200 MBq SPECT (2 mSv ED). Cleared by phagocytosis into the reticuloendothelial cells, where it is retained. Spleen is demonstrated as well as liver.

Equipment

1. Gamma-camera
2. Low-energy general purpose collimator (high-sensitivity collimator for flow studies).

Patient preparation

None.

Technique

1. ^{99m}Tc-colloid is administered i.v.
2. With the patient supine, images are obtained after 15 min, or longer in patients with very poor clearance.

Films

500 kilocounts for first view, others for same length of time:

1. Anterior, with costal margin markers
2. Posterior
3. Left lateral
4. Right lateral.

Additional techniques

1. A first-pass dynamic flow study may be performed to improve differential diagnosis of liver masses:
   a. The fasted patient is positioned supine with the camera anterior or posterior depending upon analysis method to be employed[1]
   b. A fast bolus injection of ^{99m}Tc-colloid is given using the Oldendorf technique (see p. 16) if the patient has good veins
   c. 1-s images are collected on computer for 60 s
   d. Analysis of regional time-activity curves may be performed to provide an index of liver arterial and portal perfusion[1]
   e. Static images are acquired as above.
2. SPECT may be used for assessment of diffuse liver disease[2] and to improve detection of small and deep-seated lesions.

Aftercare

None.

Complications

None.

References

1. Britten, A.J., Fleming, J.S., Flowerdew, A.D.S., et al. (1990) A comparison of three indices of relative hepatic perfusion derived from dynamic liver scintigraphy. *Clin. Phys. Physiol. Meas.* **11**, 45–51.
2. Delcourt, E., Vanhaeverbeek, M., Binon, J.P., et al. (1992) Emission tomography for assessment of diffuse alcoholic liver disease. *J. Nucl. Med.* **33**, 1337–1345.

Further reading

Harding, L.K. & Notghi, A. (1998) Gastrointestinal tract and liver. In: Sharp, P.F., Gemmell,

H.G. & Smith, F.W. (eds) *Practical Nuclear Medicine*, pp. 188–190. Oxford: Oxford University Press.

Harding, L.K. & Robinson, P.J.A. (1990) Liver disease. In: *Clinician's Guide to Nuclear Medicine: Gastroenterology*, pp. 49–79. London: Churchill Livingstone.

DYNAMIC RADIONUCLIDE HEPATOBILIARY IMAGING (CHOLESCINTIGRAPHY)

RN

Indications

1. Suspected acute cholecystitis[1]
2. Assessment of gallbladder, common bile duct and sphincter of Oddi function[2,3]
3. Assessment of neonatal jaundice where biliary atresia is considered[4]
4. Suspected bile leaks after trauma or surgery.[5]

Contraindications

None.

Radiopharmaceuticals

^{99m}Tc-trimethylbromo-iminodiacetic acid (TBIDA) or other iminodiacetic acid (IDA) derivative; 80 MBq typical (1 mSv ED), 150 MBq max (2 mSv ED).

These ^{99m}Tc-labelled IDA derivatives are rapidly cleared from the circulation by hepatocytes and secreted into bile in a similar way to bilirubin.[6] A number have been developed with similar kinetics, but the later ones such as TBIDA have high hepatic uptake and low urinary excretion, giving better visualization of the biliary tract at high bilirubin levels than the early agents.

Equipment

1. Gamma-camera
2. Low-energy general purpose collimator.

Patient preparation

1. Nil by mouth for 4–6 h.
2. For the investigation of biliary atresia, infants are given phenobarbitone orally 5 mg kg^{-1} day^{-1} in two divided doses for 3–5 days prior to the study to enhance hepatic excretion of radiopharmaceutical.[1]

Technique

The imaging protocol depends upon the clinical question being asked. A dynamic study should be performed where it is important to visualize the progress of the bile in detail, e.g. post-surgery:

1. The patient lies supine with the camera anterior and the liver at the top of the field of view.
2. The radiopharmaceutical is injected i.v.

Films

1. 1-min 128×128 dynamic images are acquired for 45 min.
2. If the gallbladder and duodenum are not seen, static images are obtained at intervals up to 4–6 h.
3. Right lateral and oblique views may be useful if a bile leak is suspected or to distinguish the gallbladder from duodenal activity.
4. If no bowel activity is seen by 4–6 h and it is important to detect any flow of bile at all, e.g. in suspected biliary atresia, a 24-h image should be taken.

Additional techniques

Cholecystokinin (CCK) and morphine provocation[2]

Pharmacological intervention can be used in combination with TBIDA scanning to improve diagnosis of diseases affecting the gallbladder, common bile duct or sphincter of Oddi. CCK causes gallbladder contraction and sphincter of Oddi relaxation. An i.v. infusion of CCK is given over 2–3 min when the gallbladder is visualized 30–45 min after TBIDA administration. Dynamic imaging is continued for a further 30–40 min.

Quantitative measures of gallbladder ejection fraction and emptying rate can be calculated. It has been suggested that a slow CCK infusion over 30–60 min may improve specificity.[7]

Morphine causes sphincter of Oddi contraction. In a clinical setting of suspected acute cholecystitis, if the gallbladder is not observed by 60 min, an infusion of 0.04 mg kg^{-1} over 1 min can be given and imaging continued for a further 30 min. Continued non-visualization of the gallbladder up to 90 min is considered to confirm the diagnosis.

More recently, morphine provocation has found success in diagnosis of elevated sphincter of Oddi basal pressure.[3]

Quantitative analysis

Some investigators have calculated liver function parameters from dynamic studies, e.g. to attempt to differentiate between transplant rejection and hepatocyte dysfunction.[8]

Aftercare

None.

Complications

Monitor for adverse reactions to CCK and morphine.

References

1. Harding, L.K. & Robinson, P.J.A. (1990) Hepatobiliary studies: bile reflux, jaundice and acute cholecystitis. In: *Clinician's Guide to Nuclear Medicine: Gastroenterology*, pp. 31–48. London: Churchill Livingstone.
2. Krishnamurthy, S. & Krishnamurthy, G.T. (1996) Cholecystokinin and morphine pharmacological intervention during ^{99m}Tc-HIDA cholescintigraphy: a rational approach. *Semin. Nucl. Med.* **26**, 16–24.
3. Thomas, P.D., Turner, J.G., Dobbs, B.R., et al. (2000) Use of ^{99m}Tc-DISIDA biliary scanning with morphine provocation for detection of elevated sphincter of Oddi basal pressure. *Gut* (in press).
4. Johnston, G.S., Rosenbaum, R.C., Hill, J.L., et al. (1985) Differentiation of jaundice in infancy: an application of radionuclide biliary studies. *J. Surg. Oncol.* **30**, 206–208.
5. Rayter, Z., Tonge, C., Bennett, C., et al. (1991) Ultrasound and HIDA: scanning in evaluating bile leaks after cholecystectomy. *Nucl. Med. Commun.* **12**, 197–202.
6. Krishnamurthy, G.T. & Turner, F.E. (1990) Pharmacokinetics and clinical application of technetium 99m-labelled hepatobiliary agents. *Semin. Nucl. Med.* **20**, 130–149.
7. Ziessman, H.A. (1999) Cholecystokinin cholescintigraphy: victim of its own success? *J. Nucl. Med.* **40**, 2038–2042.
8. Merion, R.M., Campbell, D.A. Jr, Dafoe, D.C., et al. (1988) Observations on quantitative scintigraphy with deconvolutional analysis in liver transplantation. *Transplant. Proc.* **20 (suppl. 1)**, 695–697.

Further reading

Harding, L.K. & Notghi, A. (1998) Gastrointestinal tract and liver. In: Sharp, P.F., Gemmell, H.G. & Smith, F.W. (eds) *Practical Nuclear Medicine*, 2nd edn, pp. 190–193. Oxford, Oxford University Press.

MRI OF THE LIVER   MRI

Focal lesions may be identified on most pulse sequences. However, multiple sequences are usually necessary for confident tissue characterisation. Common pulse sequences are:

T1-WEIGHTED SPIN-ECHO (SE)

T1-weighted spoiled gradient echo (GRE)

SPGR (GE Medical Systems) or FLASH (Siemens). This can replace the conventional spin-echo sequence for patients who are able to suspend respiration.

Magnetization-prepared T1-weighted GRE

A further breath-hold technique with very short sequential image acquisition.

T2-WEIGHTED SE

T2-weighted fast spin-echo (FSE; General Electric) or turbo spin-echo (TSE; Siemens)

Compared with conventional T2-weighted SE images, FSE/TSE images show (a) fat with higher signal intensity, (b) reduced magnetic susceptibility effects which are of advantage in patients with embolization coils, IVC filters etc., but disadvantageous after injection of superparamagnetic oxide contrast agent and (c) increased magnetization transfer which may lower signal intensity for solid liver tumours.

Fat suppression

1. Decreases the motion artefact from subcutaneous and intra-abdominal fat
2. Increases the dynamic range of the image
3. Improves signal-to-noise and contrast-to-noise ratios of focal liver lesions.

Short tau inversion recovery (STIR)

Also suppresses fat, which has a short T1 relaxation time. Other tissues with short T1 relaxation (haemorrhage, metastases and melanoma) are also suppressed.

Gadolinium-enhanced T1-weighted

These probably do not increase sensitivity for focal abnormalities but may improve tissue characterization. When used in conjunction with spoiled GRE sequences it is possible to obtain images during the arterial phase (ideal for metastatic disease and hepatocellular carcinoma), portal phase (hypovascular malignancies) and equilibrium phase (cholangiocarcinoma, slow-flow haemangiomas and fibrosis).

MR Angiography

Contrast-enhanced spoiled GRE images give improved images compared with 2D time-of-flight (TOF) sequences.

Further reading

Hahn, P.F. & Saini, S. (1998) Liver-specific MR imaging contrast agents. *Radiol. Clin. N. Am.* **36 (2)**, 287–297.

Siegelman, E.S. & Outwater, E.K. (1998) MR imaging techniques of the liver. *Radiol. Clin. N. Am.* **36 (2)**, 263–286.

THE INVESTIGATION OF JAUNDICE

The aim is to separate haemolytic causes of jaundice from obstructive jaundice or hepatocellular jaundice. Clinical history and examination are followed by biochemical tests of blood and urine and haematological tests.

IMAGING INVESTIGATIONS

Obstructive jaundice

US is the primary imaging modality and achieves accuracy figures of 95% for the level of obstruction and 88% for the cause.[1] Dilated ducts suggest obstructive jaundice. The bile ducts, gallbladder and pancreas should be examined to determine the level and cause of obstruction. ERCP or, if that is not possible, PTC are often required to confirm the cause of the obstruction. They may also offer the opportunity for therapy. If the suspected cause is tumour, a CT scan to assess the pancreas and related lymph nodes is often required. In some cases, angiography is used to exclude involvement of the mesenteric and portal veins prior to surgery.

In some cases due to high bile duct tumours PTC may be required as well as ERCP to fully evaluate the bile ducts.

Non-obstructive jaundice

When US shows no dilated ducts and hepatocellular jaundice is suspected, liver biopsy is considered. There may be other US evidence of parenchymal liver disease or signs of portal hypertension.

If obstructive jaundice is still suspected despite the US result, then ERCP or PTC is required. Extrahepatic obstruction may be present in the absence of duct dilatation,[2] and patients with primary sclerosing cholangitis or widespread intrahepatic metastases may have obstruction without duct dilatation.

References

1. Gibson R.N., Yeung, E., Thompson, J.N. et al. (1986) Bile duct obstruction: radiologic evaluation of level, cause and tumour resectability. *Radiology* **160**, 43–47.
2. Muhletaler, C.A., Gerlock, A.J., Fleischer, A.C. & James, A.E. (1980) Diagnosis of obstructive jaundice with non-dilated bile ducts. *Am. J. Roentgenol.* **134**, 1149–1152.

THE INVESTIGATION OF LIVER TUMOURS

Investigation falls into three stages:

1. Detection
2. Characterization of the tumour
3. Assessment for surgical resection or staging for chemotherapy.

The clinical context and proposed management course usually determine the extent of investigation. Liver metastases are much commoner than primary liver cancers. Benign haemangiomas are also common, being present in 5–10% of the population. Other benign liver tumours are uncommon.

The clinical data correlated with the radiological investigations usually enable the character of a liver tumour to be determined with a high degree of probability. This can be confirmed with image-guided or surgical biopsy when appropriate. Some surgeons are averse to preoperative biopsy because of the small risk of disseminating malignant cells and the possibility of misleading sampling error.[1] If biopsy is performed, it is often important to sample the 'normal' liver as well as the lesion. The presence of, for example, cirrhosis may have a major impact on management.

Hepatic resection is an established procedure for the management of hepatic metastases and primary liver tumours. Various imaging methods are used to assess the number and location of tumours. Variation in imaging equipment makes comparison of sensitivities of techniques difficult. A recent study[2] gave the following results:

	Sensitivity
Contrast-enhanced CT	68%
MRI	63%
US	53%

However, at present, CT arterial portography (CTAP) and intraoperative US are the most sensitive techniques for detecting liver tumours, with sensitivities of 91% and 96%, respectively.[3,4]

US

Widely used for general screening for metastases and often the first modality to detect an unsuspected focal liver lesion.

CT[5,6]

There are various techniques. Used for general screening and staging. The remainder of the abdomen and chest may also be imaged for full staging.

The duration of a helical scan is determined by the breath-holding ability of the patient, while the length (volume) of tissue scanned can be adjusted by increasing pitch beyond the usual 1:1 (extended helical scanning). The majority of out patients can hold their breath for 30 s. A typical helical protocol for the liver using a single breath hold is:

Table increment	8 mm
Slice thickness	8 mm
Reconstruction interval	4 mm
Scan time	24 s (= image volume length 19.2 cm; adequate for most livers)

There is little evidence to support the continued use of the non-contrast-enhanced CT scan (NCECT), particularly if biphasic imaging is employed, unless diffuse liver diseases such as haemo-chromatosis and cirrhosis are under investigation. (Triple-phase CT = NCECT + dual-phase CT.)

LOCM or HOCM (300)	150 ml at 3 ml s^{-1} (single-phase imaging)
	150 ml at 4 ml s^{-1} (dual-phase imaging)
	scanning is commenced manually after the start of the injection or triggered by a software package (e.g. Smart Prep; General Electric).

Single-phase contrast-enhanced CT (CECT)

This is the technique for the majority of routine liver CT imaging. The liver is imaged during the peak of parenchymal enhancement, i.e. when contrast medium-laden portal venous blood is perfusing the liver. This begins about 60 s after the start of a bolus injection.

Dual-phase (biphasic) CECT

The fast imaging times of helical CT enable the liver to be scanned twice after a single bolus injection of contrast medium.

Most liver tumours receive their blood supply from the hepatic artery, unlike the hepatic parenchyma, which receives 80% of its blood supply from the portal vein. Thus liver tumours (particularly hypervascular tumours) will be strongly enhanced during the arterial phase (beginning 20 s after the start of a bolus injection) but of similar density to enhanced normal parenchyma during the portal venous phase.

Haemangiomas show a characteristic 'fill-in' on delayed scans. After the initial dual- or triple-phase protocol, delayed images at 5 and 10 min are obtained through the lesion.

ANGIOGRAPHY

May provide diagnostic characterization of various tumours, including haemangioma, hepatoma and focal nodular hyperplasia. It is also used to provide a 'road map' to plan surgery.

Arteriography is a pre-requisite for *Lipiodol-enhanced CT*. Follow-up CT scans are obtained 7–10 days after the injection of 7–10 ml of Lipiodol through the hepatic arterial catheter. This may show small hepatoma nodules not visualized by standard CT or US.

Arteriography is also a pre-requisite for CT arterial portography, a technique usually limited to potential candidates for surgical resection of tumour. A 5-F catheter is left with its tip positioned in the superior mesenteric artery and the patient is transferred immediately to the CT scanner. A pump injector is used to deliver 100–150 ml of LOCM 300 at 1–2 ml s^{-1}. An intra-arterial injection of 40 mg papaverine hydrochloride may be given prior to the pump injection to increase portal vein flow. Scanning is commenced 10–20 s after initiation of the pump injection and contiguous 10-mm slices are taken through the liver using a fast scan mode. Normal hepatic tissue is perfused by the portal vein, whereas tumours obtain their blood supply predominantly from the hepatic artery. Consequently, they appear as low density on CTAP. This is the most sensitive method of preoperative liver metastasis detection with spatial display of their segmental distribution. If the hepatic artery arises from the superior mesenteric artery (SMA), there may be confusing hepatic arterial enhancement.

MRI

With modern equipment, liver lesions are readily detected, at least as well as with CT, but its true role has yet to be clarified. The characteristics of some tumours may be determined (see page 131).

RADIONUCLIDE SCANS

Standard colloid scans are of little value because defects are non-specific. Uptake of isotope in focal nodular hyperplasia may distinguish this condition from other liver tumours. Labelled red cell scans may confirm haemangioma with a high degree of specificity. Radionuclide bone scans may be required for staging possible bony spread of hepatocellular carcinoma.

IMAGE-GUIDED BIOPSY

When clinically justified, US or CT-guided biopsy is possible for virtually any liver lesion that can be imaged. Vascular lesions such as haemangioma are best approached through normal liver to reduce the risk of bleeding.

INTRAOPERATIVE TECHNIQUES

Laparoscopy is now widely used in surgical practice. Intraoperative US may detect intrahepatic lesions not palpable at laparotomy. Laparoscopic US is not widely available but may ultimately prove the favoured surgical staging technique.

References

1. Pain, J.A., Karani, J. & Howard, E.R. (1991) Pre-operative radiological and clinical assessment of hepatic tumours – is biopsy necessary? *Clin. Radiol.* **44**, 181–182.
2. Wernecke, K., Rummeny, E., Bongartz, G., et al. (1991) Detection of hepatic masses in patients with carcinoma: comparative sensitivities of sonography, CT and MR imaging. *Am. J. Roentgenol.* **157**, 731–739.
3. Soyer, P. Levesque, M., Elias, D., et al. (1992) Detection of liver metastases from colo-rectal cancer: comparison intraoperative ultrasound during arterial portography. *Radiology* **183**, 541–544.
4. McGrath, F.P., Malone, D.E., Dobranowski, J., et al. (1993) Editorial. CT Portography and delayed high dose iodine CT. *Clin. Radiol.* **47**, 1–6.
5. Bluemke, D.A., Soyer, P. & Fishman, E.K. (1995) Helical (spiral) CT of the liver. *Radiol. Clin. N. Am.* **33 (5)**, 863–886.
6. Kemmerer, S.R., Mortele, K.J. & Ros, P.R. (1998) CT scan of the liver. *Radiol. Clin. N. Am.* **36 (2)**, 247–261.

PANCREATITIS

US is the first-line investigation but in acute pancreatitis the presence of a sentinel loop will often obscure the pancreas and prevent good visualization. Even if the pancreas is seen, it can appear normal in acute pancreatitis. The gallbladder and biliary tree should always be examined in the fasted patient to exclude the presence of gallstones which may be causing the pancreatitis.

CT is the next investigation. It should be performed initially without oral or i.v. contrast enhancement to look for the presence of calcification within the pancreas itself and to look for small gallstones, which can be obscured by the presence of oral contrast medium. Scans of the pancreas should then be obtained during dynamic incremental scanning following rapid infusion of intravenous contrast medium (100 ml of LOCM 300–350). This will enable identification of non-perfused areas of pancreas, and the presence of pseudocysts, abscesses and phlegmons should be sought.

PANCREATIC PSEUDOCYSTS

Initial investigation should be with US. It should be remembered that pseudocysts can occur anywhere in the abdomen or pelvis and can even be found in the thorax. The spleen and left kidney provide acoustic windows to visualize the region of the tail of the pancreas.

CT scanning may also be performed if bowel loops prevent adequate visualization. It should always be performed prior to radiologically guided intervention to prevent drainage of a pseudoaneurysm. (During ultrasonography supposed fluid collections can be interrogated with colour or duplex Doppler.)

Further reading

Freeny, P.C. (ed.) (1989) Radiology of the pancreas. *Radiol. Clin. N. Am.* **27 (1)**.
Jones, S.N. (1991) Editorial. The drainage of pancreatic fluid collections. *Clin. Radiol.* **43**, 153–155.

PANCREATIC CARCINOMA

First-line investigation is usually US. Having diagnosed a pancreatic mass, local extension should be determined with special reference to the portal vein; patency should be verified with duplex or colour flow Doppler. Other features to be ascertained are encasement of vessels, relationship of tumour to inferior vena cava, spread to adjacent bowel, regional lymphadenopathy and any distant metastases. If the mass is easily visible on US it can be used to guide biopsy.

If US fails to diagnose a lesion or suggests that surgery is possible, CT should be performed either to identify a focal pancreatic lesion or to confirm surgical resectability.

HELICAL CT OF THE PANCREAS

A typical protocol is as follows:

1. The bowel is outlined with dilute barium, water-soluble contrast medium or water.
2. Contiguous 5-mm non-helical scans to localize the pancreas.
3. Post-contrast scan *from* bottom of pancreas *to* top of liver during a single breath-hold.

Table increment	5 mm
Slice thickness	5 mm
Reconstruction interval	4 mm
Scan time	30 s (= image volume length 15 cm)
LOCM or HOCM 300	150 ml at 3 ml s^{-1}
	scanning is commenced manually at 60 s after the start of the injection or triggered by a software package (e.g. Smart Prep; General Electric).

When the patient presents with jaundice, ultrasound is usually followed by ERCP. If surgery is not planned, endoscopic stenting may be performed to relieve the jaundice.

Angiography is performed in some cases prior to surgery to exclude encasement of the portal and superior mesenteric veins, but contrast-enhanced CT and MRI show excellent correlation with conventional angiography in many series.

MRI OF THE PANCREAS

Typical sequences in the axial plane include:

1. *T1-weighted fat-suppressed spin-echo.* Normal pancreas hyperintense to normal liver.
2. *T1-weighted spoiled gradient-echo (GRE)* (SPGR, GE Medical Systems; FLASH, Siemens). Normal pancreas isointense to normal liver.
3. *Gadolinium-enhanced T1-weighted spoiled GRE.* Images are obtained immediately after the injection of contrast medium, after 45 s, after 90 s and after 10 min. Normal pancreas hyperintense to normal liver and adjacent fat on early images, fading on later images.

Further reading

Freeny, P.C. (1989) Radiologic diagnosis and staging of pancreatic ductal adenocarcinoma. *Radiol. Clin. N. Am.* **27**, 121–128.

Thompson, J.N. (1990) Diagnosing cancer of the pancreas. *Br. Med. J.* **301**, 775–776.

Zeman, R.K., Silverman, P.M., Ascher, S.M., et al. (1995) Helical (spiral) CT of the pancreas and biliary tract. *Radiol. Clin. N. Am.* **33 (5)**, 887–902.

ZOLLINGER–ELLISON SYNDROME

Caused by a gastrin-secreting tumour, usually within the pancreas or adjacent duodenum. 60% are malignant and may metastasize. Gastrinoma may be associated with parathyroid adenoma or pituitary adenoma in multiple endocrine neoplasia syndrome. Gastrinoma may present with recurrent severe peptic ulceration and is diagnosed by elevated gastrin levels in association with an elevated basal acid output.

Barium studies (or endoscopy) may show thickened gastric and duodenal folds and ulceration continuing beyond the first part of the duodenum. Having confirmed the tumour by elevated gastrin levels, investigations are directed at localization of the tumour before surgery. US and CT may show a larger tumour in the pancreas or duodenum and indicate liver or nodal metastases if present. Selective pancreatic angiography and transhepatic pancreatic venous sampling have been more likely to localize a small primary tumour. Intraoperative US shows great promise in demonstrating the tumour, and endoscopic US is also likely to be effective.

Further reading

Rossi, P., Allison, D.J., Bezzi, M., et al. (1989) Endocrine tumours of the pancreas. *Radiol. Clin. N. Am.* **27**, 129–161.

5 Urinary tract

Methods of imaging the urinary tract

1. Plain films, including tomography
2. Excretion urography
3. Micturating cystourethrography
4. Ascending urethrography
5. Retrograde pyeloureterography
6. Percutaneous renal puncture
7. Arteriography
8. Venography – including renal vein sampling
9. US
10. Radionuclide imaging
    - static
    - dynamic
    - radionuclide cystography – direct and indirect
11. CT
12. MRI.

EXCRETION UROGRAPHY

Indications

Suspected urinary tract pathology.

Contraindications

See p. 4 – general contraindications to water-soluble contrast media.

Dehydration is contraindicated in the following situations:

1. Renal failure
2. Myeloma
3. Infancy.

Contrast medium

HOCM or LOCM 370 are acceptable but the following 'high-risk' groups should receive LOCM:

1. Infants and small children and the elderly
2. Those with renal and/or cardiac failure
3. Poorly hydrated patients
4. Patients with diabetes, myelomatosis or sickle-cell anaemia
5. Patients who have had a previous severe contrast medium reaction with LOCM or those with a strong allergic history.

Adult dose

50 ml.

Paediatric dose

1 ml kg^{-1}.

Patient preparation

1. No food for 5 h prior to the examination. Dehydration is not necessary and does not improve image quality.
2. Patients should, preferably, be ambulant for 2 h prior to the examination to reduce bowel gas.
3. The routine administration of bowel preparation fails to improve the diagnostic quality of the examination and its use makes the examination more unpleasant for the patient.
4. If the examination is to be performed on a patient who has previously had a severe contrast medium reaction, consideration should be given to administering methyl prednisolone 32 mg orally 12 and 2 h prior to injection of contrast medium in addition to ensuring that a LOCM is used.

Preliminary film

1. Supine, full-length AP of the abdomen, in inspiration. The lower border of the cassette is at the level of the symphysis pubis and the X-ray beam is centred in the mid-line at the level of the iliac crests.

The position of overlying opacities may be further determined by:

2. Supine AP of the renal areas, in expiration. The X-ray beam is centred in the mid-line at the level of the lower costal margin.
3. 35% posterior oblique views, or
4. tomography of the kidneys at the level of a third of the AP diameter of the patient (approx. 8–11 cm) The optimal angle of swing is 25–40°.

The examination should not proceed further until these films have been reviewed by the radiologist and deemed satisfactory.

Technique

The median antecubital vein is the preferred injection site because flow is retarded in the cephalic vein as it pierces the clavipectoral fascia. A 19-G needle is advanced up the vein to reduce the risk of a perivenous injection and the injection is given rapidly as a bolus to maximize the density of the nephrogram.

Upper arm or shoulder pain may be due to stasis of contrast medium in the vein. This is relieved by abduction of the arm.

Films

1. *Immediate film*. AP of the renal areas. This film is exposed 10–14 s after the injection (arm-to-kidney time). It aims to show the nephrogram, i.e. the renal parenchyma opacified by contrast medium in the renal tubules.
2. *5-min film*. AP of the renal areas. This film is taken to determine if excretion is symmetrical and is invaluable for assessing the need to modify technique, e.g. a further injection of contrast medium if there has been poor initial opacification.

   A compression band is now applied around the patient's abdomen and the balloon positioned midway between the anterior superior iliac spines, i.e. precisely over the ureters as they cross the pelvic brim. The aim is to produce better pelvicalyceal distension. Compression is contraindicated:
   a. after recent abdominal surgery
   b. after renal trauma
   c. if there is a large abdominal mass
   d. when the 5-min film shows already distended calyces.

3. *15-min film*. AP of the renal areas. There is usually adequate distension of the pelvicalyceal systems with opaque urine by this time. Compression is released when satisfactory demonstration of the pelvicalyceal system has been achieved.
4. *Release film*. Supine AP abdomen. This film is taken to show the whole urinary tract. If this film is satisfactory, the patient is asked to empty their bladder.
5. *After micturition film*. Based on the clinical findings and the radiological findings on the earlier films, this will be either a full-length abdominal film or a coned view of the bladder with the tube angled 15° caudad and centred 5 cm above the symphysis pubis. The principal value of this film is to assess

bladder emptying, to demonstrate a return to normal of dilated upper tracts with relief of bladder pressure, to aid the diagnosis of bladder tumours, to confirm ureterovesical junction calculi and, uncommonly, to demonstrate a urethral diverticulum in females.

Additional films

1. 35° posterior obliques of the kidneys, ureters or bladder.
2. Tomography – when there are confusing overlying shadows.
3. 30° caudad angulation of the tube for the renal area. This may throw a faecal laden transverse colon clear of the kidneys.
4. Prone abdomen – may provide better visualization of the ureters by making them more dependent.
5. Delayed films – may be necessary for up to 24 h after injection in cases of obstructive uropathy.

The infant

Excretion urography is seldom indicated in this age group; US, with or without radionuclide imaging, is the preferred imaging modality. As in all paediatric work the technique should be flexible to suit the problem. The radiologist should inspect each film and decide on any modification of technique before the next film. A typical basic film sequence is:

a. a 2-min film of the renal areas
b. a 5-min film of the renal areas
c. a 15-min full-length abdominal film.

Abdominal compression is not used.

Excretion of contrast medium during the first month of life is delayed and prolonged. Optimum visualization of the upper urinary tract may not occur until 1–3 h. Therefore, if the initial 2- and 5-min films show little opacification, further films at 1, 2 and 3 h may provide more information than multiple films in the first hour.

The older child

Again, radiation dose should be minimized by the use of ultrasound and radionuclides in preference to radiography.

The adult film sequence is used.

Excessive bowel gas may interfere with satisfactory visualization of the kidneys. A fizzy drink will produce a gas-filled stomach, which acts as a window through which the kidneys can be seen. If the gas-filled stomach is not large enough to reveal the right kidney, the patient can be turned into the RPO position.

An important indication for excretion urography in children is evaluation of diurnal enuresis where an ectopic ureter is a possibility which has not be excluded or confirmed by other imaging modalities. The position of the distal ureters is best documented by obtaining spot films on a fluoroscopy unit with the child in a 30° oblique position.

Excretory micturating cystourethrography

This technique is used when further information is required regarding the urethra or the act of micturition. However, opacification is not as great as when contrast medium is instilled retrogradely. Excretion urography is performed in the usual manner and when the bladder is full, spot films are taken of the bladder and urethra during micturition. (See p. 157 for details of positioning, etc.)

Complications

Due to the contrast medium

See Chapter 2.

Due to the technique

Incorrectly applied abdominal compression may produce intolerable discomfort or hypotension.

PERCUTANEOUS RENAL PUNCTURE

Indications

1. *Renal cyst puncture.* At autopsy 50% of those over 50 years have grossly detectable renal cysts. 4.5% of all patients undergoing excretion urography have asymptomatic renal lesions but only 2.5% of these will be primary malignant tumours.[1] Using strict diagnostic criteria, US or CT are very accurate in diagnosing the uncomplicated renal cyst which does not need further evaluation.[2,3] Nevertheless, approximately 5% of all renal lesions will be of indeterminate aetiology on initial US or CT examination. Indications for cyst puncture, therefore, include:
   a. indeterminate mass
   b. US and CT results inconclusive or conflicting
   c. calcification within a cyst wall.

Clinical signs or symptoms may not correlate with the diagnosis of a simple cyst and the following are also indications for cyst puncture:

d. unexplained haematuria with an apparent cyst
e. unexplained fever with an apparent cyst.

Therapeutic indications for cyst puncture are:

f. to relieve local symptoms attributable to a cyst.

2. *Antegrade pyelography*
   a. when other less invasive imaging modalities fail to delineate the cause and/or level of an obstruction
   b. when retrograde pyelography is unsuccessful or not possible, e.g. internal ureteral diversion
   c. to facilitate renal pressure/flow studies. This is performed when other modalities, particularly diuretic renography, have failed to demonstrate whether the dilated upper urinary tract is truly obstructed.
3. Prior to, or as part of, *percutaneous nephrostomy* (see p. 150).

Contraindications

1. As for water-soluble contrast medium in the radiographic method (see p. 4).
2. Bleeding diathesis.
3. The possibility of renal hydatid disease.

Contrast medium

1. For preliminary visualization of the kidneys – as for excretion urography.
2. To outline the pelvicalyceal system or renal cyst – any HOCM or LOCM 200. Volume is dependent on the size of the cyst of collecting system.

Equipment

1. Fluoroscopy unit, US machine or CT scanner
2. Overcouch tube
3. 22-G needle, e.g. Chiba or Greenburg.

Patient preparation

1. As for excretion urography if this method is used to outline the kidney.
2. Confirm normal blood coagulation.

3. Nervous patients may need sedation; children will need general anaesthesia.

Preliminary film

Supine AP of the renal area for the radiographic method.

Technique

Insertion of the needle can be controlled by three imaging methods:

1. Ultrasonography
2. CT
3. Fluoroscopy.

RENAL CYST PUNCTURE

1. The patient is placed in the prone position. A radiolucent pad is placed under the abdomen to limit anterior movement of the kidney.
2. The cyst is located indirectly after opacification of the kidneys with i.v. contrast medium or directly with US or CT. The optimum site for puncture is marked on the skin.
3. The skin and subcutaneous tissues are infiltrated with 1% lignocaine.
4. The needle is passed directly into the lesion during suspended respiration. Intermittent fluoroscopy, US or CT is used to monitor the path of the needle. The combined use of US and fluoroscopy is often very helpful.[4] The needle may be deflected around the cyst and, if this happens, it will be necessary to advance it into the cyst with a quick thrust.
5. The stilette is removed and the cyst contents aspirated and examined
   a. biochemically – fat, protein
   b. bacteriologically   as clinically indicated
   c. cytologically.

Simple cyst fluid is clear and straw-coloured. Some authors have suggested that if such fluid is aspirated then no further investigation is necessary.[5,6] If no fluid can be aspirated, the position of the needle can be confirmed with US or CT, and adjustment of position made. If the procedure is performed with fluoroscopy only, the needle is withdrawn until fluid is obtained. If that is unsuccessful, a further attempt at puncture is made.

Modification of technique

1. If after correct needle placement, either no fluid or only grossly haemorrhagic aspirate is obtained then it can be presumed that the mass is solid in nature. Cytological examination of the aspirate is most important as there is a 25% chance of carcinoma being present.[7]

ANTEGRADE PYELOGRAPHY

1. The needle is introduced as for cyst puncture but directed through the renal parenchyma into a minor calyx. This reduces the risk of laceration of the pelvis and extravasation of urine.
2. Contrast medium is introduced until the level of obstruction is outlined.

Films

1. AP
2. both 35° posterior obliques.

Contrast medium should be removed from an obstructed pelvis to prevent the development of chemical pyelitis.

RENAL PRESSURE/FLOW STUDY

1. Vesicoureteric reflux should already have been excluded.
2. Catheters in the bladder and rectum are used to measure true intravesical pressure. Following antegrade puncture of the renal pelvis, the needle is connected to equipment that will infuse saline and measure intrapelvic pressure. *Absolute* intrapelvic pressure and *relative* pressure (bladder pressure subtracted from renal pressure) can be recorded during the infusion.
3. In the normal urinary tract, infusion at a rate of 10 ml min^{-1} produces a relative pressure in the renal pelvis less than 13 cm H_2O. Pressures greater than 20 cm H_2O indicate obstruction while those in the range 14–20 cm H_2O are equivocal.[8]

Aftercare

Chest radiograph to exclude a pneumothorax or haemo-pneumothorax.[9]

Complications

Major (1%), minor (10%).[10]

Due to the contrast medium

1. Contrast medium can be absorbed from the intact renal pelvis and give rise to adverse reactions.
2. Chemical pyelitis from prolonged contact of contrast medium with the obstructed pelvis.

Due to the technique

1. Perirenal and intrarenal haemorrhage
2. Haematuria
3. Pneumothorax
4. Infection – new or an exacerbation by puncture of a pyonephrosis
5. Pain
6. Urinoma
7. Arteriovenous fistula
8. Puncture of adjacent organs.

References

1. Lang, E.K. (1980) Roentgenologic approach to the diagnosis and management of cystic lesions of the kidney: is cyst exploration mandatory? *Urol. Clin. N. Am.* **7**, 677–688.
2. Pollack, H.M., Banner, M.P., Arger, P.H. et al. (1982) The accuracy of gray-scale renal ultrasound in differentiating cystic neoplasms from benign cysts. *Radiology* **143**, 741–745.
3. McClennan, B.L., Stanley, R.J., Melson, G.L. et al. (1979) CT of the renal cyst: Is cyst aspiration necessary? *Am. J. Roentgenol.* **133**, 671–675.
4. Raskin, M.M., Roen, S.A. & Serafini, A.N. (1974) Renal cyst puncture: combined fluoroscopic and ultrasonic technique. *Radiology* **113**, 425–427.
5. Stewart, B.H. & Pasalis, J.K. (1976) Aspiration and cytology in the evaluation of renal mass lesions. *Cleve. Clin. Q.* **43**, 1–6.
6. Levine, S.R., Emmet, J.L. & Woolner, L.B. (1964) Cyst and tumour occurring in the same kidney. *J. Urol.* **91**, 8–9.
7. Ainsworth, W.L. & Vest, S.A. (1951) The differential diagnosis between renal tumours and cysts. *J. Urol.* **64**, 740–749.
8. Whitaker, R.H. (1979) An evaluation of 170 diagnostic pressure flow studies in the upper urinary tract. *J. Urol.* **121**, 602–604.
9. Jeans, W.D., Penry, J.N. & Roylance, J. (1972) Renal puncture. *Clin. Radiol.* **23**, 298–311.
10. Lang, E.K. (1977) Renal cyst puncture and aspiration: a survey of complications. *Am. J. Roentgenol.* **128**, 723–727.

Further reading

Pfister, R. & Newhouse, J. (1979) Interventional percutaneous pyeloureteral techniques. I Antegrade pyelography and ureteral perfusion. II Percutaneous nephrostomy and other procedures. *Radiol. Clin. N. Am.* **17**, 341–363.
Sandler, C.M., Houston, G.K., Hall, J.T. & Morettin, L.B. (1986) Guided cyst puncture and aspiration. *Radiol. Clin. N. Am.* **24**, 527–537.

PERCUTANEOUS NEPHROSTOMY

The introduction of a drainage catheter into the collecting system of the kidney.

Indications

1. Obstructive uropathy
2. Prior to percutaneous nephrolithotomy
3. Ureteric fistulae; external drainage may allow closure.

Contraindications

Uncontrolled bleeding diathesis.

Contrast medium

As for percutaneous renal puncture.

Equipment

1. Puncturing needle (18-G); Longdwell, or equivalent.
2. Drainage catheter: at least 7-F pigtail with multiple side holes.
3. Guide-wires: conventional angiographic and Lunderquist.
4. US and/or fluoroscopy.

Patient preparation

1. Fasting for 4 h
2. Premedication
3. Prophylactic antibiotic
4. Surgical backup in view of clinical workup, possible complications and further management
5. The patient should empty the bladder just prior to the procedure.

Technique

Patient position

With the patient lying in the prone position on the fluoroscopic table, a foam pad or non-opaque pillow is placed under the abdomen so that the kidney lies in a fixed posterior position. An oblique position with the kidney to be punctured raised is sometimes used.

Identifying the collecting system

1. Real-time US may be used to identify the renal pelvis for antegrade pyelography and to determine the plane of definitive

puncture of the collecting system. With a biopsy needle attachment, a real-time US probe may be used to guide the puncturing needle into the collecting system.
2. Excretion urography, if adequate residual function.
3. Antegrade pyelography.

Site/plane of puncture

A point on the posterior axillary line is chosen below the twelfth rib. Having identified the mid/lower pole calyces with contrast/US, the plane of puncture is determined. This will be via the soft tissues and renal parenchyma, in which plane vessels around the renal pelvis will be avoided and the drainage catheter will gain some purchase on the renal parenchyma. The drainage catheter is also more comfortable for the patient in this plane, and is less likely to be kinked when he/she lies supine.

Techniques of puncture, catheterization

The skin and soft tissues are infiltrated with local anaesthetic using a spinal needle. Puncture may then be made using one of the following systems (depending on preference):

1. An 18-G sheathed needle, a cyst puncture or a Longdwell needle, in conjunction with the Seldinger technique for catheterization. Upon successful puncture a J guide-wire is inserted and coiled within the collecting system; the sheath is then pushed over the wire, which is exchanged for a more rigid Lunderquist wire. If possible the guide-wire is manipulated into the ureter. Dilatation is then performed to 1-F greater than the size of the drainage catheter, which is then inserted. During all manipulation, care must be taken not to kink the guide-wire within the soft tissues. A substantial amount of guide-wire should be maintained within the collecting system so that position is not lost and if kinking does occur, then the kinked portion of the wire can be withdrawn outside the skin.
2. *The Cope needle system*, using a 21-G puncturing needle that takes a special guide-wire. This affords a single puncture with a fine needle, leading on to eventual catheterization.
3. *The trocar-cannula system*, in which direct puncture of the collecting system is made with the drainage catheter already assembled over a trocar. On removal of the trocar the drainage catheter is pushed further into the collecting system.

Having successfully introduced a catheter, the latter is securely fixed to the skin and drainage commenced.

Aftercare

1. Bed rest for 12 h
2. Both blood pressure and temperature half-hourly for 6 h
3. Urine cultures and sensitivity.

Complications

1. Unsuccessful drainage
2. Haemorrhage
3. Perforation of the collecting system
4. Septicaemia.

PERCUTANEOUS NEPHROLITHOTOMY

The removal of renal calculi through a nephrostomy tract. Often reserved for large complicated calculi which are unsuitable for extracorporeal shock wave lithotripsy.

Indications

1. Removal of renal calculi.
2. Disintegration of large renal calculi.

Contraindications

Uncontrolled bleeding diathesis.

Contrast medium

As for percutaneous renal puncture.

Equipment

1. Puncturing needle (18-G): Longdwell or equivalent.
2. Guide-wires, including J-angiographic and Lunderquist.
3. Tract dilating equipment; Teflon dilators (from 7-F to 30-F), metal coaxial dilators or a special angioplasty balloon catheter.
4. Fluoroscopy facilities with rotating C arm if possible.

Patient preparation

1. Full discussion between radiologist/urologist concerning indications, etc.
2. Admission on the day prior to the procedure. A general anaesthetic is usually required.
3. Coagulation screen.

4. Two units of blood cross matched.
5. Antibiotic cover.
6. Premedication.
7. Bladder catheterization, as large volumes of irrigation fluid will pass down the ureter during a prolonged procdure.

Technique

Patient position

As for a percutaneous nephrostomy (see p. 150).

Methods of opacification of the collecting system

1. Excretion urography.
2. Retrograde ureteric catheterization; distension of the collecting system may be achieved. In addition, a retrograde catheter in the ureter will prevent large fragments of stone passing down the ureter.
3. Antegrade pyelography; this also enables distension of the collecting system.

Puncture of the collecting system

A lower pole posterior calyx is chosen if the calculus is situated in the renal pelvis. Otherwise the calyx in which the calculus is situated must be punctured. Special care must be taken if puncturing above the twelfth rib because of the risk of perforating the diaphragm and pleura. Puncture is in an oblique plane from the posterior axillary line through the renal parenchyma. Puncture of the selected calyx is made using either a rotating C-arm fluoroscopic facility or rocking the patient to determine the depth of the calyx in relation to the needle tip. On successful puncture a J guide-wire is inserted through the sheath and as much wire as possible is guided into the collecting system. The sheath is then pushed over the wire, which is exchanged for a more rigid Lunderquist wire. If possible, the wire is manipulated into the ureter. At this stage full dilation may be performed (single stage) or a nephrostomy tube left in situ with dilatation later (two-stage procedure).

Dilatation

This is carried out under general anaesthesia. It is performed using Teflon dilators from 7-F to 30-F which are introduced over the guide-wire. Alternatively, metal coaxial dilators or a special angioplasty balloon (10 cm long) are used. A sheath is inserted over the largest dilator or balloon and through the sheath lumen removal of the calculus or disintegration is performed.

Removal/disintegration

Removal of calculi of less than 1 cm is possible using a nephro-scope and forceps. Larger calculi must be disintegrated using an ultrasonic or electrohydraulic disintegrator.

Aftercare

1. Usually determined by the anaesthetist/urologist.
2. Plain radiograph of renal area to ensure that all calculi/fragments have been removed.

Complications

Immediate

1. Failure of access, dilatation or removal.
2. Perforation of the renal pelvis on dilatation.
3. Haemorrhage. Less than 3% of procedures should require transfusion. Rarely, balloon tamponade of the tract or embolization may be required.
4. Damage to surrounding structures, i.e. diaphragm, colon, spleen and liver.
5. Problems related to the irrigating fluid, i.e. haemolysis.

Delayed

1. Aneurysm of an intrarenal artery.

RETROGRADE PYELOURETEROGRAPHY

Indications

1. Demonstration of the site, length, lower limit and, if possible, the nature of an obstructive lesion.
2. Demonstration of the pelvicalyceal system after an unsatisfactory excretion urogram. Seldom necessary with modern imaging methods.

Contraindications

Acute urinary tract infection.

Contrast medium

HOCM or LOCM 150–200, i.e. not too dense to obscure small lesions, 10 ml.

Equipment

Fluoroscopy unit.

Patient preparation

As for surgery.

Preliminary film

Full-length supine AP abdomen when the examination is performed in the X-ray department.

Technique

In the operating theatre

The surgeon catheterizes the ureter via a cystoscope and advances the ureteric catheter to the desired level. Contrast medium is injected under fluoroscopic control and spot films exposed.

In the X-ray department

1. With ureteric catheter(s) in situ, the patient is transferred from the operating theatre to the X-ray department.
2. Urine is aspirated and under fluoroscopic control contrast medium is slowly injected. About 3–5 ml are usually enough to fill the pelvis but the injection should be terminated before this if the patient complains of pain or fullness in the loin.
3. If there is pelviureteric junction obstruction, the contrast medium in the pelvis is aspirated. The films are examined and if satisfactory, the catheter is withdrawn, first to 10 cm below the renal pelvis, and then to lie just above the ureteric orifice.

About 2 ml of contrast medium are injected at each of these levels and films taken.

Films

Using the undercouch tube:

1. supine PA of the ureter
2. both 35° anterior obliques of the ureter.

NB: The catheter may be left in the pelvis to drain a pelviureteric obstruction. In this case withdrawal ureterograms are not possible.

Aftercare

1. Post-anaesthetic observations
2. Prophylactic antibiotics may be used.

Complications

Due to the anaesthetic

Complications of general anaesthesia.

Due to the contrast medium

1. Contrast medium can be absorbed from the intact renal pelvis, giving rise to adverse reactions. However, the risks are much less than with excretion urography.
2. Chemical pyelitis – if there is stasis of contrast medium.
3. Extravasation due to overdistension of the pelvis. This is usually asymptomatic but may result in pain, fever and rigors.

Due to the technique

1. Introduction of infection.
2. Mucosal damage to the ureter.
3. Perforation of the ureter or pelvis by the catheter.

MICTURATING CYSTOURETHROGRAPHY

Indications

1. Vesicoureteric reflux
2. Study of the urethra during micturition
3. Abnormalities of the bladder
4. Stress incontinence.

Contraindications

Acute urinary tract infection.

Contrast medium

HOCM or LOCM 150.

Equipment

1. Fluoroscopy unit with spot film device and tilting table
2. Video recorder
3. Jaques or Foley catheter. In small infants a fine (5–7-F) feeding tube is adequate.

Patient preparation

The patient micturates prior to the examination.

Preliminary film

Coned view of the bladder, using the undercouch tube.

Technique

To demonstrate vesico-ureteric reflux

1. This indication is almost exclusively confined to children.
2. The patient lies supine on the X-ray table. Using aseptic technique a catheter, lubricated with Hibitane 0.05% in glycerine, is introduced into the bladder. Residual urine is drained. Contrast medium is slowly dripped in and bladder filling is observed by intermittent fluoroscopy. It is important that initial filling is monitored by fluoroscopy in case the catheter is in the distal ureter (thereby mimicking vesico-ureteric reflux) or vagina.
3. Any reflux is recorded on spot films.
4. The catheter should not be removed until the radiologist is convinced that the patient will micturate or until no more contrast medium will drip into the bladder. The examination is expedited if the catheter remains in situ until micturition commences and then is quickly withdrawn. Small feeding tubes do not obstruct micturition.
5. Older children and adults are given a urine receiver but smaller children should be allowed to micturate onto absorbent pads on which they can lie. Children can lie on the table but adults will probably find it easier to micturate while standing erect.
6. In infants and children with a neuropathic bladder, micturition may be accomplished by suprapubic pressure.
7. Spot films are taken during micturition and any reflux recorded. A video recording may be useful. The lower ureter is best seen in the anterior oblique position of that side. Boys should micturate in the LAO position, with right hip and knee flexed, or in the RAO position, with left hip and knee flexed, so that spot films can be taken of the *entire* urethra.
8. Finally, a full-length view of the abdomen is taken to demonstrate any reflux of contrast medium that might have occurred unnoticed into the kidneys and to record the post-micturition residue.

To demonstrate a vesico-vaginal or recto-vesical fistula

As above, but films are taken in the lateral position.

To demonstrate stress incontinence

Initially the technique is as for demonstrating vesico-ureteric reflux. The catheter is left in situ until the patient is in the erect position.

Films

These should include sacrum and symphysis pubis because bony landmarks are used to assess bladder neck descent.
1. Lateral bladder
2. Lateral bladder, straining
The catheter is then removed.
3. Lateral bladder during micturition.

Aftercare

1. No special aftercare is necessary, but patients and parents of children should be warned that dysuria, possibly leading to retention of urine, may rarely be experienced. In such cases a simple analgesic is helpful and children may be helped by allowing them to micturate in a warm bath.
2. Most children will already be receiving antibiotics for their recent urinary tract infection. However, if reflux is demonstrated in a child who is not receiving antibiotics, they should be prescribed.

Complications

Due to the contrast medium

1. Adverse reactions may result from absorption of contrast medium by the bladder mucosa.
The risk is small when compared with excretion urography.
2. Contrast medium-induced cystitis.

Due to the technique

1. Acute urinary tract infection.
2. Catheter trauma – may produce dysuria, frequency, haematuria and urinary retention.
3. Complications of bladder filling, e.g. perforation from overdistension – prevented by using a non-retaining catheter, e.g. Jaques.
4. Catheterization of vagina or an ectopic ureteral orifice.
5. Retention of a Foley catheter.

Further reading

Jeffcoate, T.N.A. (1958) Urethrocystography in the female. *J. Fac. Radiol.* **2**, 127–134.
McAlister, W.H., Cacciarelli, A. & Shackelford, G.D. (1974) Complications associated with cystography in children. *Radiology* **111**, 167–172.

ASCENDING URETHROGRAPHY IN THE MALE

Indications

1. Strictures
2. Urethral tears
3. Congenital abnormalities
4. Periurethral or prostatic abscess
5. Fistulae or false passages.

Contraindications

1. Acute urinary tract infection
2. Recent instrumentation.

Contrast medium

HOCM or LOCM 200–300, 20 ml. Pre-warming the contrast medium will help reduce the incidence of spasm of the external sphincter.

Equipment

1. Tilting radiography table with fluoroscopy unit and spot film device
2. Foley catheter or penile clamp, e.g. Knutsson's.

Patient preparation

None.

Preliminary film

Coned supine PA of bladder base and urethra.

Technique

1. The patient lies supine on the X-ray table.
2. Using aseptic technique the penile clamp is applied or the tip of the catheter is inserted so that the balloon lies in the fossa navicularis and its balloon is inflated with 1–2 ml of water. Contrast medium is injected under fluoroscopic control and films taken in the following positions:
   a. 30° LAO, with right leg abducted and knee flexed
   b. supine PA
   c. 30° RAO, with left leg abducted and knee flexed.
3. Ascending urethrography should be followed by micturating cystourethrography or excretory micturating cystourethrography to demonstrate the proximal urethra. Occasionally a urethral

fistula or periurethral abscess is seen only on the voiding examination; reflux of contrast medium into dilated prostatic ducts is also better seen during micturition.

Aftercare

None.

Complications

Due to the contrast medium

Adverse reactions are rare.

Due to the technique

1. Acute urinary tract infection
2. Urethral trauma
3. Intravasation of contrast medium, especially if excessive pressure is used to overcome a stricture.

Further reading

McCallum, R.W. (1979) The adult male urethra. Normal anatomy, pathology and method of urethrography. *Radiol. Clin. N. Am.* **17 (2)**, 227–244.

RENAL ARTERIOGRAPHY

Indications

1. Renal artery stenosis
2. Renal tumour prior to embolization or rarely for diagnosis
3. Kidney donor
4. Haematuria of unknown cause.

Contrast medium

Selective renal artery injection

LOCM 300, 10 ml at 5 ml s^{-1}, or by hand injection.

Flush aortic

LOCM 370, 50 ml at 12 ml s^{-1}.

Equipment

1. Digital fluoroscopy unit
2. Pump injector
3. Catheters
   a. selective injection – Sidewinder or Cobra
   b. flush aortic injection – pigtail (see Fig. 8.3).

Technique

Flush aortography

Femoral artery puncture. The catheter is placed proximal to the renal vessels (i.e. approx. T12) and AP and oblique (10° raise on the side of interest) runs are performed (the oblique run demonstrating the renal origins). Selective catheterization may overlook a stenosis at the origin of the renal artery or convert a stenosis into an occlusion, but is occasionally required to define better the renal vasculature.

Renal tumours

Selective catheterization more accurately defines the anatomy and tumour vessels may be shown better after the administration of 5 µg of adrenaline. The adrenaline is injected into the renal artery over 30 s, the catheter is then quickly flushed with saline and 10 ml of contrast medium is injected by hand.[1]

Donor kidneys

A flush aortogram is performed to count the number of renal vessels and to ensure normality of the contralateral kidney. Selective injection may occasionally be required to accurately number the renal arteries.

ULTRASOUND OF THE URINARY TRACT IN ADULTS

US

Indications

1. Suspected renal mass lesion
2. Suspected renal parenchymal disease
3. Possible renal obstruction
4. Haematuria
5. Renal cystic disease
6. Renal size measurement
7. To facilitate accurate needle placement in interventional procedures
8. Prostatism
9. Bladder volume before and after micturition
10. Bladder tumour.

Contraindications

None.

Patient preparation

None – unless full bladder is required.

Equipment

3.5–5 MHz transducer.

Technique

1. Patient supine, right and left anterior oblique positions or prone for kidneys. The kidneys are scanned longitudinally and transversely. The right kidney may be scanned through the liver and posteriorly in the right loin. The left kidney is harder to visualize anteriorly unless the spleen is large, but can be visualized from the left loin.
2. The length of the kidney measured by US is smaller than that measured at excretion urography because there is no geometric magnification and no change in size related to contrast-induced osmotic diuresis. With US measurement, care must be taken to ensure that the true longitudinal diameter is scanned. The mean length of the normal adult right kidney is 10.7 cm and the left 11.1 cm (range 9–12 cm).
3. The bladder is scanned suprapubically in transverse and longitudinal planes. Measurements taken of three diameters before and after micturition enable an approximate volume to be calculated.

ULTRASOUND OF THE URINARY TRACT IN CHILDREN

US

The availability of high-resolution real-time US has revolutionized the investigation of paediatric renal disease during the last decade. It demonstrates anatomy without the necessity for adequate renal function but, because it gives no functional information, it is the ideal complement to nuclear medicine imaging. It should be stressed that the technique is only as good as the effort put in to obtain the images.

Indications (after Lebowitz, 1985)[1]

1. Urinary tract infection – to document scarring, elicit signs of acute upper tract infection and to exclude an underlying structural abnormality.

2. An abdominal or pelvic mass. Ultrasonography will demonstrate the relationship of the mass to other organs, its possible site of origin and its characteristics, i.e. solid or cystic and the presence of calcification.

3. Renal failure – to differentiate medical from surgical causes.

4. Abnormal antenatal US – to confirm or refute an antenatal diagnosis of hydronephrosis or multicystic dysplasia. The role of US should be to help in the efficient planning of the postnatal management before infection occurs and plasma creatinine rises, rather than to provoke antenatal intervention. It must be remembered that, because urine output falls rapidly after birth when compared with in utero, US on day 1 may show considerably less pelvicalyceal dilatation than was observed on the antenatal scans. Further follow-up scans are mandatory.

5. To determine the site of obstruction when excretion urography or renography have failed to determine the exact level.

6. To evaluate a kidney not visualized by other modalities.

7. Conditions associated with a high likelihood of renal abnormalities, e.g. imperforate anus and genital anomalies. The most frequently found abnormalities are a single or ectopic kidney.

8. Conditions which predispose to renal tumours – Beckwith–Wiedemann syndrome, hemihypertrophy and aniridia. Periodic screening is necessary.

9. Screening of family members for genetically linked renal diseases, e.g. dominant polycystic renal disease.

10. Periodic follow-up of kidneys which are at risk of deterioration, e.g. children with myelomeningocele or urinary diversion. Patients on chronic dialysis have a high incidence of acquired cystic disease and may develop adenomas or adenocarcinomas.

11. To assess the patency of the IVC in patients with Wilms' tumour.

12. To assess residual bladder volume.

13. To facilitate the accurate placement of needles for renal biopsy, antegrade pyelography, percutaneous nephrostomy, cyst aspiration and drainage of perinephric collections.

When assessing possible renal disease by ultrasonography, a number of normal 'variants' may be confused with disease. These include increased parenchymal echogenicity in the neonatal period, echo-poor papillae which may mimic dilated calyces and persistent fetal lobulation, hepatic and splenic impressions and parenchymal junctional lines which may mimic scarring.

Equipment

3.5–7.5 MHz transducer – dependent on age.

Patient preparation

Full bladder. Patients with an indwelling catheter should have this clamped 1 h before the examination is scheduled.

Technique

1. Begin by examining the bladder, because contact of the transducer and jelly against the skin may promote bladder emptying. You may have only one chance to image the bladder.
2. It may be necessary to examine uncooperative children while they sit on a carer's lap. Otherwise the technique is as for adults.
3. If possible the kidneys are examined in full inspiration or with the child being asked to 'push the tummy out'.

References

1. Lebowitz, R.L. (1985) Pediatric uroradiology. *Pediatr. Clin. N. Am.* **32**, 1353–1362.

STATIC RENAL SCINTIGRAPHY   RI

Indications

1. Assessment of individual renal function
2. Investigation of urinary tract infections, particularly in children[1]
3. Assessment of reflux nephropathy
4. Investigation of horseshoe, solitary or ectopic kidney
5. Space-occupying lesions.

Contraindications

None.

Radiopharmaceuticals

^{99m}Tc-*dimercaptosuccinic acid (DMSA)*, 80 MBq max (0.7 mSv ED).

Bound to plasma proteins and cleared by tubular absorption. Retained in the renal cortex, with uptake of 40–65% of injected dose within 2 h, and no significant excretion during the imaging period.

Equipment

1. Gamma-camera
2. Low-energy high resolution collimator.

Patient preparation

None.

Technique

1. The radiopharmaceutical is administered i.v.
2. Images are acquired at any time 1–6 h later. Imaging in the first hour is to be avoided because of free ^{99m}Tc in the urine.

Images

1. Posterior, right and left posterior oblique views, 256×256 resolution, 300–500 000 counts.
2. Zoomed or pinhole views may be useful in children.

Additional images

Anterior – in suspected pelvic or horseshoe kidney and severe scoliosis, or if relative function is to be calculated by geometric mean method.

Analysis

1. Relative function is best calculated from the geometric mean of posterior and anterior computer images. A single posterior view is often used, but this requires assumptions about kidney depth, unless depth information is available to enable attenuation correction.
2. Absolute uptake can be estimated if required with additional information on patient and kidney size from lateral images.

Additional techniques

1. SPECT
2. ^{99m}Tc-mercaptoacetyltriglycine (MAG-3) (max. 100 MBq, 0.7 mSv ED) may be considered as a possible alternative to DMSA; it gives inferior kidney visualization, but has the advantage of additional dynamic assessment of excretion in the same study and a lower radiation dose.[2,3]

3. Fast dynamic frames with motion correction may be useful to reduce movement artefact, particularly in young children.

Aftercare

None.

Complications

None.

References

1. Piepsz, A., Blaufox, M.D., Gordon, I., et al. (1999) Consensus on renal cortical scintigraphy in children with urinary tract infection. Scientific Committee of Radionuclides in Nephrourology. *Semin. Nucl. Med.* **29**, 160–174.
2. Pickworth, F.E., Vivian, G.C., Franklin, K., et al. (1992) $^{99}Tc^m$-mercapto acetyl triglycine in paediatric renal tract disease. *Br. J. Radiol.* **65**, 21–29.
3. Gordon, I., Anderson, P.J., Lythgoe, M.F., et al. (1992) Can technetium-99m-mercaptoacetyltriglycine replace technetium-99m-dimercaptosuccinic acid in the exclusion of a focal renal defect? *J. Nucl. Med.* **33**, 2090–2093.

Further reading

Blaufox, M.D. (1991) Procedures of choice in renal nuclear medicine. *J. Nucl. Med.* **32**, 1301–1309.
O'Reilly, P.H., Shields, R.A. & Testa, H.J. (1986) *Nuclear Medicine in Urology and Nephrology*, 2nd edn. London: Butterworths.

DYNAMIC RENAL SCINTIGRAPHY   R

Indications[1]

1. Diagnosis of obstructed vs. non-obstructed dilatation[2]
2. Diagnosis of renal artery stenosis[3]
3. Assessment of perfusion in acute renal failure
4. Assessment of renal function following drainage procedures to the urinary tract
5. Demonstration of vesicoureteric reflux
6. Assessment of renal transplantation
7. Renal trauma.

Contraindications

None.

Radiopharmaceuticals

1. ^{99m}Tc-*MAG-3*, 100 MBq max (0.7 mSv ED), (200 MBq max (1 mSv ED) for first-pass blood flow imaging). Highly protein-

bound, so mainly cleared by tubular secretion (80%) with only around 20% glomerular filtration (mean normal clearance is approx. 370 ml min^{-1}). Good quality images due to fast clearance and greater kidney/background ratio than ^{99m}Tc-diethylene triamine pentacetic acid (DTPA), therefore better for poor renal function, although more expensive. Now the radiopharmaceutical of choice due to best image quality.

2. ^{99m}Tc-DTPA, 150 MBq typical (1 mSv ED), 300 MBq max (2 mSv ED), (800 MBq max (5 mSv ED) for first-pass blood flow imaging). Cleared by glomerular filtration (mean normal clearance is approx. 120 ml min^{-1}). Lower kidney/background ratio than MAG-3 or hippuran, so poorer image quality and noisier clearance curves. Cheap and widely available.

3. ^{123}I-orthoiodohippurate (hippuran), 20 MBq max (0.2 mSv ED). Almost entirely cleared by tubular secretion (mean normal clearance is approx. 500 ml min^{-1}). High kidney/background ratio, but image quality is limited by the recommended maximum activity. For many years the gold standard, but high cost and limited availability due to ^{123}I being a cyclotron product.

Equipment

1. Gamma-camera
2. Low-energy general purpose collimator.

Patient preparation

1. The patient should be well hydrated with around 500 ml of fluid immediately before administration of tracer.
2. The bladder should be voided before injection.

Technique[2]

1. The patient lies supine or sits reclining with their back against the camera.
2. The radiopharmaceutical is injected i.v. and image acquisition is started simultaneously.
3. Perform dynamic 128×128 acquisition with 10–15 s frames for 30–40 min. (For quantitative perfusion studies, e.g. in the transplanted kidney, 1–2-s frames over first minute are acquired.)
4. If poor excretion is seen from one or both kidneys after 10–20 min, a diuretic (frusemide 40 mg) is administered slowly during imaging. Imaging should be continued for at least a further 15 min. Since maximum diuresis does not occur

until 15 min after administration of frusemide, as an alternative it may be given 15 min before the radiopharmaceutical (the so-called 'F – 15' renogram) which can be useful after equivocal standard 'F + 20' studies.
5. If significant retention in the kidneys is apparent at the end of the imaging period, ask the patient to void and walk around for a minute, then take a further short image.

Films

All posterior.
Hard copy: 2–5-min images for duration of study.

Analysis

The following information is produced using standard computer analysis:

1. Background-subtracted kidney time-activity ('renogram') curves.
2. Relative function figures.

Additional figures are sometimes calculated:

3. Perfusion index, especially in renal transplant assessment.
4. Parenchymal and whole kidney transit times.

Additional techniques

1. Pre- and 1 h post-captopril (25–50 mg) study for diagnosis of renal artery stenosis. The patient should ideally stop diuretic and ACE inhibitor medication 3–5 days prior to the test.[3]
2. Indirect micturating cystography following renography to demonstrate vesicoureteric reflux. The bladder must not have been emptied and the kidneys should be reasonably clear of activity. Continuous dynamic 5-s images are acquired for 2 min before and up to 3 min after micturition, with generation of bladder and kidney time-activity curves.[4]
3. Glomerular filtration rate (GFR) measurement and individual kidney GFR with DTPA studies by taking blood samples for counting. Similarly, effective renal plasma flow (ERPF) measurement with hippuran and a MAG-3 clearance index may be obtained.[5]
4. The images obtained with MAG-3 can be analysed for the presence of renal scarring and there is good correlation with the results obtained with DMSA (MAG-3 is 80% tubular secreted). DMSA remains the gold standard for cortical

scarring because of the higher information density and ability to obtain multiple projections, but simultaneous renal clearance information can be gained with MAG-3.[6,7]

5. With the appropriate computer software and fast-frame acquisition, compressed images may be generated to demonstrate and quantify ureteric peristalsis and show reflux (best with MAG-3 or hippuran),[1,8] although the technique has not yet found a widely accepted clinical role.

Aftercare

1. The patient is warned that the effects of diuresis may last a couple of hours. The patient may feel faint because of hypotension when adopting the erect posture at the end of the procedure.
2. After captopril administration, blood pressure monitoring under medical supervision should be carried out until back to normal.
3. Normal radiation safety precautions (see Chapter 1).

Complications

None, except after captopril, when care must be taken in patients with severe vascular disease to avoid hypotension and renal failure.

References

1. Woolfson, R.G. & Neild, G.H. (1997) The true clinical significance of renography in nephro-urology. Eur. J. Nucl. Med. **24**, 557–570.
2. O'Reilly, P., Aurell, M., Britton, K., et al. (1996) Consensus on diuresis renography for investigating the dilated upper urinary tract. J. Nucl. Med. **37**, 1872–1876.
3. Taylor, A., Nally, J., Aurell, M., et al. (1996) Consensus report on ACE inhibitor renography for detecting renovascular hypertension. J. Nucl. Med. **37**, 1876–1882.
4. Chapman, S.J., Chantler, C., Haycock, G.B., et al. (1988) Radionuclide cystography in vesicoureteric reflux. Arch. Dis. Child. **63**, 650–651.
5. Blaufox, M.D., Aurell, M., Bubeck, B., et al. (1996) Report of the radionuclides in nephrourology committee on renal clearance. J. Nucl. Med. **37**, 1883–1890.
6. Gordon, I., Anderson, P.J., Lythgoe, M.F., et al. (1992) Can Technetium-99m-mercaptoacetyltriglycine replace technetium-99m-dimercaptosuccinic acid in the exclusion of a focal renal defect? J. Nucl. Med. **33**, 2090–2093.
7. Pickworth, F.E., Vivian, G.C., Franklin, K., et al. (1992) [99]Tc[m]-mercapto acetyl triglycine in paediatric renal tract disease. Br. J. Radiol. **65**, 21–29.
8. Lepej, J., Kliment, J., Horák, V., et al. (1991) A new approach in radionuclide imaging to ureteric peristalsis using [99]Tc[m]-MAG-3 and condensed images. Nucl. Med. Commun. **12**, 397–407.

Further reading

Woolfson, R.G. & Neild, G.H. (1998) Renal nuclear medicine: can it survive the millennium? Nephrol. Dial. Transplant. **13**, 12–14.

Britton, K.E., Brown, N.J. & Nimmon, C.C. (1996) Clinical renography: 25 years on. *Eur. J. Nucl. Med.* **23**, 1541–1546.

Cosgriff, P.S., Lawson, R.S. & Nimmon, C.C. (1992) Towards standardisation in gamma camera renography. *Nucl. Med. Commun.* **13**, 580–585.

Smith, F.W. & Gemmell, H.G. (1998) The urinary tract. In: Sharp P.F., Gemmell, H.G. & Smith, F.W. (eds) *Practical Nuclear Medicine*, pp. 214–234. Oxford: Oxford University Press.

DIRECT RADIONUCLIDE MICTURATING CYSTOGRAPHY

RN

Indications

Vesicoureteric reflux.

Contraindications

Acute urinary tract infection.

Radiopharmaceuticals

^{99m}Tc-*pertechnetate*, 25 MBq max (0.3 mSv ED), adminstered into the bladder. Some pertechnetate is absorbed in the urinary tract and gastric activity may be seen.

Equipment

1. Gamma-camera
2. Low-energy general purpose collimator
4. Sterile saline infusion
5. Commode or plastic urinal
6. Screens for patient privacy.

Patient preparation

The patient micturates prior to the investigation.

Technique[1]

This examination is most frequently performed on children. Direct radionuclide cystography is considered to be at least as sensitive as conventional X-ray micturating cystourethrography (MCU) for the detection of vesicoureteric reflux.[1–3] It enables continuous imaging and quantification of bladder, ureter and kidney activity to be performed and delivers a much smaller radiation dose than conventional cystography.

The technique requires catheterization and is similar to that for MCU except that:

1. ^{99m}Tc-pertechnetate is administered using one of two methods:
   a. diluted in 500 ml sterile saline solution at body temperature and then infused into the bladder via the catheter
   b. injected directly into the bladder via the catheter and continuously diluted with sterile saline solution infusion at body temperature.
2. During infusion, the patient lies supine with the gamma-camera posterior. Ensure that both kidneys, ureters and bladder are in the field of view for all imaging. Dynamic image acquisition is performed for the duration of bladder filling at 5–10 s per frame with a 128×128 matrix size to demonstrate any reflux during this phase.
3. When the bladder is as full as tolerable, the infusion is stopped but imaging is continued for a further 30 s. The patient then sits in front of the gamma-camera on a commode or child's plastic urinal.
4. Dynamic imaging with 5–10-s frames is performed during micturition, continuing for 2–5 min after to evaluate bladder re-filling. If the patient is capable, the embarrassment of the procedure may be reduced by giving them a remote control to start computer acquisition just before they micturate, and leaving them in private.

Analysis

1. Time–activity curves are produced from regions over the bladder, kidneys and ureters.
2. If the voided volume is measured, residual and reflux volumes can be calculated.[4]
3. Viewing the image set cinematically may aid identification of reflux.
4. Images may be summed to highlight any reflux episodes.

Additional techniques

1. If vesico-ureteric reflux is not seen during a single filling and voiding cycle, the sensitivity of the test may be improved by immediately repeating the procedure.[5] The first voiding is performed if possible without removing the catheter, and re-filling is commenced shortly after.
2. Indirect radionuclide cystography may be performed after conventional radionuclide renography[6] (see 'Dynamic renal scintigraphy', p. 166).
3. Intrarenal reflux has been investigated with delayed imaging of radiocolloid reflux at 5 and 20 h.[3]

Aftercare

As for conventional cystography.

Complications

As for conventional cystography.

References

1. Mandell, G.A., Eggli, D.F., Gilday, D.L., et al. (1997) Procedure guideline for radionuclide cystography in children. *J. Nucl. Med.* **38**, 1650–1654.
2. Van den Abbeele, A.D., Treves, S.T., Lebowitz, R.L. et al. (1987) Vesicoureteral reflux in asymptomatic siblings of patients with known reflux: Radionuclide cystography. *Pediatrics* **79**, 147–156.
3. Rizzoni, G., Perale, R., Bui, F., et al. (1986) Radionuclide voiding cystography in intrarenal reflux detection. *Ann. Radiol.* **29**, 415–420.
4. Gelfand, M.J. (1988) Nuclear cystography. In: Gelfand, M.J. & Thomas, S.R. (eds) *Effective Use of Computers in Nuclear Medicine*, pp. 402–411. New York: McGraw-Hill.
5. Fettich, J.J. & Kenda, R.B. (1992) Cyclic direct radionuclide voiding cystography: Increasing reliability in detecting vesicoureteral reflux in children. *Pediatr. Radiol.* **22**, 337–338.
6. Bower, G., Lovegrove, F.T., Geijsel, H., et al. (1985) Comparison of 'direct' and 'indirect' radionuclide cystography. *J. Nucl. Med.* **26**, 465–468.

Further reading

Treves, S.T., Gelfand, M. & Willi, U.V. (1995) Vesicoureteric reflux and radionuclide cystography. In: Treves, S.T. (ed) *Pediatric Nuclear Medicine*, 2nd edn, pp 411–429. New York: Springer-Verlag.

HELICAL (SPIRAL) CT OF THE KIDNEYS

RENAL PARENCHYMA

A typical protocol to identify parenchymal disease utilizes a three-phase breath-hold examination:

Collimation	3–5 mm
Pitch	1:1 or 1.5:1
Reconstruction interval	3 mm
Scan time	30 s
First Phase	Unenhanced scan
Second (Cortical) Phase	LOCM or HOCM (300); 120 ml at 3 ml s^{-1} scanning is commenced manually at 30 s after the start of the injection or triggered by a software package (e.g. Smart Prep, General Electric)

Third (Cortical & Medullary) Phase
                              100 s after the start of the injection
In some situations when it is necessary to image contrast medium in the collecting system, a fourth phase may be acquired:
Fourth Phase   5 min after the start of the injection.

RENAL ANGIOGRAPHY

Indication

1. Renal artery stenosis
2. Assessment of living related renal transplant donors.

A suitable protocol is as follows:

1. 30- or 40-s breath hold
2. Unenhanced scan with 10-mm collimation and pitch 2:1 to localize the area of interest
3. Post-contrast scan using 5-mm collimation, 5 mm s^{-1} table speed, pitch 1:1
4. LOCM (300) at 4–5 ml s^{-1} for the duration of the scan
5. The onset of scanning is determined manually from sequential scans after a test dose or using commercially available bolus tracking techniques e.g. Smart Prep (General Electric), usually 15–25 s
6. Image reconstruction by
   a. multiplanar and curved reformations
   b. threshold-shaded surface display
   c. maximum intensity projection (MIP)
   d. volume rendering.

Further reading

Rubin, G.D. & Silverman, S.G. (1995) Helical (spiral) CT of the retroperitoneum. *Radiol. Clin. N. Am.* **33 (5)**, 903–932.

6 Reproductive system

Methods of imaging the female reproductive system

1. US (transabdominal/transvaginal)
2. Plain abdominal film
3. Hysterosalpingography
4. CT
5. MRI
6. Arteriography (including embolization of fibroids).

Methods of imaging the scrotum and testes

1. US
2. MRI
3. Radionuclide imaging
4. Arteriography
5. Venography (including embolization of varices).

Further reading

Clements, R., Griffiths, G.J., Peeling, W.B. & Conn, I.G. (1991) Transrectal ultrasound of the ejaculatory apparatus. *Clin. Radiol.* **44**, 240–244.
Demas, B.E., Hricak, H. & McClure, R.D. (1991) Varicoceles. Radiologic diagnosis and treatment. *Radiol. Clin. N. Am.* **29**, 619–627.
Fowler, R. (1990) Review. Imaging the testis and scrotal structures. *Clin. Radiol.* **41**, 81–85.

HYSTEROSALPINGOGRAPHY

Indications

1. Infertility
2. Recurrent miscarriages
3. Following tubal surgery
4. Assessment of the integrity of a Caesarean uterine scar.

Contraindications

1. Pregnancy

2. A purulent discharge on inspection of the vulva or cervix, or diagnosed PID in the preceding 6 months
3. Recent dilatation and curettage or abortion, or immediately post-menstruation. This applies only to oily contrast medium because of the risk of intravasation
4. Contrast sensitivity.

Contrast medium

Oily contrast medium is no longer recommended.

HOCM or LOCM 300. Volume 10–20 ml.

LOCM have no advantage[1] with regard to image quality or side-effects but the nonionic dimer, iotrolan, is associated with a lower incidence and decreased severity of delayed pain.[2]

Equipment

1. Fluoroscopy unit with spot film device
2. Vaginal speculum
3. Vulsellum forceps
4. Uterine cannula, Leech-Wilkinson cannula, olive or 8-F paediatric Foley catheter.

Patient preparation

1. The patient should abstain from intercourse between booking the appointment and the time of the examination unless she uses a reliable method of contraception, *or* the examination can be booked between the fourth and tenth days in a patient with a regular 28-day cycle.
2. Apprehensive patients may need premedication.

Preliminary film

Coned PA view of the pelvic cavity.

Technique

1. The patient lies supine on the table with knees flexed, legs abducted and heels together.
2. Using aseptic technique the operator inserts a speculum and cleans the vagina and cervix with chlorhexidine.
3. The anterior lip of the cervix is steadied with the vulsellum forceps and the cannula is inserted into the cervical canal. If a Foley catheter is used, there is usually no need to grasp the cervix with the vulsellum forceps.
4. Care must be taken to expel all air bubbles from the syringe

and cannula, as these would otherwise cause confusion in interpretation. Contrast medium is injected slowly under intermittent fluoroscopic control.
5. Spasm of the uterine cornu may be relieved by i.v. glucagon.

NB: Opiates increase pain by stimulating smooth muscle contraction.

Films

Using the undercouch tube:

1. As the tubes begin to fill.
2. When peritoneal spill has occurred and with all the instruments removed.

Aftercare

1. It must be ensured that the patient is in no serious discomfort nor has significant bleeding before she leaves.
2. The patient must be advised that she may have bleeding per vaginam for 1–2 days and pain may persist for up to 2 weeks.

Complications

Due to the contrast medium

1. Allergic phenomena – especially if contrast medium is forced into the circulation.

Due to the technique

1. Pain may occur at the following times:
   a. using the vulsellum forceps
   b. during insertion of the cannula
   c. with tubal distension proximal to a block
   d. with distension of the uterus if there is tubal spasm
   e. with peritoneal irritation during the following day, and up to 2 weeks.
2. Bleeding from trauma to the uterus or cervix.
3. Transient nausea, vomiting and headache.
4. Intravasation of contrast medium into the venous system of the uterus results in a fine lace-like pattern within the uterine wall. When more extensive, intravasation outlines larger veins. It is of little significance when water-soluble contrast media are used. The following factors predispose to intravasation:
   a. direct trauma to the endometrium
   b. timing of the procedure near to menstruation
   c. timing of the procedure within a few days after curettage

        d. tubal occlusion because of the high pressures generated within the uterine cavity

        e. uterine abnormalities, e.g. uterine tuberculosis, carcinoma and fibroids.

5. Infection – which may be delayed. Occurs in up to 2% of patients and more likely when there is a previous history of pelvic infection.

6. Abortion. The operator must ensure that the patient is not pregnant.

References

Davies, A.C., Keightley, A., Borthwick-Clark, A. & Walters, H.L. (1985) The use of low-osmolarity contrast medium in hysterosalpingography: comparison with a conventional contrast medium. *Clin. Radiol.* **36**, 533–536.

Brokensha, C. & Whitehouse, G. (1991) A comparison between iotrolan, a non-ionic dimer, and a hyperosmolar contrast medium, Urografin, in hysterosalpingography. *Br. J. Radiol.* **64**, 587–590.

ULTRASOUND OF THE FEMALE REPRODUCTIVE SYSTEM

Indications

1. Pelvic mass
2. Pregnancy – normal and suspected ectopic
3. Precocious puberty
4. Delayed puberty
5. Assessment of tubal patency
6. In assisted fertilization techniques.

Contraindications

None.

Patient preparation

1. Transabdominal – full bladder
   Transvaginal – empty bladder
2. Patient consent.[1]

It is always advisable to have a chaperone.

Equipment

5–10-MHz transducers.

Colour Doppler is useful in the assessment of tubal patency and in monitoring follicular development. It may also be used in differentiating malignant from benign ovarian masses.[2]

Contrast medium

Galactose monosacharride microparticles (Echovist) is a specific contrast agent employed in the assessment of tubal patency; spillage of the microparticles into the peritoneal cavity infers patency.

References

1. General Medical Council (1999) *Seeking Patients' Consent: the Ethical Considerations.* London: General Medical Council.
2. Kurjak, A., Shalan, H., Kupesic, S., et al. (1994) An attempt to screen asymptomatic women for ovarian and endometrial cancer with transvaginal color and pulsed Doppler sonography. *J. Ultrasound. Med.* **13**, 295–301.

ULTRASOUND OF THE SCROTUM   US

Indications

1. Suspected testicular tumour
2. Suspected epididymo-orchitis
3. Hydrocoele
4. Acute torsion. In boys or young men in whom this clinical diagnosis has been made and emergency surgical exploration is planned, ultrasound should not delay the operation. Although colour Doppler may show an absence of vessels in the ischaemic testis, it is possible that partial untwisting resulting in some blood flow could lead to a false negative examination
5. Suspected varicocoele
6. Scrotal trauma.

Contraindications

None.

Patient preparation

Consent.

Equipment

7.5–10 MHz transducer. Linear array for optimum imaging. Stand-off may be helpful in some cases.

Technique

1. Patient supine with legs together. Some operators support the scrotum on a towel draped beneath it or in a gloved hand.
2. Both sides are examined with longitudinal and transverse scans enabling comparison to be made.
3. Real-time scanning enables the optimal oblique planes to be examined.
4. In comparing the 'normal' with the 'abnormal' side, the machine settings should be optimized for the normal side, especially for colour Doppler. They should not be changed until both sides have been compared.

Further reading

Bree, R.L. & Hoang, D.T. (1996) Scrotal Ultrasound. In: Dunnick N.R. (ed) Advances in Uroradiology II. *Radiol. Clin. N. Am.* **34**, 1183–1205.

Cook, J.L. & Dewbury, K. (2000) The changes seen on high resolution ultrasound in orchitis. *Clin. Radiol.* **55**, 13–18.

Sidhu, P.S. (1999) Clinical and imaging features of testicular torsion: role of ultrasound. *Clin. Radiol.* **54**, 343–352.

MRI OF THE REPRODUCTIVE SYSTEM

Artefacts

Artefact from small bowel peristalsis and to a lesser extent colonic peristalsis can occasionally be a problem in the pelvis and glucagon may be used to minimize this. Respiratory artefact is less of a problem in the pelvis than in the upper and mid abdomen. However, if this is a problem, then scanning the patient prone or with a compression band over the pelvis can help to minimize this artefact. Respiratory gating can be used, but there is a time penalty.

Pulse sequences

For midline structures (uterus, cervix and vagina) sagittal T1-weighted and T2-weighted spin-echo sequences can be augmented with further axial sequences as required. Inclined axial images perpendicular to the long axis of the uterus or the long axis of the cervix are helpful for uterine and cervical abnormalities respectively.

The ovaries may be assessed with axial and coronal T1-weighted and T2-weighted spin-echo sequences.

Perfusion imaging of the uterus can be used to assess the effectiveness of uterine fibroid therapy.

MRI is also used in pelvimetry to avoid radiation dose.

Further reading

Baker, L.L., Hajek, P.C., Burkhard, T.K., et al. (1987a) Magnetic resonance imaging of the scrotum: normal anatomy. *Radiology* **163**, 89–92.

Baker, L.L., Hajek, P.C., Burkhard, T.K., et al. (1987b) Magnetic resonance imaging of the scrotum: pathology. *Radiology* **163**, 93–98.

Smith, R.C., Reinhold, C., McCauley, T.R., et al. (1992) Multicoil high resolution fast spin echo MR imaging of the female pelvis. *Radiology* **184**, 671–675.

7 Respiratory system

Methods of imaging the respiratory system

1. Plain films
2. Radionuclide imaging (V/Q scans)
3. CT
4. US (for pleural disease)
5. MRI
6. Bronchography.

Further reading

Klein, J.S. (ed) (2000) Interventional Chest Radiology. *Radiol. Clin. N. Am.* **38 (2)**.
Macklem P.T. (1998) New methods of imaging the respiratory system. *Respirology* **3**, 101–102.

Methods of imaging pulmonary embolism

1. *Plain film chest radiograph*. The initial chest radiograph is often normal. Numerous signs have been described in association with pulmonary embolism but, overall, the chest radiograph is neither specific nor sensitive.
2. *Ventilation/perfusion (V/Q) radionuclide scanning*. The technique is described later in this chapter. Interpretation of V/Q images is not clear-cut and there are a number of causes for the typical V/Q mismatch. Diagnostic criteria developed divide results into normal, low-probability, intermediate (or indeterminate) and high-risk groups. Specificity and sensitivity are such that, if the criteria place the images in the normal group, pulmonary embolism is virtually excluded and if the images fit the criteria for high risk it is very likely (85–90%). In the intermediate risk group specificity is poor and pulmonary angiography may be required.
3. *Doppler* of leg veins to confirm deep vein thromboses.
4. *Spiral CT* of the chest to diagnose central pulmonary emboli.
5. *Pulmonary arteriography* (Chapter 8) is the 'gold standard' and will detect most pulmonary emboli.

Further reading

PIOPED Investigators. (1990) Value of ventilation/perfusion scanning in acute pulmonary embolism. *JAMA* **263**, 2753–2759.

Robinson, P.J. (1989) Lung scintigraphy. *Clin. Radiol.* **40**, 557–560.

RADIONUCLIDE LUNG VENTILATION/PERFUSION (V/Q) IMAGING

Indications

1. Suspected pulmonary embolism[1]
2. Assessment of perfusion and ventilation abnormalities, e.g. in congenital cardiac or pulmonary disease
3. Quantitative assessment of right-to-left shunting (perfusion only).[2]

Contraindications (to perfusion imaging)

1. Right-to-left shunt – because of the risk of cerebral emboli.
2. Severe pulmonary hypertension.

Neither of these are absolute contraindications (indeed, perfusion imaging can be used for assessment of shunts), and it may be considered acceptable to reduce the number of particles administered in these cases.

Radiopharmaceuticals

Perfusion

1. ^{99m}Tc-macroaggregated albumin (MAA), 100 MBq max (1 mSv ED), SPECT: 200 MBq (2 mSv ED).
2. Labelled albumin particles 10–100 μm in diameter which occlude small lung vessels (< 0.5% of total capillary bed).

Ventilation

1. ^{81m}Kr (Krypton) gas, 6000 MBq max (0.2 mSv ED). Generator-produced agent of choice with a short $T_{1/2}$ of 13 s and a γ-energy of 190 keV. Simultaneous dual isotope ventilation and perfusion imaging is possible because of different γ-energy to ^{99m}Tc. Wash-in and wash-out studies are not possible. Expensive and limited availability.
2. ^{99m}Tc-Technegas, 40 MBq max (0.6 mSv ED).[3,4] Labelled carbon particles, 5–20 nm in size. No simultaneous ventilation and perfusion imaging. Longer residence time in lungs than aerosols, so SPECT and respiration-gated studies possible. Similar diagnostic efficacy to krypton. Expensive dispensing system.

3. ^{99m}Tc-DTPA, aerosol, 80 MBq max (0.4 mSv ED). No simultaneous ventilation and perfusion imaging. Cheap and readily available alternative to krypton, but less suitable in patients with chronic obstructive airways disease or chronic asthma because clumping of aerosol particles is likely.

4. ^{133}Xe (xenon) gas, 400 MBq max (0.4 mSv ED) diluted in 10 litres and re-breathed for 5 min.[5] Long $T_{1/2}$ of 5.25 days and a γ-energy of 81 keV. Ventilation must precede perfusion study because low γ-energy would be swamped by scatter from ^{99m}Tc. Wash-in and wash-out studies are possible. Discharged gas must be dealt with safely. Poor quality images, but cheap and widely available.

Equipment

1. Gamma-camera, preferably multi-headed for SPECT
2. Low-energy general purpose collimator
3. Gas dispensing system and breathing circuit for ventilation
4. Foam wedges for oblique positioning.

Patient preparation

1. For ventilation, familiarization with breathing equipment.
2. A current chest X-ray is required to assist with interpretation.
3. For breast feeding women, express and save milk before test, then express and discard for 12 h afterwards.

Technique

Perfusion

1. The injection may be given in the supine, semirecumbent or sitting position (NB: MAA particle uptake is affected by gravity).
2. The syringe is shaken to prevent particles settling.
3. A slow i.v. injection is given directly into a vein (particles will stick to a plastic cannula) over about 10 s. Avoid drawing blood into the syringe as this can cause clumping.
4. The patient must remain in position for 2–3 min while the particles become fixed in the lungs.
5. Imaging may begin immediately, preferably in the sitting position.

Ventilation

^{81m}Kr gas

This is performed at the same time as the perfusion study, either by dual isotope acquisition or swapping energy windows at each patient position.

1. The patient is positioned to obtain identical views to the perfusion images.
2. The patient should be asked to breathe normally through the mouthpiece.
3. The air supply attached to the generator is turned on and imaging commenced.
4. Continue until 300–400 000 counts per view have been collected.

^{99m}Tc-DTPA aerosol

This scan is performed before the perfusion study, which may follow immediately unless there is clumping of aerosol particles in the lungs, in which case it is delayed for 1–2 h.

1. A DTPA kit is made up with approx. 600 MBq ^{99m}Tc per ml (volume dependent upon aerosol equipment).
2. ^{99m}Tc-DTPA is drawn into a 5 ml syringe with 2 ml air.
3. ^{99m}Tc-DTPA is injected into the nebulizer and flushed through with air.
4. The patient is positioned initially with their back to the camera, sitting if possible.
5. The nose-clip is placed on the patient who is asked to breathe normally through the mouthpiece.
6. The air supply is turned on to deliver a rate of 10 l min^{-1}.
7. When the count rate reaches around 1000 counts s^{-1}, the air supply is turned off.
8. The patient should continue to breathe through the mouthpiece for a further 15 s.
9. The nose-clip is removed and the patient given a mouth wash.
10. Imaging is commenced.

Images

300–400 000 counts, 128×128 matrix.

Anterior, posterior, left and right posterior obliques.

Since perfusion and ventilation images are directly compared, it is important to have identical views for each. Foam wedges between the patient's back and the camera assist accurate oblique positioning.

Additional techniques

1. SPECT imaging appears to significantly improve the specificity of the technique by reducing the number of intermediate probability scans.[6]

2. Standardized interpretation of images can improve the clinical effectiveness of V/Q scans, and criteria have been published which are widely used.[7]

Aftercare

None.

Complications

1. Care should be taken when injecting MAA not to induce respiratory failure in patients with severe pulmonary hypertension. In these cases, inject very slowly.

References

1. Maki, D.D., Gefter, W.B. & Alavi, A. (1999) Recent advances in pulmonary imaging. *Chest* **116**, 1388–1402.
2. Grimon, G., André, L., Raffestin, B., et al. (1994) Early radionuclide detection of intrapulmonary shunts in children with liver disease. *J. Nucl. Med.* **35**, 1328–1332.
3. James, J.M., Herman, K.J., Lloyd, J.J. et al. (1991) Evaluation of $^{99m}Tc^m$ Technegas ventilation scintigraphy in the diagnosis of pulmonary embolism. *Br. J. Radiol.* **64**, 711–719.
4. Howarth, D.M., Lan, L., Thomas, P.A., et al. (1999) ^{99m}Tc Technegas ventilation and perfusion lung scintigraphy for the diagnosis of pulmonary embolus. *J. Nucl. Med.* **40**, 579–584.
5. Gray, H.W. (1998) The lung. In: Sharp, P.F., Gemmell, H.G. & Smith, F.W. (eds) *Practical Nuclear Medicine*, pp. 159–175. Oxford: Oxford University Press.
6. Corbus, H.F., Seitz, J.P., Larson, R.K., et al. (1997) Diagnostic usefulness of lung SPET in pulmonary thromboembolism: an outcome study. *Nucl. Med. Commun.* **18**, 897–906.
7. Freitas, J.E., Sarosi, M.G., Nagle, C.C., et al. (1995) Modified PIOPED criteria used in clinical practice. *J. Nucl. Med.* **36**, 1573–1578.

Further reading

Robinson, P.J.A. (1996) Ventilation-perfusion lung scanning and spiral computed tomography of the lungs: competing or complementary modalities? *Eur. J. Nucl. Med.* **23**, 1547–1553.
White, P.G., Hayward, M.W.J. & Cooper, T. (1991) Ventilation agents – what agents are currently used? *Nucl. Med. Commun.* **12**, 349–352.

SPIRAL CT IN THE DIAGNOSIS OF PULMONARY EMBOLI

CT

Technique

1. Unenhanced scan of thorax – to detect any other clinical abnormality which might account for symptoms.
2. Enhanced scan of pulmonary arterial system

    a. Volume of contrast medium – 150 ml (20 ml of this is used as a test, to determine the delay required between starting the injection and commencing imaging)
    b. Delay – usually 15 s (see above)
    c. Rate of injection – 4 ml s^{-1}
    d. Collimation – 3 mm
    e. Pitch – 1.8
    f. Start point – just above the aortic arch
    g. End point – the lowest hemidiaphragm.

Further reading

Remy-Jardin, M., Artaud, D., Fribourg, M. & Beragi, J.P. (1998) Spiral CT of pulmonary emboli: diagnostic approach, interpretative pitfalls and current indications. *Eur. Radiol.* **8**, 1376–1390.

CT OF THE RESPIRATORY SYSTEM

Indications

1. To exclude metastatic disease.
2. In the assessment of masses.
3. In the assessment of diffuse infiltrative lung disease (high resolution CT).
4. Arterial assessment (pulmonary emboli, aortic dissection).

Technique of high resolution scans

1. Patient lies prone.
2. 1-mm slices at 15-mm to 20-mm intervals in full inspiration.
3. Image reconstruction using 'bone' algorithm, i.e. high-resolution algorithm.
4. Maximize spatial resolution using smallest field of view possible.

CT-GUIDED LUNG BIOPSY

Indications

1. Investigation of a pulmonary opacity when other diagnostic techniques have failed to make a diagnosis.
2. Investigation of a new chest lesion in a patient with a known malignancy.

3. To obtain material for culture when other techniques have
    failed to identify the causative organism in a patient with
    persistent consolidation.

NB: Central lesions are best biopsied trans-bronchially.

Contraindications

1. Bleeding diathesis, or concurrent administration of
    anticoagulants
2. Contralateral pneumonectomy
3. Presence of bullae
4. Suspected hydatid disease
5. Suspected vascular lesion
6. Seriously impaired respiratory function such that a
    pneumothorax could not be tolerated.

Equipment

1. Biopsy needle – there are several types available, e.g. 19-G
    Temno cutting needle.
2. Full resuscitation equipment including a chest drain.

Patient preparation

1. Premedication with diazepam may be required. However, the
    patient must remain cooperative so that a consistent breathing
    pattern can be maintained during the procedure.
2. The procedure may be performed on an outpatient basis, but a
    bed should be available in case of complications.
3. Clotting screen.

Aftercare

1. Chest X-ray in expiration.
2. Patients with pre-existing impairment of respiratory function
    are best admitted overnight.

Complications

1. Pneumothorax in 20%. However, a chest drain is necessary in
    only a small minority (about 1%). The incidence of
    pneumothorax is increased if:
    a. The operator is inexperienced
    b. Larger bore needles are used
    c. There is an increased number of punctures
    d. Small or central lesions are biopsied
    e. The needle traverses a fissure.

2. Local pulmonary haemorrhage (10%).
3. Haemoptysis (2–5%).
4. Other complications, such as implantation of malignant cells along the needle track, spread of infection and air embolism, are all extremely rare.

Further reading
Klein, J.S., & Zarka, M.A. (1997) Transthoracic needle biopsy: an overview. *J. Thorac. Imaging* **12**, 232–249.

BRONCHOGRAPHY

Indications
1. Bronchiectasis
2. To demonstrate the site and extent of bronchial obstruction.

Contraindications
1. Acute respiratory infection
2. Poor respiratory reserve.

Contrast medium
LOCM – most recently new non-ionic dimer agents, e.g. iotrolan 300, have been advocated for the purpose, but iohexol can be used.
2–3 ml iotrolan 300 per lung segment, maximum 25 ml per patient.

Equipment
1. Overcouch tube
2. Fluoroscopy unit.

Patient preparation
1. Chest physiotherapy
2. Nothing by mouth for 6 h
3. Treat purulent sputum with appropriate antibiotic therapy
4. Premedication with atropine 0.6 mg and morphine 10 mg
5. Asthmatics should have steroid prophylaxis and salbutamol preoperatively.

Preliminary film
Chest: PA and lateral

Technique

In the past, using the more viscous contrast agents such as Dionosil, various techniques were described to introduce contrast into the bronchial tree. The low osmolar contrast agents are not so viscous and satisfactory coating is more difficult. The preferred method is direct injection via the bronchoscope.

For children

A catheter may be passed via an endotracheal tube with the child anaesthetized.

Films

1. Spot views are taken of the lobe or segment being examined. Timing is critical as the viscosity of the medium is such that any delay will result in inadequate coating.
2. Chest PA at 4 h to exclude complications.

Aftercare

1. Chest physiotherapy
2. Nil by mouth until the anaesthetic has worn off.

Complications

1. Slight impairment in respiratory function – drop in Sa_{O_2} during procedure and fall in FEV_1 and FVC at 4 h.
2. Bronchospasm – well recognized with bronchoscopy alone and particularly in asthmatic individuals.
3. Minor symptoms of headache, nausea, vomiting and a sensation of heat or flushing have been reported.

Further reading

Flower, C.D.R. & Schneerson, J.M. (1984) Bronchography via the fibreoptic bronchoscope. *Thorax* **35**, 260–263.
Morcos, S.K., Anderson, P.B., Clout, C., et al. (1990) Suitability and tolerance of Iotrolan 300 in bronchography via the fibreoptic bronchoscope. *Thorax* **45**, 628–629.

PULMONARY ARTERIOGRAPHY

Indication

Demonstration of pulmonary emboli and other peripheral abnormalities, e.g. arteriovenous malformations.

Contrast medium

LOCM 370; 0.75 ml kg^{-1} at 18–20 ml s^{-1} (max. 40 ml).

Equipment

1. Fluoroscopy unit on a C- or U-arm, with digital subtraction facilities if possible
2. Pump injector
4. Catheter:
   a. pigtail (coiled end, end hole and 12 side holes; Fig. 8.3)
   b. NIH (no end hole, six side holes; Fig. 8.2).

Technique

Seldinger technique via the right femoral vein. The NIH catheter is introduced via an introducer sheath. The catheter tip is sited, under fluoroscopic control, to lie 1–3 cm above the pulmonary valve.

Additional techniques

1. If the entire chest cannot be accommodated on one field of view, the examination can be repeated by examining each lung. The catheter is advanced to lie in each main pulmonary artery in turn. For the right lung the patient, or the tube, is turned 10° LPO and for the left lung 10° RPO.
2. 40° caudal-cranial view. This view is optimal for the visualization of the bifurcation of the right and left pulmonary arteries, the pulmonary valve, annulus and trunk. With this manoeuvre the pulmonary trunk is no longer foreshortened and is not superimposed over its bifurcation.

Complications

See p. 221.

BRONCHIAL STENTING

Indications

1. Compression/stricture (particularly secondary to malignant disease)
2. Fistulae/dehiscence with the oesophagus or pleural cavity
3. Tracheobronchomalacia (relative indication).

Stents

1. Polymers, e.g. Dumon
2. Metallic, e.g. Palmaz
3. Covered, e.g. covered Wallstent
4. Hybrid, e.g. Orlowski.

For malignant disease, polymer or covered stents should be used to prevent tumour in-growth.

Complications

1. Migration
2. Mucostasis
3. Obstruction
4. Mechanical failure
5. Perforation.

Further reading

Becker, H.D. (1995) Stenting the central airways. *J. Broncholo.* **2**, 98–106.

MRI OF THE RESPIRATORY SYSTEM   MRI

MRI only has a limited role in assessing the respiratory system as the susceptibility artefact from the large volume of air makes imaging the lungs difficult. The mediastinum is well assessed by MRI due to the ability to image in the coronal plane. Fast sequences and cardiac gating may be used to minimize motion artefacts. However, CT is more widely available and also gives excellent imaging of the mediastinum.

In future, MR pulmonary angiography may have a role to play in assessing pulmonary emboli, but at present spiral CT scanning is the preferred method due to the availability and ease of performance.

Further reading

Mai, V.M., Knight-Scott, J. & Berr, S.S. (1999) Improved visualisation of the human lung in 1H MRI using multiple inversion recovery for simultaneous suppression of signal contributions from fat and muscle. *Magn. Reson. Med.* **41**, 866–870.

Shepard, J.O. & McLoud, T.C. (1991) Imaging the airways. Computed tomography and magnetic resonance imaging. *Clin. Chest Med.* **12**, 151–168.

8 Heart

Methods of imaging the heart

1. Chest radiography
2. Fluoroscopy
3. Angiocardiography
4. Echocardiography, including the transoesophageal technique
5. Radionuclide imaging
   a. ventriculography
   b. myocardial perfusion imaging
   c. acute myocardial infarction imaging
6. CT
7. MRI.

ANGIOCARDIOGRAPHY

Usually performed simultaneously with cardiac catheterization, in which pressures and oximetry are measured in the cardiac chambers and vessels that are under investigations. The right heart, left heart and great vessels are examined together or alone, depending on the clinical problem.

Indications

1. Congenital heart disease and anomalies of the great vessels
2. Valve disease
3. Myocardial disease and ventricular function.

Contrast medium

LOCM 370 (see Table 8.1).

Equipment

1. Biplane fluoroscopy and cine radiography, preferably digital and preferably with C-arms to facilitate axial projections

Table 8.1   Volumes of contrast media in angiocardiography

	Injection site	
	Ventricle	Aorta or pulmonary artery
Adult	1 ml kg^{-1} at 18–20 ml s^{-1}	0.75 ml kg^{-1} at 18–20 ml s^{-1} (max. 40 ml)
Child		
First year	1.5 ml kg^{-1} ⎫ injected	⎫
2–4 years	1.2 ml kg^{-1} ⎬ over	⎬ 75% of the ventricular volume
5 years	1.0 ml kg^{-1} ⎭ 1–2 s	⎭

In general, hypoplastic or obstructed chambers require smaller volumes and flow rates and large shunts require greater volumes and flow rates of contrast medium.

2. Pressure recording device
3. ECG monitor
4. Blood oxygen analyser
5. Catheter
   a. For pressure measurements and blood sampling: Cournand (Fig. 8.1), 4–7-F
   b. For angiocardiography: NIH (Fig. 8.2) or pigtail (Fig. 8.3), 5–8-F.

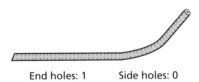

End holes: 1   Side holes: 0

Figure 8.1   Cournand catheter.

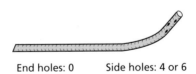

End holes: 0   Side holes: 4 or 6

Figure 8.2   NIH catheter.

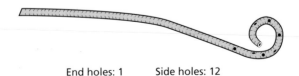

End holes: 1   Side holes: 12

Figure 8.3   Pigtail catheter.

Technique

1. Right-sided cardiac structures and pulmonary arteries are examined by introducing a catheter into a peripheral vein. In babies the femoral vein may be the only vein large enough to take the catheter. If an atrial septal defect is suspected, the femoral vein approach offers the best chance of passing the catheter into the left atrium through the defect.
2. In adults the right antecubital or basilic vein may be used. The cephalic vein should not be used because it can be difficult to pass the catheter past the site where the vein pierces the clavipectoral fascia to join the axillary vein. The catheter, or introducer, is introduced using the Seldinger technique. (The NIH catheter must be introduced via an introducer as there is no end hole for a guide-wire.)
3. In children it is usually possible to examine the left heart and occasionally the aorta by manipulating a venous catheter through a patent foramen ovale. In adults the aorta and left ventricle are studied via a catheter passed retrogradely from the femoral artery.
4. The catheter is manipulated into the appropriate positions for recording pressures and sampling blood for oxygen saturation. Following this, angiography is performed.

Films

1. The recording of cardiac images is now most commonly performed using digital subtraction angiography at 30 frames per s.
2. Angled views which place the pathological lesion at right-angles to the X-ray beam increase diagnostic accuracy in angiocardiography. The first principle of axial cineangiography is axial alignment of the heart, i.e. aligning the X-ray beam perpendicular to the long axis of the heart (Fig. 8.4). The second principle involves rotation of the direction of the X-ray beam so as to profile those areas of heart under examination. For modern equipment with movable C-arms it is possible to achieve correct positioning by moving the equipment alone without disturbing the patient.
4. Useful views are:
    a. *40° caudal-cranial (sitting up) view.* This manoeuvre places the pulmonary trunk and its bifurcation perpendicular to the X-ray beam. Because these structures are no longer foreshortened, this projection is ideal for demonstrating the pulmonary trunk, pulmonary valve, annulus and bifurcation into right and left pulmonary arteries.

b. *40° cranial/40° LAO (hepatoclavicular or four-chamber) view*. This view places the beam perpendicular to the long axis of the heart and aligns the atrial septum and posterior interventricular septum parallel to the beam.

c. *Long axial 20° RAO (long axial oblique) view*. With a C-arm arrangement, the lateral tube and image intensifier is angled 25–30° cranially, to align with the long axis of the heart, and 20° RAO.

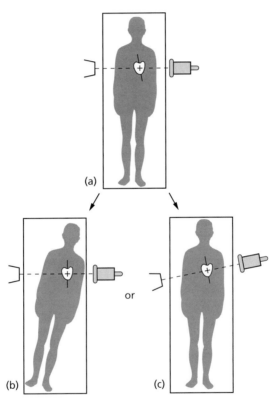

Figure 8.4   Principles of axial angiography. Alignment of the heart perpendicular to the X-ray beam.

CORONARY ARTERIOGRAPHY

Indications

1. Diagnosis of the presence and extent of ischaemic heart disease

2. After revascularization procedures
3. Congenital heart lesions.

Contrast medium

LOCM 370, 8–10 ml given as a hand injection for each projection.

Equipment

1. Digital angiography with C-arm
2. Pressure recording device and ECG monitor
3. Judkins (Fig. 8.5) or Amplatz (Fig. 8.6) catheters – the left and right coronary artery catheters are of different shape.

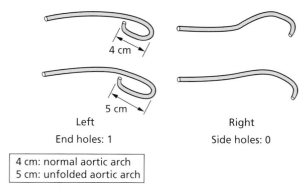

Left	Right
End holes: 1	Side holes: 0

4 cm: normal aortic arch
5 cm: unfolded aortic arch

Figure 8.5   Judkins' coronary artery catheters.

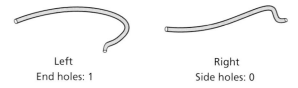

Left	Right
End holes: 1	Side holes: 0

Figure 8.6   Amplatz coronary artery catheters.

Patient preparation

1. As for routine arteriography.
2. β-blockers are stopped 48 h prior to the procedure.

Preliminary film

Chest X-ray.

Technique

The catheter is introduced using the Seldinger technique and advanced until its tip lies in the ostium of the coronary artery.

Films

Angiography (30 frames s^{-1}) is performed in the following positions:

Right coronary artery

1. 60° LAO
2. 30° RAO
3. Right lateral.

Left coronary artery

1. 30° RAO
2. 60° LAO
3. Left lateral.

Additional projection

The left main stem coronary artery may appear foreshortened in the above three projections. If so, the 40° caudal–cranial view should be performed.

Coronary arteriography may be preceded by left ventricular angiography, in the 30° RAO position, to assess left ventricular function.

Complications

In addition to the general complications discussed in Chapter 9, patients undergoing coronary arteriography are particularly liable to:

1. Sudden death
2. Myocardial infarction
3. Arrhythmias.

RADIONUCLIDE VENTRICULOGRAPHY

Indications

Gated blood-pool study

1. Evaluation of ventricular function, particularly left ventricular ejection fraction (LVEF).[1]
2. Assessment of myocardial reserve in coronary artery disease.
3. Cardiomyopathy, including the effects of cardiotoxic drugs.

First pass radionuclide angiography

1. Evaluation of right ventricular ejection fraction (RVEF).[2]
2. Detection and quantification of intracardiac shunts.[3]

Contraindications

Significant arrhythmias may make gated blood-pool imaging impossible.

Radiopharmaceuticals

^{99m}Tc-in-vivo-labelled red blood cells, 800 MBq max (8 mSv ED).

Before radiolabelling with ^{99m}Tc-pertechnetate, the red blood cells are 'primed' with an injection of stannous pyrophosphate. The stannous ions reduce the pertechnetate and allow it to bind to the pyrophosphate which adsorbs on to the red blood cells.

Equipment

1. Gamma-camera: small field of view preferable for optimal positioning. High count rate capability required for first pass studies.
2. Low-energy general purpose collimator.
3. Imaging computer, preferably with list-mode acquisition or multi-gated acquisition (MUGA).
4. ECG monitor with gating pulse output.

Patient preparation

1. An i.v. injection of 'cold' stannous pyrophosphate (20 μg kg^{-1}) is given directly into a vein 20–30 min before the pertechnetate injection. (Injection via a plastic cannula will result in a poor label.)
2. Three ECG electrodes are placed in standard positions to give a gating signal.

Technique

Gated blood-pool study

1. Patient supine
2. The ECG trigger signal is connected
3. i.v. injection of ^{99m}Tc-pertechnetate
4. One min is allowed for the bolus to equilibrate before computer acquisition is commenced (see 'Films' below).

List mode is best, where individual events are stored as their x, y coordinates along with timing and gating pulses. This allows maximum flexibility for later manipulation and framing of data. Around 5 million counts should be acquired. However, MUGA mode is adequate, and is still the most commonly used. In this, the start of an acquisition cycle is usually triggered by the R wave of the patient's ECG. A series of 16–32 fast frames are then recorded before the next R wave occurs. Each of these has very few counts in from a single cycle, so every time the R wave trigger arrives, another set of frames is recorded and summed with the first. The sequence continues until 100–200 kilo-counts per frame have been acquired in about 4–7 min. Some degree of arrhythmia can be tolerated using the technique of 'buffered bad beat rejection', where cardiac cycles of irregular length are rejected and the data not included in the images. The length of time to acquire an image set increases as the proportion of rejected beats rises.

First pass radionuclide angiography

This can provide additional information on right ventricular function and intracardiac shunts, although only from one view unless a multi-headed camera or biplanar collimator is available.

1. Positioning depends upon the clinical question. For ventricular function evaluation, the patient lies supine with the camera against the chest in the RAO 30° position for best visualization of the right atrium and ventricle, or the LAO 35–45° position for best visualization of the left ventricle. A caudal tilt of 15–30° may improve separation of the ventricles. For assessment of shunting, the camera is positioned anteriorly.

2. The ECG trigger signal is connected.

3. The validity of the first pass study is dependent on the quality of the bolus injection. For RVEF assessment, the ^{99m}Tc-pertechnetate is injected over approximately 3 s (too tight a bolus will not provide sufficient cardiac cycles for evaluation; too slow an injection will result in poor image statistics before circulation through the lung capillary bed and left side of the heart). However, for shunt quantification,[3] ^{99m}Tc-pertechnetate is injected in as tight a bolus as possible by using the Oldendorf or similar technique (see Chapter 1).

4. Gated list-mode computer acquisition is started as the bolus is released. Although the first pass usually takes a maximum of 10–15 s, it is advisable to continue data acquisition for up to 50 s in case of slow bolus arrival. (If list mode is not available, a short-frame dynamic study with 20 frames s^{-1} or faster on a 64×64 matrix may be used, although it is unlikely that gating information will be able to be stored, so calculation of RVEF will be sub-optimal.[2] For shunt assessment, a rate of 2 frames s^{-1} is reasonable.)

5. A gated blood-pool study follows, as above.

Images

Gated blood-pool study

A number of views may be recorded, depending on the clinical problem:

1. LAO 35–45° with a 15–30° caudal tilt, chosen to give best separation between left and right ventricles. Patient supine. This view is sufficient if only LVEF is required.
2. Anterior, patient supine.
3. LPO, chosen to give best separation between atria and ventricles. Patient in right lateral decubitus position.

Analysis

Gated blood-pool study

1. The LVEF is calculated.[1]
2. Systolic, diastolic, phase and amplitude images are generated.
3. The frames can be displayed in cine mode to give good visualization of wall motion.

First pass study

1. The RVEF can be calculated.[2]
2. Serial images can be produced showing the sequence of chamber filling.
3. A time–activity curve from the pulmonary region can be used for quantitative assessment of a shunt.[3]
4. LVEF may be calculated, although the gated blood pool study provides a more reliable method.
5. Chamber transit times may be calculated.

Additional techniques

1. Gated blood-pool imaging can be carried out during controlled exercise with appropriate precautions to assess ventricular functional reserve. Leg exercise using a bed-mounted bicycle ergometer is the method of choice. Shoulder restraints and hand grips help to reduce upper body movement during imaging.[4] For patients unable to exercise effectively, stress with dobutamine infusion may be useful.[5] Dobutamine increases cardiac contractility by stimulating the β_1 receptors. Under continuous monitoring, the dose is incrementally increased from 5 to 20 $\mu g\ kg^{-1}\ min^{-1}$, infusing each dose for 8 min. The infusion is stopped when S-T segment depression of > 3 mm, any ventricular arrhythmia, systolic blood pressure

> 220 mmHg, attainment of maximum heart rate, or any side-effects occur. An alternative method of stress is with ventricular pacing, gradually increasing the rate up to maximum predicted heart rate.

2. With gated SPECT using the myocardial perfusion imaging agents ^{99m}Tc-MIBI and ^{99m}Tc-tetrofosmin (see 'Radionuclide Myocardial Perfusion Imaging'), it is possible to combine ventriculography and perfusion scans in a single study.[6,7]

Aftercare

1. Monitor recovery from exercise
2. Normal radiation safety precautions (see Chapter 1).

Complications

Exercise test

1. Induction of angina
2. Cardiac arrhythmias
3. Cardiac arrest.

References

1. Walton, S. (1998) Radionuclide ventriculography. In: Sharp, P.F., Gemmell, H.G. & Smith, F.W. (eds) *Practical Nuclear Medicine*, pp. 146–153. Oxford: Oxford University Press.
2. Rezai, K., Weiss, R., Stanford, W., et al. (1991) Relative accuracy of three scintigraphic methods for determination of right ventricular ejection fraction: a correlative study with ultrafast computed tomography. *J. Nucl. Med.* **32**, 429–435.
3. Arheden, H., Holmqvist, C., Thilen, U., et al. (1999) Left-to-right cardiac shunts: comparison of measurements obtained with MR velocity mapping and with radionuclide angiography. *Radiology* **211**, 453–458.
4. Tamaki, N., Fischman, A.J. & Strauss, H.W. (1991) Radionuclide imaging of the heart. In: Maisey, M.N., Britton, K.E. & Gilday, D.L. (eds) *Clinical Nuclear Medicine*, 2nd edn, pp. 1–40. London: Chapman & Hall.
5. Konishi, T., Koyama, T., Aoki, T., et al. (1990) Radionuclide assessment of left ventricular function during dobutamine infusion in patients with coronary artery disease: Comparison with ergometer exercise. *Clin. Cardiol.* **13**, 183–188.
6. Yoshioka, J., Hasegawa, S., Yamaguchi, H., et al. (1999) Left ventricular volumes and ejection fraction calculated from quantitative electrocardiographic-gated ^{99m}Tc-tetrofosmin myocardial SPECT. *J. Nucl. Med.* **40**, 1693–1698.
7. Anagnostopoulos, C., Underwood, S.R. (1998) Simultaneous assessment of myocardial perfusion and function: how and when? *Eur. J. Nucl. Med.* **25**, 555–558.

RADIONUCLIDE MYOCARDIAL PERFUSION IMAGING

RN

Indications

1. Diagnosis and assessment of extent and severity of myocardial ischaemia or infarction
2. Assessment of myocardial viability
3. Evaluation of prognosis
4. Evaluation of effects of angioplasty and bypass surgery on myocardial perfusion with pre- and post-intervention imaging.

Contraindications

1. Unstable angina
2. Frequent ventricular arrhythmias at rest
3. Contraindications to pharmacological stress agent
4. Third-degree heart block
5. Severe valvular disease, especially aortic valve stenosis.

Radiopharmaceuticals

1. *^{99m}Tc-methoxyisobutylisonitrile (MIBI or sestamibi)*,[1] 300 MBq max (4 mSv ED) for planar imaging, 400 MBq max (5 mSv ED) for SPECT (or 1000 MBq max. for the total of two injections in single day rest-exercise protocols). Cationic complex with myocardial uptake in near proportion to coronary blood flow but minimal redistribution. There is also, normally, liver uptake and biliary excretion, which can cause inferior wall artefacts on SPECT if care is not taken. Separate injections are required for stress/rest studies, but image timing is flexible due to minimal redistribution.
2. *^{99m}Tc-tetrofosmin (Myoview)*[2] (activity and radiation dose as for MIBI). Similar uptake characteristics and diagnostic efficacy to MIBI but with easier preparation.
3. *^{201}Tl-thallous chloride*, 80 MBq max. (18 mSv ED).[3] (A clinical decision may be made to increase dose to 120 MBq in obese patients.) Thallium is a potassium analogue with initial rapid myocardial uptake in near proportion to coronary blood flow, and subsequent washout and redistribution. Hence, unlike the ^{99m}Tc agents, same-day stress and rest redistribution studies can be performed with a single injection. With principal photon energies of 68–72 and 167 keV and $T_{1/2}$ of 73 h, it is not ideal for imaging and gives a higher radiation

dose than the newer ^{99m}Tc alternatives. Formerly the most widely used myocardial perfusion agent, it is increasingly being replaced by ^{99m}Tc agents. However, many still consider ^{201}Tl to be a superior agent for assessment of myocardial viability and hibernation, with either re-injection at rest or a separate day rest-redistribution study giving the greatest sensitivity.

4. $^{18}FDG + blood\ flow\ PET$. The gold standard for viability assessment, but not widely available.[4]

Equipment

1. SPECT-capable gamma-camera, preferably dual-headed (planar imaging is possible but greatly inferior)
2. Low-energy high-resolution, general purpose or specialized cardiac collimators
3. Pharmacological stressing agent (adenosine or dobutamine) or exercise equipment, e.g. bicycle ergometer or treadmill
4. Nitroglycerin (tablets or sublingual spray) to enhance resting uptake of ischaemic but viable segments
5. 12-lead ECG monitor
6. Resuscitation facilities including defibrillator
7. Aminophylline to reverse possible severe bronchospasm after adenosine infusion
8. Lignocaine to reverse serious arrhythmias caused by dobutamine infusion
9. Medical supervision during stress study.

Patient preparation

1. Nil by mouth or light breakfast 4–6 h prior to test. Avoid caffeine for 24 h.
2. Cessation of cardiac medication on the day of the test if possible. β-blockers can be continued and adenosine stress used.

Technique

The principal of the technique is to compare myocardial perfusion under conditions of pharmacological stress or physical exercise, with perfusion at rest. Diseased but patent arterial territories will show lower perfusion under stress conditions than healthy arteries, but will show relatively improved perfusion at rest. Infarcted tissue will show no improvement at rest. Hence, prognostic information on the likelihood of adverse cardiac events and the benefits of revascularization can be gained.[5]

Stress regime

Pharmacological stress is becoming increasingly widely used instead of physical exercise.[6] The optimal stress technique aims to maximize coronary arterial flow. The gold standard is now pharmacological stress with adenosine infusion (0.14 mg kg^{-1} min^{-1} for 6 min), in combination with light exercise to reduce side-effects.[7,8] Adenosine is a potent coronary vasodilator without rate-related effects, so is not arrhythmogenic. It reproducibly increases coronary artery flow by more than maximal physical exercise (which anyway often cannot be achieved in this group of patients). It has a short biological half-life of 8–10 s, so most side-effects are reversed simply by discontinuing infusion.

Stressing with adenosine has now largely replaced dipyridamole, which will not be discussed here.

There are circumstances where adenosine is contraindicated, e.g. asthma, second-degree heart block or systolic blood pressure < 100 mmHg. Dobutamine stress may be employed in these circumstances.[9] Dobutamine acts as a β_1 receptor agonist, increasing contractility and heart rate. Under continuous monitoring, the dose is incrementally increased from 5 to 20 µg kg^{-1} min^{-1}, infusing each dose for 8 min. The infusion is terminated when S-T segment depression of > 3 mm, any ventricular arrhythmia, systolic blood pressure > 220 mmHg, attainment of maximum heart rate, or any side-effects occur.

^{99m}Tc-MIBI or tetrofosmin rest/stress test

Because MIBI and tetrofosmin have minimal redistribution, separate injections are needed for stress and rest studies. Two-day protocols are optimal, but it is often more convenient to perform both studies on the same day. A number of groups have shown that this is possible without significantly degrading the results, most effectively when the resting study is performed first.[10]

2-Day protocol

1. Initiate pharmacological stress or exercise.
2. 400 MBq MIBI or tetrofosmin is administered i.v. at maximal stress, continuing the stress protocol for 1 min post-injection to allow uptake in the myocardium.
3. 10–30 min post-injection, a milky drink or similar is given to promote biliary clearance; high fluid intake will dilute bowel contents.
4. Images are acquired 30–60 min post-injection. If there is excessive liver uptake or activity in small bowel close to the heart, imaging should be delayed by a further 30–60 min.

5. Depending on the clinical situation, if the stress scan is completely normal the patient may not need to return for the rest scan.[11]

6. Preferably 2–7 days later, the patient returns for a resting scan.

7. Glyceryl trinitrate (GTN) (two 0.3 mg tablets) or equivalent sublingual spray is given to improve blood flow to ischaemic but viable segments.[12,13]

8. Immediately, 400 MBq MIBI or tetrofosmin i.v. is administered and proceed as for stress imaging, but image at 60–90 min after injection.

1-Day protocol (stress/rest)

1. Initiate pharmacological stress or exercise; 250 MBq MIBI or tetrofosmin i.v. is administered at maximum stress.

2. Image 30–60 min later.

3. A minimum of 3 h after first injection, GTN is administered as above, followed by 750 MBq MIBI or tetrofosmin. (If a longer period is available between injections, the activity of the second injection may be reduced.)

4. Image 60–90 min later.

[201]Tl stress/rest test

Since ^{201}Tl redistributes after injection, stress/rest studies can be performed with a single injection. However, stress image timing is more critical.

1. Initiate pharmacological stress or exercise.

2. Administer 80 MBq [201]Tl i.v. at maximal stress, continuing the stress protocol for 1 min post-injection to allow uptake in the myocardium.

3. Image after 5 min.

4. Image at rest 3–4 h after redistribution period, during which time patients should not eat.

5. If fixed defects are present in exercise and rest images and assessment of viability and hibernation is required, either:

    a. Administer a second smaller dose of 40 MBq ^{201}Tl, giving GTN pre-injection, and image 20–30 min later. If defects still persist, image again at 18–24 h. A significant number (around 30%) of fixed defects at 3–4 h will show reversibility.[14]

    b. Perform a separate day rest-redistribution study with 80 MBq ^{201}Tl after GTN, and imaging at 20–30 min and 3–4 h.

Images

SPECT

1. Position patient as comfortably as possible with their arms above their head (or at least the left arm) if possible. SPECT images may be severely degraded by patient movement, so attention should be paid to keeping the patient very still. If this proves impossible in some cases, planar images may be taken.
2. For the ^{99m}Tc agents, check for activity in bowel loops close to the inferior wall of the heart. This can cause artefacts in the reconstructed images, so if significant activity is seen, delay the imaging to give greater time for clearance.
3. 180° orbit from RAO 45° to LPO 45°, elliptical if possible. With modern dual-headed systems, this can be achieved with the heads at 90° to each other to minimize the amount of camera rotation required.
4. Matrix size and zoom to give a pixel size of 3–4 mm.
5. 30–40 projections, with a total imaging time of about 30 min for single and 15 min for dual-head systems.
6. View the projections as a cine before the patient leaves the department. If available, perform software motion correction. If there is significant movement that cannot be corrected, repeat imaging. Beware 'diaphragmatic creep', particularly on ^{201}Tl patients breathless after exercise, where the average position of the diaphragm changes as they recover.

Analysis

1. Short, vertical long and horizontal long axis views are reconstructed, taking care to use the same orientation for stress and rest image data sets (modern systems have automatic alignment software).
2. Two-dimensional circumferential profile or 'bull's-eye' polar maps may be generated.[15]

Additional techniques

1. Gated SPECT is now practicable on modern dual-head cameras, and with special software (e.g. Cedars Sinai QGS package) can provide additional information on ventricular wall motion, ejection fraction and chamber volume.[16] It can also improve specificity by reducing artefactual defects caused by regional myocardial motion and wall thickening.[17]
2. Bull's-eye maps can be compared to normal databases and displayed quantitatively in terms of severity and extent of relative underperfusion.[18]

3. Attenuation and scatter correction using scanning transmission line sources are now available on most modern dual-headed systems. This technique can also improve diagnostic specificity by correcting attenuation artefacts and thereby increasing the normalcy rate.[19] However, algorithms are still being improved, so at present it is wise to view the attenuation-corrected and uncorrected images together to identify possible introduced artefacts.

4. The combination of rest ^{201}Tl and exercise ^{99m}Tc MIBI or tetrofosmin can be used to assess both ischaemia and viability.[20]

Aftercare

1. Monitoring of patient post-exercise.
2. Normal radiation safety precautions (see Chapter 1).

Complications

1. Induction of angina
2. Cardiac arrhythmias, particularly after dobutamine. Lignocaine may be given to reverse effects
3. Cardiac arrest
4. Bronchospasm after adenosine. Aminophylline may be administered to reverse severe side-effects (75–100 mg i.v. given slowly, then up to 250 mg if symptoms persist).

References

1. Santana-Boado, C., Candell-Riera, J. & Castell-Conesa, J., et al. (1998) Diagnostic accuracy of technetium-99m-MIBI myocardial SPECT in women and men. *J. Nucl. Med.* **39**, 751–755.
2. Azzarelli, S., Galassi, A.R., Foti, R., et al. (1999) Accuracy of ^{99m}Tc-tetrofosmin myocardial tomography in the evaluation of coronary artery disease. *J. Nucl. Cardiol.* **6**, 183–189.
3. Beller, G.A. (1994) Myocardial perfusion imaging with thallium-201. *J. Nucl. Med.* **35**, 674–680.
4. Jadvar, H., Strauss, H.W. & Segall, G.M. (1999) SPECT and PET in the evaluation of coronary artery disease. *Radiographics* **19**, 915–926.
5. Verani, M.S. (1999) Stress myocardial perfusion imaging versus echocardiography for the diagnosis and risk stratification of patients with known or suspected coronary artery disease. *Semin. Nucl. Med.* **29**, 319–329.
6. Travain, M.I. & Wexler, J.P. (1999) Pharmacological stress testing. *Semin. Nucl. Med.* **29**, 298–318.
7. Takeishi, Y., Takahashi, N., Fujiwara, S., et al. (1998) Myocardial tomography with technetium-99m-tetrofosmin during intravenous infusion of adenosine triphosphate. *J. Nucl. Med.* **39**, 582–586.
8. Amanullah, A.M., Berman, D.S., Erel, J., et al. (1998) Incremental prognostic value of adenosine myocardial perfusion single-photon emission computed tomography in women with suspected coronary artery disease. *Am. J. Cardiol.* **82**, 725–730.

9. Verani, M.S. (1994) Dobutamine myocardial perfusion imaging. *J. Nucl. Med.* **35**, 737–739.
10. Borges-Neto, S., Coleman, R.E. & Jones, R.H. (1990) Perfusion and function at rest and treadmill exercise using technetium-99m-sestamibi: comparison of one- and two-day protocols in normal volunteers. *J. Nucl. Med.* **31**, 1128–1132.
11. Lavalaye, J.M., Shroeder-Tanka, J.M., Tiel-van Buul, M.M., et al. (1997) Implementation of technetium-99m MIBI SPECT imaging guidelines: optimizing the two-day stress-rest protocol. *Int. J. Card. Imaging* **13**, 331–335.
12. Flotats, A., Carrio, I., Estorch, M., et al. (1997) Nitrate administration to enhance the detection of myocardial viability by technetium-99m tetrofosmin single-photon emission tomography. *Eur. J. Nucl. Med.* **24**, 767–773.
13. Thorley, P.J., Sheard, K.L., Wright, D.J., et al. (1998) The routine use of sublingual GTN with resting ^{99}Tc^m-tetrofosmin myocardial perfusion imaging. *Nucl. Med. Commun.* **19**, 937–942.
14. Pieri, P., Abraham, S.A., Katayama, H., et al. (1990) Thallium-201 myocardial scintigraphy: single injection, re-injection, or 24-hour delayed imaging? *J. Nucl. Med.* **31**, 1390–1396.
15. Garcia, E.V., Van Train, K., Maddahi, J., et al. (1985) Quantification of rotational thallium-201 myocardial tomography. *J. Nucl. Med.* **26**, 17–26.
16. Yoshioka, J., Hasegawa, S., Yamaguchi, H., et al. (1999) Left ventricular volumes and ejection fraction calculated from quantitative electrocardiographic-gated ^{99m}Tc-tetrofosmin myocardial SPECT. *J. Nucl. Med.* **40**, 1693–1698.
17. Anagnostopoulos, C. & Underwood, S.R. (1998) Simultaneous assessment of myocardial perfusion and function: how and when? *Eur. J. Nucl. Med.* **25**, 555–558.
18. Schwaiger, M., Melin, J. (1999) Cardiological applications of nuclear medicine. *Lancet* **354**, 661–666.
19. Hendel, R.C., Berman, D.S., Cullom, S.J., et al. (1999) Multicenter trial to evaluate the efficacy of correction for photon attenuation and scatter in SPECT myocardial perfusion imaging. *Circulation* **99**, 2742–2749.
20. Kim, Y., Goto, H., Kobayashi, K., et al. (1999) A new method to evaluate ischemic heart disease: combined use of rest thallium-201 myocardial SPECT and Tc-99m exercise tetrofosmin first pass and myocardial SPECT. *Ann. Nucl. Med.* **13**, 147–153.

ACUTE MYOCARDIAL INFARCTION IMAGING   RN

Indications

Diagnosis of recent myocardial infarction, especially when standard tests are inconclusive.[1]

Contraindications

None.

Radiopharmaceuticals

1. *^{111}In-antimyosin monoclonal antibody (Myoscint)*, 80 MBq max (19 mSv ED). Accumulates on myosin exposed by damaged cell membranes in acute infarcts within 48 h of

administration. Significant uptake occurs with administration as early as a few hours or up to 2 weeks after onset of infarction, making the timing of the investigation less critical than for pyrophosphate. Better localization in necrotic infarct centres than pyrophosphate and no bone uptake. Need to wait 24–48 h before imaging. Available commercially, and has replaced pyrophosphate as the agent of choice.

2. ^{99m}Tc-pyrophosphate, 600 MBq max (3 mSv ED). Considered to form a complex with calcium in damaged myocardium. Localizes best in 2–3-day-old infarcts, but there is some variability making optimal timing difficult. There is greater uptake in the ischaemic area around the margins of an infarct than in the infarct itself, producing a 'doughnut' shape in large regions of infarction. It also localizes in bone, so rib uptake interferes with planar images.

Equipment

1. Gamma-camera, with SPECT for pyrophosphate, mobile if patient cannot be moved from coronary care unit.
2. Low-energy general purpose collimator for ^{99m}Tc, medium-energy collimator for ^{111}In.

Patient preparation

None.

Technique

^{111}In-antimyosin

1. Give i.v. injection slowly over 30–60 s up to 2 weeks after suspected infarction.
2. Image 24 and 48 h later.

^{99m}Tc-pyrophosphate

1. Give i.v. injection 2–3 days after suspected infarction.
2. Image 3 h later.

Images

Patient supine, 5 min per view:

1. Anterior
2. LAO 45°
3. Left lateral or LAO 70°
4. SPECT imaging with pyrophosphate will improve sensitivity and localization of infarcts, in particular by removing overlying bone uptake of pyrophosphate.

Aftercare

Normal radiation safety precautions (see Chapter 1).

Complications

None.

Reference

1. Khaw, B.A. (1999) The current role of infarct avid imaging. *Semin. Nucl. Med.* **29**, 259–270.

9 Arterial system

INTRODUCTION TO CATHETER TECHNIQUES

The basic technique of arterial catheterization is also applicable to veins.

Patient preparation

1. The patient will need admission to hospital as careful preparation before and observation after the procedure will be required. With the introduction of smaller diameter catheters, day case admission may be all that is needed for routine peripheral angiography using 3–5-F catheters and some simple angioplasty cases.
2. If the patient is taking anticoagulants, he should be monitored to ensure that they are within their therapeutic 'window'.
3. The radiologist should see the patient on the ward prior to the examination in order to:
   a. explain the procedure
   b. obtain informed consent
   c. examine the patient, with special reference to blood pressure and peripheral pulses as a baseline for post-arteriographic problems.

Puncture sites

1. Femoral artery – most frequently used
2. Brachial artery – a high approach is preferable (see p. 220)
3. Axillary artery
4. Aorta – of historical interest only.

Equipment for the Seldinger technique

Needles

The technique of catheter insertion via double-wall needle puncture and guide-wire is known as the Seldinger technique.[2] The original Seldinger needle consisted of three parts:

1. An outer thin-walled blunt cannula
2. An inner needle
3. A stilette.

Many radiologists now prefer to use modified needles:

1. Double-wall puncture with a two-piece needle consisting of a bevelled central stilette and an outer tube.
2. Single-wall puncture with a simple sharp needle (without a stilette) with a bore just wide enough to accommodate the guide-wire.

Guide-wires

These consist of two central cores of straight wire around which is wound a tightly coiled wire spring (Fig. 9.1). The ends are sealed with solder. One of the central core wires is secured at both ends – a safety feature in case of fracturing. The other is anchored in solder at one end, but terminates 5 cm from the other end, leaving a soft flexible tip. Some guide-wires have a movable central core so that the tip can be flexible or stiff. Others have a J-shaped tip which is useful for negotiating tortuous vessels and selectively catheterizing vessels. The size of the J-curve is denoted by its radius in millimetres. Guide-wires are polyethylene coated but may be coated with a thin film of Teflon to reduce friction. Teflon, however, also increases the thrombogenicity, although this can be countered by using heparin-bonded Teflon. The most common sizes are 0.035 and 0.038 inches diameter. A more recent development is hydrophilic wires. These are very slippery with excellent torque and are useful in negotiating narrow tortuous vessels. They require constant lubrication with saline.

Catheters

Most catheters are manufactured commercially, complete with end hole, side holes, preformed curves and Luer Lok connection. They are made of Dacron, Teflon, polyurethane or polyethylene. Details of the specific catheter types are given with the appropriate technique.

Some straight catheters may be shaped for specific purposes by immersion in hot sterile water until they become malleable, forming the desired shape and then fixing the shape by cooling in cold sterile water.

For the average adult a 100-cm catheter with a 145-cm guide-wire is suitable for reaching the aortic branches from a femoral puncture.

The introduction of a catheter over a guide-wire is facilitated

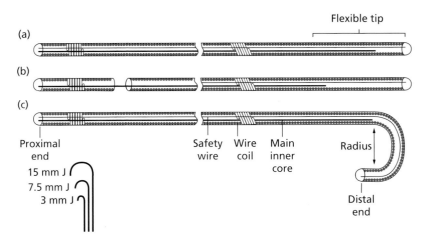

Figure 9.1 Guide-wire construction. (a) Fixed core, straight. (b) Movable core, straight. (c) Fixed core, J-curve.

by dilatation of the track with a dilator (short length of graded tubing).

If the patient has a large amount of subcutaneous fat in the puncture area, catheter control will be better if passed through an introducer set, and this is also indicated where it is anticipated that catheter exchange may be required.

Taps and connectors

These should have a large internal diameter that will not increase resistence to flow and Luer Loks which will not come apart during a pressure injection.

FEMORAL ARTERY PUNCTURE

This is the most frequently used puncture site providing access to the left ventricle, aorta and all its branches. It also has the lowest complication rate of the peripheral sites.

Relative contraindications

1. Blood dyscrasias
2. Femoral artery aneurysm
3. Marked tortuosity of the iliac vessels may prevent further advancement of the guide-wire or catheter. In such a case, high brachial artery puncture may be necessary. The clinical question may be answered by contrast enhanced CT or MR angiography.

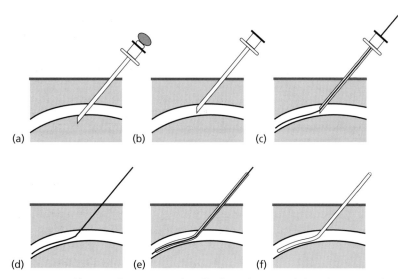

Figure 9.2 Seldinger technique. (a) Both walls of vessel punctured. (b) Stilette removed. Needle withdrawn so that bevel is within the lumen of the vessel and blood flows from the hub. (c) Guide-wire inserted through needle. (d) Needle withdrawn, leaving guide-wire in situ. (e) Catheter threaded over wire. (f) Guide-wire withdrawn.

Technique (Fig. 9.2)

1. The patient lies supine on the X-ray table. Both femoral arteries are palpated and if pulsations are of similar strength the side opposite to the symptoms is chosen. The reasoning for this is that this leaves the symptomatic groin untouched so that future surgery in this region is not made more hazardous. If all else is equal, then the right side is technically easier (for right-handed operators).

2. Before beginning, the appropriate catheter and guide-wire are selected and their compatibility checked by passing the guide-wire through the catheter and needle.

3. Using aseptic technique, local anaesthetic is infiltrated either side of the artery down to the periosteum. A 5 mm transverse incision is made over the artery to avoid binding of soft tissues on the catheter. In thin patients the artery may be very superficial and, to avoid injury to it, a position is chosen and the skin reflected laterally before making the incision.

4. The actual point of puncture of the femoral artery must be considered. The femoral artery arches medially and posteriorly as it becomes the external iliac artery. Attempts to puncture the

artery cephalad to the apex of the arch will result in either failure to puncture the artery or puncture of the artery deep in the pelvis at a point where haemostasis cannot be secured by pressure. Correct puncture is made at the apex of the arch with the needle directed 45° to the skin surface and slightly medially.

5. The artery is immobilized by placing the index and middle fingers of the left hand on either side of the artery, and the needle is held in the right hand. The needle is advanced through the soft tissues until transmitted pulsations are felt. Both walls of the artery are punctured with a stab (single-wall puncture increases the risk of intimal dissection). The stilette is removed, and the needle hub is depressed so that it runs more parallel to the skin and then withdrawn until pulsatile blood flow indicates a satisfactory puncture. Poor flow may be due to:
   a. femoral vein puncture
   b. the end of the needle lying sub-intimally
   c. hypotension – due to vasovagal reaction during the puncture
   d. atherosclerosis.

6. When good flow is obtained the guide-wire is inserted through the needle and advanced gently up the artery whilst screening. When it is in the descending aorta the needle is withdrawn over the guide-wire, keeping firm pressure on the puncture site to prevent bleeding. The guide-wire is then wiped clean with a wet sponge and the catheter threaded over it. For 5-F and greater diameter catheters, particularly those which are curved, a dilator is recommended of a size matched to the catheter. The catheter is advanced up the descending aorta, under fluoroscopic control, and when in a satisfactory position the guide-wire is withdrawn.

7. The catheter is connected via a two-way tap to a syringe of heparinized saline (2500 units in 500 ml of 0.9% saline), and flushed. Flushing should be done rapidly otherwise the more distal catheter holes will remain unflushed. Continuous flushing from a bag of heparinized saline or intermittent flushing throughout the procedure must be undertaken.

8. At the end of the procedure the catheter is withdrawn and compression of the puncture site should be maintained for 5 min. If continued bleeding becomes a concern, consideration should be given to neutralizing the effects of heparin by giving protamine sulphate, 1 mg for each 100 units of heparin.

Aftercare

1. Bed rest – if a 5-F system (or less) is used on a day-case basis, then this should be for at least 4 h.

   Larger catheters require longer bed rest and observation.
2. Careful observation of the puncture site.
3. Pulse and blood pressure observation half-hourly for 4 h and then 4-hourly for the remainder of 24 h, if the larger catheter systems are used.

HIGH BRACHIAL ARTERY PUNCTURE

Indications

As for femoral artery puncture, but as this approach is associated with a higher incidence of complications, it should only be used if femoral artery puncture is not possible.

Contraindications

1. Atherosclerosis of the axillary or subclavian arteries
2. Subclavian artery aneurysm.

Technique

Good accounts are given by Gaines and Reidy[1] and Watkinson and Hartnell.[2]

1. The patient lies on the X-ray table with his arm in supination. The peripheral pulses are palpated and the brachial artery localized approx. 10 cm above the elbow.
2. A small incision is made in the skin, 1–2 cm distal to the selected point of arterial puncture.
3. A single-wall puncture needle is used, with an acute angle of entry into the artery.
4. A straight, soft-tipped guide-wire is introduced when good pulsatile flow is obtained.
5. A 5-F pigtail catheter is introduced over the guide-wire and its pigtail formed in the aorta.
6. At the end of the procedure the catheter tip is straightened using the guide-wire and then removed. This reduces the risk of intimal damage and flap formation during withdrawal of the catheter.

AXILLARY ARTERY PUNCTURE

Indications

As for femoral artery puncture, but this approach is associated with a higher incidence of complications and should only be used if femoral or high brachial artery puncture is not possible.

Contraindications

1. Atherosclerosis of the axillary or subclavian arteries
2. Subclavian artery aneurysm.

Technique

1. The patient lies supine on the X-ray table with his arm fully abducted. The puncture point is just distal to the axillary fold, which is infiltrated with local anaesthetic.
2. A small incision is made in the skin, 1–2 cm distal to the point of the arterial puncture.
3. The needle is directed more horizontally than the femoral approach and along the line of the humerus.
4. Following satisfactory puncture the remainder of the technique is as for femoral artery catheterization.

GENERAL COMPLICATIONS OF CATHETER TECHNIQUES

Due to the anaesthetic

See Chapter 1.

Due to the contrast medium

See Chapter 2.

Due to the technique

Angiography is an invasive procedure and complications are to be expected. However, the majority of these are minor, e.g. groin haematoma. Recommended upper limits for complication rates have been produced by the Society of Cardiovascular and Interventional Radiology (SCVIR)[1] and been supported by the The Royal College of Radiologists.[2] These rates are included in the following discussion.

Local

The most frequently encountered complications occur at the puncture site. The incidence of complications is lowest with the femoral puncture site.

1. *Haemorrhage/haematoma.* The commonest complication, small haematomas occurring in up to 20% of examinations and large haematomas in up to 4%. The SCVIR threshold for haematomas requiring transfusion, surgery or delayed discharge is < 3.0%. Haematoma formation is greater with interventional procedures which employ larger catheters, more

frequent catheter changes and heparin or thrombolytic agents. Haematoma formation is also greater when the femoral artery is punctured high because of inadequate compression of the artery following catheter removal.

2. *Arterial thrombus.* May be due to:
   a. stripping of thrombus from the catheter wall as it is withdrawn
   b. trauma to the vessel wall.

Factors implicated in increased thrombus formation are:

a. large catheters
b. excessive time in the artery
c. many catheter changes
d. inexperience of the radiologist
e. polyurethane catheters, because of their rough surface.

The incidence is decreased by the use of:

a. heparin-bonded catheters
b. heparin-bonded guide-wires
c. flushing with heparinized saline.

3. *Infection at the puncture site.*
4. *Damage to local structures*, especially the brachial plexus during axillary artery puncture.
5. *Pseudoaneurysm.* Rare. SCVIR threshold < 0.5%. Presents as a pulsatile mass at the puncture site, usually 1–2 weeks after arteriography and is due to communication between the lumen of the artery and a cavity within an organized haematoma. Arterial puncture below the common femoral artery bifurcation increases the risk of this complication. Some may require surgical repair.
6. *Arteriovenous fistula.* Rare. SCVIR threshold < 0.1%. More common at the femoral puncture site when puncture is below the common femoral artery bifurcation because at this level the vein lies posterior to the artery and both are punctured in the standard double-wall technique.

Distant

1. *Peripheral embolus* from the stripped catheter thrombus. Emboli to small digital arteries will resolve spontaneously; emboli to large arteries may need surgical embolectomy. SCVIR threshold < 0.5%.
2. *Atheroembolism.* More likely in old people. J-shaped guide-wires are less likely to dislodge atheromatous plaques.

3. *Air embolus.* May be fatal in a coronary or cerebral artery. It is prevented by:
   a. ensuring that all taps and connectors are tight
   b. always sucking back when a new syringe is connected
   c. ensuring that all bubbles are excluded from the syringe before injecting
   d. keeping the syringe vertical, plunger up, when injecting.
4. *Cotton fibre embolus.* Occurs when syringes are filled from a bowl containing swabs. This very bad practice is prevented by:
   a. separate bowls of saline for flushing and wet swabs, or preferably
   b. a closed system of perfusion.

   May also occur when a guide wire is wiped with a dry gauze pad.
5. *Artery dissection*, due to entry of the catheter, guide-wire or contrast medium into the subintimal space. It is recognized by resistance to movement of the guide-wire or catheter, increased resistance to injection of contrast medium or subintimal contrast medium. The risk of serious dissection is reduced by:
   a. not using a single-wall needle with a long bevel
   b. using floppy J-shaped guide-wires
   c. using catheters with multiple side holes
   d. employing a test injection prior to a pump injection
   e. careful and gentle manipulation of catheters.
6. *Catheter knotting.* More likely during the investigation of complex congenital heart disease. Non-surgical reduction of catheter knots is discussed by Thomas and Sievers.[3] Surgical removal after withdrawal of the knotted end to the groin may be only solution in some cases.
7. *Catheter impaction*
   a. In a coronary artery produces cardiac ischaemic pain.
   b. In a mesenteric artery produces abdominal pain.

   There should be rapid wash-out of contrast medium after a selective injection.
8. *Guide-wire breakage.* More common in the past and tended to occur 5 cm from the tip, where a single central core terminates.
9. *Bacteraemia/septicaemia.* Rarely of any clinical significance.

References

1. Spies, J.B., Bakal, C.W., Burke, D.R., et al. (1993) Standard for diagnostic arteriography in adults. *J. Vasc. Intervent. Radiol.* **4**, 385–395.

2. *Standards in Vascular Radiology*. (1999) London: The Royal College of Radiologists.
3. Thomas, H.A. & Sievers, R.E. (1979) Nonsurgical reduction of arterial catheter knots. *Am. J. Roentgenol.* **132**, 1018–1019.

Further reading

Ray, C.E. Jr. & Kaufman, J.A. (1996) In: Ansell, G., Bettmann, M.A., Kaufman, J.A., et al. (eds) *Complications in Diagnostic Imaging and Interventional Radiology*, pp 303–316. Oxford: Blackwell Science.

ASCENDING AORTOGRAPHY

Indications

1. Aortic aneurysm or dissection (echocardiography, CT with intravenous contrast enhancement, and MRI can also be used to demonstrate a dissection).
2. Atheroma at the origin of the major vessels.
3. Aortic regurgitation (echocardiography is more sensitive and less invasive if available).
4. Congenital heart disease – particularly the demonstration of congenital or iatrogenic aorto-pulmonary shunts and coarctation.
5. Aortic trauma.

Contrast medium

LOCM 370, 0.75 ml kg^{-1} (max. 40 ml). Inject at 18–20 ml s^{-1}.

Equipment

1. Digital fluoroscopy unit with C-arm capable of 20–30 frames s^{-1}.
2. Pump injector
3. Catheter:
   a. pigtail (Fig. 8.3), or
   b. Gensini (Fig. 9.3), or
   c. NIH (Fig. 8.2).

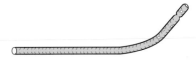

End holes: 1   Side holes: 6

Figure 9.3   Gensini catheter. Note tapered end.

Technique

1. The catheter is introduced using the Seldinger technique via the femoral artery, and its tip sited 1–3 cm above the aortic valve.
2. The patient is positioned 45° RPO to open out the aortic arch, and to show the aortic valve and the left ventricle to best advantage.
3. A test injection is performed to ensure that:
   a. the catheter is correctly placed in relation to the aortic valve (which is particularly important in the hyperkinetic heart)
   b. the catheter tip is not in a coronary artery.

Films

20–30 frames s^{-1}.

Additional films

If, on the original run, the right common carotid artery overlies the right innominate artery or an aneurysm is present on the anterior aspect of the ascending aorta, the injection is repeated with the patient positioned LPO.

ARTERIOGRAPHY OF THE LOWER LIMB

Indications

1. Arterial ischaemia
2. Trauma
3. Investigation of a mass
4. Arteriovenous malformation.

Methods

Both lower limbs

1. Catheter angiography – using a pigtail catheter introduced into the femoral artery and sited proximal to the aortic bifurcation.
3. Brachial or axillary puncture.

One lower limb

1. Using a femoral artery catheter:
   a. introduced retrogradely and sited in the ipsilateral common iliac artery
   b. introduced retrogradely from the contra-lateral side and

sited in the common iliac, external iliac or femoral artery (Sidewinder catheter)

c. introduced antegradely.

If thin 4-F catheters are used, only day case admission is necessary.

Contrast medium

All of these techniques can be performed under local anaesthesia and LOCM are, therefore, appropriate. 10–20 ml of 300 mg I ml^{-1} concentration is suitable for the examination of one limb. 50 ml of 350 mg I ml^{-1}, at a rate of 12–15 ml s^{-1}, is suitable for the catheter aortogram.

VASCULAR DILATATION

(Also known as percutaneous transluminal angioplasty or balloon dilatation.)

Indications

1. Dilatation of localized vascular stenoses, mainly of the renal, iliac, lower limb and coronary arteries.
2. Dilatation of occluded segments of vessels in selected cases.

Dilatation procedures are often combined with preparatory diagnostic angiography in the same session; the majority are done under local anaesthetic.

The procedure is often needed after lysis of arterial thrombus: this is outlined below.

Equipment

1. Digital fluoroscopy unit with C-arm capable of angiography and preferably with 'road mapping' facilities.
2. Arterial pressure measuring equipment (optional).
3. Catheters
   a. Gruntzig double-lumen dilatation catheters (these vary in length of catheter from 80 to 120 cm, in balloon length from 2 to 10 cm and in balloon diameter from 2 to 10 mm: they may also be straight, curved or of the 'sidewinder' type, and are chosen in relation to the particular lesion to be treated)

     b. van Andel dilatation catheter (a tapered, straight Teflon catheter, occasionally useful)

     c. straight Teflon or polyethylene catheters, 7-F.

5. Guide-wires

     a. 0.035- or 0.038-inch diameter wires, 145 cm long (straight), with 2-, 3- and 15-mm J-shapes; a Terumo Teflon-coated wire may be helpful for crossing tight stenoses

     b. 250-cm exchange guide-wire.

6. Streptokinase may be infused into recently thrombosed vessels, prior to dilatation. This is diluted and used with a pressure injector to infuse 5000 units h^{-1}. Recombinant tissue plasminogen activator (rTPA) may be used as an alternative, in which case 0.5 mg h^{-1} is used. Heparin, 500 units h^{-1}, may also be infused to prevent catheter thrombosis.

Technique

Principles

1. Adequate angiograms must be available before any dilatation is attempted.
2. Dilatation is always performed with the guide-wire remaining across the stenosis or occlusion until the procedure is completed.
3. Adequate vascular surgical assistance must be readily available before attempting dilatation.
4. If the history suggests that a thrombosis has occurred within the previous 3 weeks, streptokinase (or rTPA) lysis may be helpful.
5. The patient should be anticoagulated during the procedure, using 3000–5000 units of heparin.
6. The balloon diameter is selected by reference to the measured size of the normal artery on the preceding angiogram, allowing for magnification. Usually the iliac arteries take a 7-mm and the superficial femoral artery a 5-mm balloon.

Renal arteries

1. A J-guide-wire is positioned in the renal artery distal to the stenosis, from either the femoral or high brachial artery approach.
2. A balloon catheter of suitable diameter is positioned across the stenosis and distended (approx. 7 atmospheres for 1 min), after injecting 3000 units of heparin. A post-dilatation angiogram is then taken. If a residual stenosis remains, further dilatations may be necessary.

Iliac arteries

1. These are preferably dilated retrogradely from a femoral puncture on the side of the lesion.
2. If the femoral pulse is absent or difficult to feel, it may be located using a portable Doppler scanner and its position marked. The artery can then be found and fixed with a fine needle attached to a syringe. The fine needle can then be used as a guide for the Seldinger needle. (Alternatively a sidewinder catheter can be introduced from the opposite groin and a guide-wire directed over the aortic bifurcation and across the lesion.)
3. If possible, a femoral artery pressure should be measured immediately after introducing the catheter, and before a guide-wire is passed through the lesion. This is to assess the severity of the pressure gradient before and after angioplasty.
4. A 3-mm J-guide-wire is then advanced carefully through the lesion. If the lesion is eccentrically situated, it may be preferable to advance using a headhunter catheter, to inject contrast medium to position the catheter, and then to advance through the patent lumen, so avoiding possible dissection from below. If the lesion is particularly tight, a Terumo wire may be useful to negotiate the lesion.
5. A catheter is passed over the guide-wire and into the distal aorta.
6. No heparin need be injected.
7. The guide-wire is removed, to allow a pressure measurement in the aorta. It is then replaced and the catheter exchanged for a balloon catheter. After dilating the lesion, an angiogram is performed and the pressures checked to ensure that a gradient no longer exists.

Femoral arteries (common, and origins of SFA and profunda)

1. These cannot be approached by a puncture on the side of the lesion, since there is not enough room for manoeuvre.
2. The contralateral femoral artery is catheterized using a sidewinder catheter. The tip of this is positioned in the iliac artery ipsilateral to the lesion and a heavy-duty exchange guide-wire advanced down through the lesion. The catheter is then exchanged for a balloon catheter and, after injecting heparin 3000 units, the lesion is dilated and a check angiogram performed.

Superficial femoral and popliteal arteries

1. An antegrade puncture is performed (i.e. needle angled towards the feet) on the side of the lesion, the puncture site

being about 2 cm higher than normal (the highest point at which the artery can be felt).

2. A 15-mm J-guide-wire is used to select the required branch, usually the superficial femoral artery.

3. The guide-wire is advanced almost down to the lesion, and a straight Teflon or polyethylene catheter is inserted over the guide-wire to the same point. The guide-wire is then gently passed across the lesion with the catheter following. A van Andel dilatation catheter may be useful once the lesion has been traversed.

4. If the catheter becomes impacted in an occlusion, the guide-wire is removed and a little dilute contrast medium is injected. If the catheter is still in the lumen, immediate arterial filling is seen. Ten millilitres of heparinized saline should be injected, the guide-wire reintroduced, and passage of the occlusion attempted. Usually the saline will have acted as a hydrostatic dilator, and a pathway will be obtained.

   If the dilute contrast medium runs down parallel to the expected lumen, dissection has occurred. The catheter should be withdrawn into the patent lumen, and the operator should wait 5 min before trying again.

5. When the lesion has been passed the catheter is exchanged for a balloon catheter (usually 5 mm diameter), 3000 units of heparin are injected, and dilatation is performed. The distal 'run-off' should be carefully assessed on the post-dilatation films, since success is related to the adequacy of 'run-off' and it is also necessary to ensure that there has been no distal embolization.

Streptokinase lysis

1. A 5-F catheter is advanced to the site of occlusion. If possible, a guide-wire is passed across the occlusion and the catheter advanced through the thrombus, its tip being placed in the distal part of the thrombus. If this is not possible, the tip of the catheter is embedded in the proximal thrombus. The catheter is connected to a pressure injector and securely fixed to the skin to prevent accidental movement.

2. A solution of streptokinase is run in at a rate of 5000 units h^{-1}. To this solution may be added heparin, 500 units h^{-1} to prevent catheter thrombosis.

3. The patient is returned to the ward, and brought back in about 4 h for assessment, which is done by injecting a few millilitres of contrast medium, by hand, to see if lysis is taking place.

4. If lysis is seen, the catheter is withdrawn back into the remaining thrombus. If the catheter had originally been embedded in the proximal thrombus, then the external part of the catheter is cleaned and its tip advanced once again into the thrombus. This process is repeated for up to 24 h, unless no progress is seen, or unless bleeding occurs around the catheter, in which case the procedure is terminated.

5. If a stenosis is shown after the thrombus has lysed, a guide-wire is passed across the lesion and it is dilated.

NB: Streptokinase is antigenic and so may cause allergic reactions including anaphylaxis. Thus previous allergic reactions to strepto-kinase or therapy, from 5 days to 6 months previously, are a contraindication to its use. A useful, if more expensive, alternative is rTPA.

Aftercare

1. The pulses distal to the artery that has been dilated and the colour of the toes should be observed half-hourly for 4 h.
2. Aspirin 150 mg daily (for life, unless there is a contraindication).
3. Reinforcement of the need to stop smoking.

Complications

Due to technique

1. Perforation of iliac artery leading to retroperitoneal haemorrhage
2. Embolization of clot or atheroma distally, down either leg. This may be removed by suction thromboembolectomy or by surgical embolectomy
3. Occlusion of main artery
4. Occlusion of collateral artery
5. Major haematoma formation, which may suddenly develop several hours after the procedure is completed
6. Increased risk of false aneurysm formation at the puncture site.

VASCULAR EMBOLIZATION

Indications

1. To control bleeding – from the gastrointestinal and genitourinary tracts, from the lungs and after trauma.

2. To infarct or reduce the blood supply to tumours or organs.
3. To reduce or stop blood flow through arteriovenous malformations, aneurysms, fistulae or varicoceles.
4. To reduce the blood flow in priapism.

Equipment

1. Digital fluoroscopy unit with C-arm capable of angiography and preferably with 'road mapping' facilities.
2. Catheters; end hole only. Size and shape will depend on the particular problem.

Balloon occlusion catheters and co-axial catheters may also be useful.

3. Embolic materials
   a. Liquid – 50% dextrose alcohol, quick-setting glues.
   b. Particulate – gel-foam, polyvinyl-alcohol.
   c. Solid – Gianturco steel coils, detachable balloons.

The material used depends on the lesion, its site and the duration of the occlusion required. Other materials than those listed have been reported.

Patient preparation

1. As for arteriogram.
2. Some procedures and materials are painful and sedation may be needed.

Technique

Principles

1. All therapeutic occlusions are potentially dangerous: the expected gain must justify the risk.
2. Adequate angiograms must be available before commencing.
3. The operator must be an experienced angiographer.
4. The lesion must be selectively catheterized. When permanent occlusion is required, the centre of the lesion should be filled with non-absorbable material (e.g. silicone spheres, polyvinyl-alcohol) before the supplying blood vessels are occluded.
5. Reflux of embolic material is likely to occur as the blood flow slows down; injection of emboli should be done slowly with intermittent gentle injections of contrast medium to assess flow and progress.
6. It is safer to come back another day than to continue for too long.

Aftercare

1. Infarction of tissue often causes pain, and adequate pain relief should be provided.
2. Arterial clotting may be progressive, and observations on the tissues distal to the occluded vessel should be maintained for 24 h.
3. Many patients have fever for up to 10 days. However, infarcted tissue may become infected, and so antibiotics should be used with care.

Complications

1. Misplacement of emboli: this may occur without the operator being aware that it has happened.
2. There may be propagation of thrombus, with embolization to the lungs or elsewhere.
3. The infarcted tissue may become infected.

10 Venous system

Methods of imaging the venous system

1. Contrast medium venography.
2. US.
3. CT can show inferior vena cava involvement and renal vein involvement in renal cell carcinoma and Wilms' tumour.
4. MRI will show the presence or absence of flowing blood. The ability of MR to image in the plane of the vessel makes it well suited to assessing the venous system. Flow artefact can cause problems in interpretation but the use of bolus gadolinium enhancement techniques, combined with volume gradient echo imaging (with maximum intensity projection post-processing) can produce excellent visualization of the venous system. In addition, MRI can be used to 'age' thrombus and differentiate acute from chronic clot.
5. Radioisotopes. The patency of blood vessels may be examined using ^{99m}Tc-colloid or ^{99m}Tc-macroaggregated albumin (MAA) injected into a supplying vessel with fast-frame dynamic imaging. Thrombus may be imaged with ^{111}In- or ^{99m}Tc-in vitro-labelled platelets.

Further reading

Saddik, D., Frazer, C., Robins, P., et al. (1999) Gadolinium enhanced three dimensional MR portal venography. *Am. J. Roentgenol.* **172**, 413–417.

Smith F.W. (1998) Vascular and lymphatic systems. In: Sharp, P.F., Gemmell, H.G. & Smith, F.W. (eds) *Practical Nuclear Medicine*, pp. 204–212. Oxford: Oxford University Press.

Whitehouse, G.H. (1990) Editorial. Venous thrombosis and thromboembolism. *Clin. Radiol.* **41**, 77–80.

PERIPHERAL VENOGRAPHY

LOWER LIMB

Methods

Intravenous venography

Indications

1. Deep venous thrombosis
2. To demonstrate incompetent perforating veins
3. Oedema of unknown cause
4. Congenital abnormality of the venous system (rare).

Contraindications

Local sepsis.

Contrast medium

LOCM 240.

Equipment

1. Fluoroscopy unit with spot film device
2. Tilting radiography table.

Patient preparation

Elevated leg overnight if oedema is severe.

Technique

1. The patient is supine and tilted 40° head up, to delay the transit time of the contrast medium.
2. A tourniquet is applied tightly just above the ankle to occlude the superficial venous system. It is important to remember that this may also occlude the anterior tibial vein, and so its absence should not automatically be interpreted as due to a venous thrombosis.
3. A 19-G butterfly needle (smaller if necessary) is inserted into a distal vein on the dorsum of the foot. If the needle is too proximal, the contrast medium may bypass the deep veins and so give the impression of a deep venous occlusion.
4. 40 ml of contrast medium is injected by hand. The first series of spot films is then taken.
5. A further 20 ml of contrast are injected quickly whilst the patient performs a Valsalva manoeuvre to delay the transit of contrast medium into the proximal and pelvic veins. The patient is tilted quickly into a slightly head down position and the Valsalva manoeuvre is relaxed. Alternatively, if the patient is unable to Valsalva, direct manual pressure over the femoral vein whilst the table is being tilted into the head-down position will delay transit of contrast medium proximally. Films are taken 2–3 s after releasing pressure.

6. At the end of the procedure the needle should be flushed with 0.9% saline to avoid the risk of phlebitis due to stasis of contrast medium.

Films

(Collimated to include all veins)

1. AP of calf
2. Both obliques of calf (foot internally and externally rotated)
3. AP of popliteal, common femoral and iliac veins.

Aftercare

The limb should be exercised.

Complications

Due to the contrast medium

1. As for the general complications of intravascular contrast media (see p. 30).
2. Thrombophlebitis.
3. Tissue necrosis due to extravasation of contrast medium. This is rare, but may occur in patients with peripheral ischaemia.
4. Cardiac arrhythmia – more likely if the patient has pulmonary hypertension.

Due to the technique

1. Haematoma
2. Pulmonary embolus – due to dislodged clot or air.

UPPER LIMB

Methods

Intravenous venography.

Indications

1. Oedema
2. To demonstrate the site of a venous obstruction
3. SVC obstruction – see p. 238.

Contrast medium

LOCM 300.

Equipment

Fluoroscopy unit with spot film device.

Patient preparation

None.

Preliminary film

PA shoulder.

Technique

For intravenous venography

1. The patient is supine.
2. An 18-G butterfly needle is inserted into the medium cubital vein at the elbow. The cephalic vein is not used, as this bypasses the axillary vein.
3. Spot films are taken of the region of interest during a hand injection of 30 ml of contrast medium.

Aftercare

None.

Complications

Due to the contrast medium

See Chapter 2.

PERIPHERAL VARICOGRAPHY

Indications

1. To demonstrate distribution of varicose veins.
2. To demonstrate sites of communication with deep venous system.
3. Assessment of recurrent varicosity.

Contraindications

Local sepsis.

Contrast medium

LOCM 240. Volume depends on extent and volume of varicosities.

Equipment

1. Fluoroscopy unit with spot film device or 100-mm camera.
2. Tilting fluoroscopy table.

Patient preparation

None.

Technique

1. The patient lies supine and tilted 40° head up to delay washout of contrast.
2. A 19-G butterfly needle is inserted into a suitable varix below the knee.
3. 40–50 ml of contrast are injected by hand under fluoroscopic control.
4. A series of spot films is taken:
   a. AP calf and 2 obliques
   b. lateral knee – to assess the short saphenopopliteal junction.
5. If contrast filling above the knee is adequate, then further views of the thigh can be taken to demonstrate the extent of long saphenous varicosity.
6. Due to the large volume of varicose veins, it may be necessary to re-site the needle in a suitable varix above the knee to obtain adequate contrast filling of the entire system.
7. A further 40 ml of contrast are then injected and spot films taken.
   a. AP thigh and oblique – particular attention should be given to the potential sites of communication, e.g. mid-thigh perforator
   b. AP and oblique of groin – views to demonstrate the saphenofemoral junction are particularly necessary in assessing recurrent varicosity even if there has been previous saphenofemoral ligation, as recurrence at this site is common.
8. After injection and imaging is complete the veins should be flushed with saline to prevent contrast stasis and the risk of phlebitis.
9. The needles are removed and pressure applied to ensure haemostasis.

Aftercare

The limb should be exercised gently to washout any remaining contrast.

Complications

As for peripheral venography.

CENTRAL VENOGRAPHY

SUPERIOR VENA CAVOGRAPHY

Indications

1. To demonstrate the site of a venous obstruction.
2. Congenital abnormality of the venous system, e.g. left-sided superior vena cava.

Contrast medium

LOCM 370, 60 ml.

Equipment

Rapid serial radiography unit.

Patient preparation

Nil orally for 5 h prior to the procedure.

Preliminary films

PA film of upper chest and lower neck.

Technique

1. The patient is supine.
2. 18-G butterfly needles are inserted into the median antecubital vein of both arms.
3. Hand injections of contrast medium 30 ml per side, are made simultaneously, as rapidly as possible by two operators. The injection is recorded by rapid serial radiography (see 'Films' below). The film sequence is commenced after about two-thirds of the contrast medium has been injected.

NB: If the study is to demonstrate a congenital abnormality, or on the rare occasion that the opacification obtained by the above method is too poor, a 5-F catheter with side holes, introduced by the Seldinger technique, may be used.

Films

Rapid serial radiography is performed: one film per s for 10 s.

Aftercare

None, unless a catheter is used.

Complications

Due to the contrast medium

See Chapter 2.

INFERIOR VENA CAVOGRAPHY

Indications

1. To demonstrate the site of a venous obstruction, displacement or infiltration.
2. Congenital abnormality of the venous system.

Contrast medium

LOCM 370, 40 ml.

Technique

1. With the patient supine, the catheter is inserted into the femoral vein using the Seldinger technique. A Valsalva manoeuvre may facilitate vene-puncture by dilating the veins.
2. An injection of 40 ml of contrast medium is made in 2 s by the pump injector, and recorded by rapid serial radiography.

Aftercare

Pressure at venepuncture site.
Routine observations for 2 h.

Complications

Due to the contrast medium

See Chapter 2.

Due to the technique

See Chapter 9 – complications of catheter technique.

PORTAL VENOGRAPHY

Methods

1. Late-phase superior mesenteric angiography (see p. 83)
2. Trans-splenic approach (discussed below)
3. Transhepatic approach (see p. 115)
4. Paraumbilical vein catheterization.

Indications

1. To demonstrate prior to operation the anatomy of the portal system in patients with portal hypertension.
2. To check the patency of a portosystemic anastomosis.

Contrast medium

LOCM 370, 50 ml.

Equipment

1. Rapid serial radiography unit.
2. Arterial catheter (SMA approach).
3. 10-cm needle (20-G) with stilette and outer plastic sheath, e.g. Longdwell (trans-splenic approach).

Patient preparation

1. Admission to hospital. A surgeon should be informed in case complications of procedure arise (for the trans-splenic approach).
2. Clotting factors are checked.
3. Severe ascites is drained.
4. Nil orally for 5 h prior to the procedure.
5. Premedication, e.g. diazepam 10 mg orally.

Technique

Superior mesenteric angiography

See page 83.

For trans-splenic approach

1. With the patient supine, the position of the spleen is percussed or identified with ultrasound. The access point is as low as possible in the midaxillary line, usually at the level of the tenth or eleventh intercostal space.
2. The region is anaesthetized using a sterile procedure.
3. The patient is asked to hold his breath in mid-inspiration, and the needle is then inserted inwards and upwards into the spleen (about three-quarters of the length of the needle is inserted, i.e. 7.5 cm). The needle and stilette are then withdrawn, leaving the plastic cannula in situ. Blood will flow back easily if the cannula is correctly sited. The patient is then asked to breathe as shallowly as possible to avoid trauma to the spleen from excessive movement of the cannula.
4. A test injection of a small volume of contrast medium under screening control can be made to ensure correct siting of the

cannula. If it is sited outside the spleen, simple withdrawal into the body of the spleen is not acceptable, as any contrast medium subsequently injected would follow the track created by the withdrawal. Complete repuncture is necessary.

5. When the cannula is in a satisfactory position, the splenic pulp pressure may be measured with a sterile manometer. (It is normally 10–15 cm H_2O.)

6. A hand injection of 50 ml of contrast medium is made in 5 s, and recorded by rapid serial radiography. The cannula should be removed as soon as possible after the injection to minimize trauma to the spleen.

7. Occasionally a patent portal vein will fail to opacify, owing to major portosystemic collaterals causing reversed flow in the portal vein. The final arbiter of portal vein patency is direct mesenteric venography performed at operation. The maximum width of a normal portal vein is said to be 2 cm.

Films

Rapid serial radiography: One film per s for 10 s.

Aftercare

1. Blood pressure and pulse initially quarter-hourly, subsequently 4-hourly.

2. The patient must remain in hospital overnight.

Complications

Due to the contrast medium

See Chapter 2.

Due to the technique

1. Haemorrhage
2. Subcapsular injection
3. Perforation of adjacent structures (e.g. pleura, colon)
4. Splenic rupture
5. Infection
6. Pain (especially with an extracapsular injection)

Due to the catheter

See Chapter 9.

Reference

1. Rosch, J., Antonovic, R. & Dotter, C.T. (1975) Transjugular approach to the liver, biliary system, and portal circulation. *Am. J. Roentgenol.* **125**, 602–608.

Further reading

Tamura, S., Kodama, T., Kihara, Y., et al. (1992) Right anterior caudocranial oblique projection for portal venography; its indications and advantages. *Eur. J. Radiol.* **15**, 215–219.

TRANSHEPATIC PORTAL VENOUS CATHETERIZATION

Indications

To localize pancreatic hormone-secreting tumours before operation.

Contraindications

There are none specific to the technique. Ascites and hepatic cirrhosis make the procedure more difficult.

Contrast medium

LOCM 370, to demonstrate anatomy and position of catheter.

Technique

1. 5-ml samples of blood are taken at points along the splenic vein, superior mesenteric vein and first part of the portal vein. The samples are numbered sequentially, and the site from which each was taken is marked on a sketch map of the portal drainage system. Simultaneous peripheral blood samples should be obtained at the same time as each portal sample to assess changing blood levels.
2. The accuracy of sampling can be improved by selective catheterization of pancreatic veins using varying shapes of catheter.[1]

Reference

1. Reichardt, W. & Ingemansson, S. (1980) Selective vein catheterization for hormone assay in endocrine tumours of the pancreas. Technique and Results. *Acta Radiol. (Diagn.)* **21**, 177–187.

Further reading

Eustace, S., Buff, B. Kruskal, J. et al (1994) Magnetic resonance angiography in transjugular intrahepatic portosystemic stenting: comparison with contrast hepatic and portal venography. *Eur. J. Radiol.* **19**, 43–49.

ULTRASOUND VENOGRAPHY

Indications

1. Suspected deep vein thrombosis
2. Follow-up of known deep vein thrombosis
3. To guide access for interventional venous procedures.

Contraindications

None.

Patient preparation

None.

Equipment

1. 5–7.5-MHz transducer
2. Colour Doppler is helpful.

Technique

1. Patient supine with foot-down tilt. The popliteal and calf veins can be easily examined with the patient sitting with legs dependent or lying on a tilted couch with flexed knees and externally rotated hips. The femoral veins and external iliac veins are examined supine and popliteal veins may be examined with the patient prone.

2. Longitudinal and transverse scans for external iliac, femoral and popliteal veins. For tibial and peroneal veins, these may be supplemented by oblique coronal scans.

3. Each vein may be identified by real-time scanning and colour Doppler. If in any doubt it may be confirmed as a vein by the spectral Doppler tracing. A normally patient vein can be completely occluded on real time scanning by transducer pressure. This is not always possible for a superficial femoral vein in the adductor canal.

4. The normal venous signal is phasic and in the larger veins varies with respiration. Flow can be stopped by a Valsalva manoeuvre and is augmented by distal compression of the foot or calf. Acute thrombus may be non-echogenic but the vein should not fill with colour Doppler and should not be compressible. The thrombus tends to become echogenic after a few days.

5. Although this technique is less well established for the exclusion of thrombus in the calf vessels, it has been shown to have a sensitivity and specificity close to that of venography. Cannulation of a vein and injection of contrast medium can thus be avoided.

Further reading

Baxter, G.M. & Duffy, P. (1992) Calf vein anatomy and flow: implications for colour Doppler imaging. *Clin. Radiol.* **46**, 84–87.

Baxter, G.M., McKeckney, S. & Duffy, P. (1990) Colour Doppler ultrasound in deep venous thrombosis. A comparison with venography. *Clin. Radiol.* **42**, 32–36.

Dorfman, G.S. & Cronan, J.J. (1992) Venous ultrasonography. *Radiol. Clin. N. Am.* **30**, 879–894.

Rose, S.C., Zwiebell, W.J., Nelson, B.D., et al. (1990) Symptomatic lower extremity deep venous thrombosis: accuracy, limitations, and role of colour Duplex flow imaging in diagnosis. *Radiology* **174**, 639–644.

IMAGING OF DEEP VENOUS THROMBOSIS (DVT)

ULTRASOUND

Veins can be systematically examined using a combination of continuous wave, duplex and colour Doppler systems.

Continuous wave

Continuous wave Doppler assesses movement, it is difficult to be sure which vein is being examined and incomplete venous thrombus can be missed. Its overall sensitivity and specificity are not sufficiently satisfactory for it to be used in isolation.

Duplex

Duplex scanning involves a combination of pulsed Doppler and real time for direct visualization. Expansion and filling of the normal echo-free lumen can be identified but slow moving blood may be misinterpreted for thrombus. Valsalva manoeuvre will cause expansion in the normal vein but is not a totally reliable sign. Pulsed Doppler assesses flow, and enhancement due to respiratory excursion and distal venous compression suggest patency. The most reliable sign is compressibility. Direct pressure with the US probe over the vein will cause the normal vein to collapse. If thrombus is present, this will not occur.

Colour Doppler

Colour Doppler examination gives the added advantage of assessing more accurately the veins in the calf. Once identified the veins are examined for thrombus in the manner above.

CONTRAST VENOGRAPHY

This technique provides an image of the venous system. There are disadvantages. It is an invasive procedure requiring intravenous injection of contrast medium, with the attendant risks that this entails. Failure to cannulate veins occurs with swollen limbs. False negative results do occur.

RADIOISOTOPES

Thrombus may be imaged with ^{111}In- or ^{99m}Tc-in vitro-labelled platelets. Radiolabelled fibrinogen is no longer available.

IMPEDANCE PLETHYSMOGRAPHY

This technique depends on the principle of the capacity of the veins to fill and empty in response to temporary obstruction to venous outflow by occlusion of the thigh veins with a pneumatic cuff. Changes in calf volume produce changes in impedance measured by electrodes applied to the calf. The technique is demanding and requires skilled personnel. Clinical states that impair venous return, such as cardiac failure and pelvic pathology and also arterial insufficiency, produce abnormal results.

MAGNETIC RESONANCE

In some series, MRI has been shown to be as sensitive as US and venography. Using surface coils to obtain high resolution, popliteal and femoral thrombus are easy to detect but the small vessels in the calf may not be seen with certainty. A number of imaging sequences are advocated, including standard T1- and T2-weighted images and more accurately gradient-recalled acquisition in the steady state (GRASS). Recently, MRI has been advocated as a method of 'ageing' thrombus.

MRI of the arterial and venous systems is progressing rapidly, and in the future its use in the diagnosis of venous thrombosis is likely to become increasingly indicated.

Further reading

Cronan, J. (1991) Contemporary venous imaging. *Cardiovasc. Intervent. Radiol.* **14**, 87–97.
Smith F.W. (1998) Vascular and lymphatic systems. In: Sharp, P.F., Gemmell, H.G. & Smith, F.W. (eds) *Practical Nuclear Medicine*, pp. 204–212. Oxford: Oxford University Press.

11 Lymph glands, lymphatics and tumours

Methods of imaging lymph glands

1. Plain films – may show:
   a. a soft tissue mass, e.g. hilar lymph glands
   b. calcification, e.g. mesenteric glands and tuberculous glands.
2. Indirect evidence from displacement of normal structures, e.g. displacement of ureters seen during excretion urography.
3. US

Advantages
   a. Non-invasive and without risk to the patient.

Disadvantages
   a. Highly operator-dependent.
   b. Intestinal gas is a major factor in poor visualization.
4. CT

Advantages
   a. Can image all intra-abdominal glands.
   b. Technically easy to perform.

Disadvantages
   a. Internal structure of glands is not seen.
   b. Retroperitoneal glands are difficult to define if there is a paucity of retroperitoneal fat.
5. MRI.
6. Lymphography – technically difficult and superseded by US, CT and MRI.
7. Radioisotopes.

LYMPHOSCINTIGRAPHY RN

Lymphoscintigraphy now provides a more physiological and less invasive alternative to conventional lymphography. High-resolution anatomical detail is not possible.

Indications

1. Intraoperative location of the 'sentinel' node in breast carcinoma and malignant melanoma using a hand-held probe. In recent years, this has become the major indication for lymphoscintigraphy. Although still awaiting completion of long-term clinical trials, the early indications are that if the first or 'sentinel' node in the lymphatic drainage chain from the primary site is shown to have negative histology (approx 60% of cases in breast cancer), then more extensive nodal clearance and associated morbidity can be avoided.[1-4]
2. Differentiation of lymphoedema from venous oedema.
3. Assessment of lymphatic flow in lymphoedema.
4. Confirmation and assessment of lymph node metastases.

Contraindications

1. History of hypersensitivity to human albumin products.
2. Complete blockage of the lymphatic system (because of the local radiation dose at the injection sites).

Radiopharmaceuticals

1. ^{99m}Tc-nanocolloidal albumin, 40 MBq max (0.4 mSv ED) total for all injections. With a particle size < 80 nm, the colloid is injected subcutaneously and cleared from the interstitial space by lymphatic drainage.
2. A number of other colloids are used around the world for sentinel node imaging,[5] and other radiopharmaceuticals have been used for lymphoscintigraphy.[6]

Equipment

1. Gamma-camera
2. High-resolution general purpose collimator.

Patient preparation

Clean injection sites, especially on feet.

Technique

Sentinel node imaging

The optimal technique is still evolving, with discussions centring on best size of colloid particle to use, the site and volume of injection and the best design of intraoperative probe.[1,5]

1. Example protocols are:
   a. *Breast carcinoma*: Inject ^{99m}Tc-colloid in around 5 ml

      volume subdermally for palpable lesions and peritumorally under ultrasound guidance for non-palpable lesions.

   b. *Melanoma*: Inject ^{99m}Tc-colloid intradermally in a ring of locations around the melanoma site, with a volume of about 0.1 ml for each injection.

2. Static images are taken at intervals until the first node is seen. For breast cancer, take anterior and left or right lateral images with the arm raised as for surgery. Mark the skin over the node in both axes to guide surgical incision and intraoperative location with a gamma-detecting probe.

3. With effectively no background activity in the body, anatomical localization on the images is needed. A [57]Cobalt flood source (usually available for routine camera quality assurance) can be placed for a short period under the imaging couch to produce a body outline on the image.

Other sites of investigation

1. The patient lies supine for lower limb investigation, in the lithotomy position for ischiorectal injection and sitting for other sites.

2. ^{99m}Tc-colloid in 0.1–0.3 ml volume is injected subcutaneously at sites depending upon the area to be studied:

   a. Nodes below diaphragm and lower limb drainage – 1 or 2 equal injections in each foot in the first and second interdigital webbed spaces for drainage into lymphatics following the long saphenous vein, or over the lateral dorsum of the foot for lymphatics following the short saphenous vein.[6–8]

   b. Axillary nodes and upper limb drainage – 1 or 2 equal injections in each hand in the second and third interdigital webbed spaces.[9]

   c. Internal mammary chains – separate studies for each side if required because of the possibility of cross-over drainage patterns. A variety of injection sites have been used including the periosteum of the ribs, the posterior rectus sheath beside the xiphisternum and the sub-areolar region.[10]

   d. Ileopelvic lymphatic network – bilateral injections into the ischiorectal fossae adjacent to the anal margin.[11]

   e. Drainage routes from a particular region – a ring of small injections around the site of interest.[12]

3. Check that the needle is not sited in a blood vessel by aspirating before injection. If any blood appears, another site should be chosen.

4. Static images are taken of the injection site(s) immediately, followed by injection site, drainage route and liver images at intervals, e.g. 15, 30, 60, and 180 min, continuing up to 24 h or until the liver is seen. Visualization of the liver indicates patency of at least one lymphatic channel (except early liver activity within 15 min, which implies some colloid entry into blood vessels).

Analysis

If more frequent imaging or a long dynamic study is performed, time-activity curves for regions along the drainage route can be plotted and used to quantify flow impairment.[13]

Aftercare

None.

Complications

Anaphylactic reaction – rare.

References

1. Keshtgar, M.R.S., & Ell, P.J. (1999) Sentinel lymph node detection and imaging. *Eur. J. Nucl. Med.* **26**, 57–67.
2. Alazraki, N., Grant, S. & Styblo, T. (1999) Is sentinel node staging for breast cancer standard care? The role of imaging. *Nucl. Med. Commun.* **20**, 1089–1091.
3. Yudd, A.P.Y., Kempf, J.S., Goydos, J.S., et al. (1999) Use of sentinel node lymphoscintigraphy in malignant melanoma. *Radiographics* **19**, 343–353.
4. Veronesi, U., Paganelli, G., Galimberti, V., et al. (1997) Sentinel node biopsy to avoid axillary dissection in breast cancer with clinically negative lymph-nodes. *Lancet* **349**, 1864–1867.
5. Baxter, K.G. (1999) Invited commentary. *Radiographics* **19**, 354–356.
6. Kramer, E.L. (1990) Lymphoscintigraphy: radiopharmaceutical selection and methods. *Nucl. Med. Int. J. Radiat. Instrum. Part B* **17**, 57–63.
7. Rijke, A.M., Croft, B.Y., Johnson, R.A., et al. (1990) Lymphoscintigraphy and lymphedema of the lower extremities. *J. Nucl. Med.* **31**, 990–998.
8. Proby, C.M., Gane, J.N., Joseph, A.E.A., et al. (1990) Investigation of the swollen limb with isotope lymphography. *Br. J. Dermatol.* **123**, 29–37.
9. Hayes, D.F. (1990) Axillary lymphoscintigraphy for breast cancer: should we do it? Can we do it? *J. Nucl. Med.* **31**, 1835–1838.
10. Terui, S. & Yamamoto, H. (1989) New simplified lymphoscintigraphic technique in patients with breast cancer. *J. Nucl. Med.* **30**, 1198–1204.
11. Ege, G.N. & Cummings, B.J. (1980) Interstitial radio-colloid iliopelvic lymphoscintigraphy: technique, anatomy and clinical application. *Int. J. Radiat. Oncol. Biol. Phys.* **6**, 1483–1490.
12. Wanebo, H.J., Harpole, D. & Teates, C.D. (1985) Radionuclide lymphoscintigraphy with technetium 99m antimony sulfide colloid to identify lymphatic drainage of cutaneous melanoma at ambiguous sites in the head and neck and trunk. *Cancer* **55**, 1403–1413.

13. Weissleder, H. & Weissleder, R. (1988) Lymphedema: evaluation of qualitative and quantitative lymphoscintigraphy in 238 patients. *Radiology* **167**, 729–735.

Further reading

Jewkes, R.F. (1991) Lymph node scanning. In: Maisey, M.N., Britton, K.E. & Gilday, D.L. (eds) *Clinical Nuclear Medicine*, 2nd edn. pp. 503–508. London: Chapman & Hall.

RADIONUCLIDE IMAGING OF INFECTION AND INFLAMMATION

RN

Indications

Diagnosis and localization of infection and inflammation in soft tissue and bone.[1]

Contraindications

None.

Radiopharmaceuticals

1. *[111]In-labelled leucocytes*, 20 MBq max (9 mSv ED). ^{111}In-oxine, tropolonate and acetylacetonate are highly lipophilic complexes that will label leucocytes, erythrocytes and platelets. The leucocytes have to be labelled in vitro by a lengthy procedure under aseptic conditions and the labelled cell suspension reinjected.[2,3] ABO/Rh-matched donor leucocytes can be used with neutropenic patients or to reduce infection hazard in HIV-positive patients.[4] [111]In has a $T_{1/2}$ of 67 h and principal gamma emissions at 171 and 245 keV.

2. *[99m]Tc-hexamethylpropyleneamineoxime (HMPAO)-labelled leucocytes*, 200 MBq max (3 mSv ED). HMPAO is also a highly lipophilic complex which preferentially labels granulocytes. The cell-labelling technique is similar to that for ^{111}In,[2,3] but HMPAO has the advantage that kits can be stocked and used at short notice. There is more bowel uptake than with ^{111}In-labelled leucocytes, so images must be taken earlier than 4 h post-injection for diagnosis of abdominal infection.[5,6] The ^{99m}Tc label delivers a lower radiation dose than ^{111}In-labelled leucocytes and has better imaging resolution, which can, for example, help identify inflammation in small bowel.[7]

3. *[67]Ga-gallium citrate*, 150 MBq max (17 mSv ED). Localizes in inflammatory sites. Formerly the most commonly used agent, it has now largely been replaced by labelled leucocyte

imaging. It still has a role in pyrexia of unknown origin, osteomyelitis of the spine and in the immunocompromized patient.[8] There is significant bowel activity up to 72 h, so delayed imaging may be necessary for suspected abdominal infection. ^{67}Ga, with a $T_{1/2}$ of 78 h and principal γ-emissions at 93, 185 and 300 keV, delivers a higher radiation dose than ^{99m}Tc-HMPAO- and ^{111}In-labelled leucocytes, but it has the advantage of requiring no special preparation.

4. *^{99m}Tc- or ^{111}In-human immunoglobulin (HIG)*. A newer agent for which a commercial kit is available for ^{99m}Tc labelling. It has the advantage of not requiring a complex preparation procedure, but its place relative to labelled leucocytes is still a matter of debate.[1,9]

5. *^{99m}Tc-sulesomab (Leukoscan)*. This is another more recent commercial agent comprising a labelled antigranulocyte monoclonal antibody fragment. It also has a simple preparation procedure, and is finding a role in the diagnosis of orthopaedic infections.[10]

Equipment

1. Gamma camera, preferably with whole body imaging facility.
2. Low-energy high-resolution collimator for ^{99m}Tc, medium-energy for ^{111}In, medium- or high-energy for ^{67}Ga.

Patient preparation

None.

Technique

1. The radiopharmaceutical is administered i.v.
2. Image timing depends upon the radiopharmaceutical used and the suspected source of infection. Whole-body imaging may be employed for all of the radiopharmaceuticals.
   - *^{111}In-labelled white cells*. Static images are acquired at 3 and 24 h post-injection at sites determined by the clinical history. Further imaging at 48 h may prove helpful.
   - *^{99m}Tc-HMPAO-labelled white cells*. For suspected abdominal infections, image at 0.5 and 2 h, i.e. before significant normal bowel activity is seen.[5] For other sites, image at 1, 2 and 4 h. Additional 24 h images may be useful.
   - *^{67}Ga-citrate*. Images are acquired at 48 and 72 h for regions where normal bowel, urinary and blood pool activity may obscure abnormal collection sites. Later images may prove helpful in non-urgent cases. Extremities and urgent cases

may be imaged from as early as 6 h. If not contraindicated, laxatives given for 48 h post-injection will help to clear bowel activity.

Additional techniques

1. The diagnosis of bone infection may be improved by combination with three-phase radioisotope bone scanning[11,12] or bone marrow imaging.[11,13]
2. A radiocolloid scan may help to discriminate between infection in the region of the liver or spleen and normal uptake in these organs.

Aftercare

Normal radiation safety precautions (see Chapter 1).

Complications

None.

References

1. Peters, A.M. (1998) The use of nuclear medicine in infections. *Br. J. Radiol.* **71**, 252–261.
2. Peters, A.M. (1998) Infection. In: Sharp, P.F., Gemmell, H.G. & Smith, F.W. (eds) *Practical Nuclear Medicine*, pp. 285–315. Oxford: Oxford University Press.
3. Danpure, H.J. & Osman, S. (1988) A review of methods of separating and radiolabelling human leucocytes. *Nucl. Med. Commun.* **9**, 681–685.
4. O'Doherty, M.J., Revell, P., Page, C.J., et al. (1990) Donor leucocyte imaging in patients with AIDS: a preliminary report. *Eur. J. Nucl. Med.* **17**, 327–333.
5. Lantto, E.H., Lantto, T.J. & Vorne, M. (1991) Fast diagnosis of abdominal infections and inflammations with technetium-99m-HMPAO labelled leukocytes. *J. Nucl. Med.* **32**, 2029–2034.
6. Mountford, P.J., Kettle, A.G., O'Doherty, M.J., et al. (1990) Comparison of technetium-99m-HMPAO leukocytes with indium-111-oxine leukocytes for localizing intraabdominal sepsis. *J. Nucl. Med.* **31**, 311–315.
7. Peters, A.M. & Lavender, J.P. (1991) Editorial. Imaging inflammation with radiolabelled white cells; ^{99}Tc^m-HMPAO or ^{111}In? *Nucl. Med. Commun.* **12**, 923–925.
8. Palestro, C.J. (1994) The current role of gallium imaging in infection. *Semin. Nucl. Med.* **24**, 128–141.
9. Palermo, F., Boccaletto, F., Paolin, A., et al. (1998) Comparison of technetium-99m-MDP, technetium-99m-WBC and technetium-99m-HIG in musculoskeletal inflammation. *J. Nucl. Med.* **39**, 516–521.
10. Hakki, S., Harwood, S.J., Morrissey, M.A., et al. (1997) Comparative study of monoclonal antibody scan in diagnosing orthopaedic infection. *Clin. Orthopaedics* **335**, 275–285.
11. Peters, A.M. & Lavender, J.P. (1990) Editorial. Diagnosis of bone infection. *Nucl. Med. Commun.* **11**, 463–467.
12. Copping, C., Dalgliesh, S.M., Dudley, N.J., et al. (1992) The role of ^{99m}Tc-HMPAO white cell imaging in suspected orthopaedic infection. *Br. J. Radiol.* **65**, 309–312.

13. King, A.D., Peters, A.M., Stuttle, A.W.J., et al. (1990) Imaging of bone infection with labelled white blood cells: role of contemporaneous bone marrow imaging. *Eur. J. Nucl. Med.* **17**, 148–151.

Further reading

Corstens, F.H.M. & van der Meer, J.W.M. (1999) Nuclear medicine's role in infection and inflammation. *Lancet* **354**, 765–770.

GALLIUM RADIONUCLIDE TUMOUR IMAGING

Indications

1. Hodgkin's and non-Hodgkin's lymphoma: assessment of residual masses after therapy and early diagnosis of recurrence.[1,2]
2. Gallium imaging has been used with variable success in a variety of other tumours, e.g. hepatoma,[3] bronchial carcinoma,[4] multiple myeloma[5] and sarcoma.[6]

Contraindications

None.

Radiopharmaceutical

67Ga-Gallium citrate, 150 MBq max (17 mSv ED).

Highly protein-bound in plasma, mainly to transferrin. Normal accumulation is seen in the liver, bone marrow and nasal sinuses and variably in the spleen, salivary and lacrimal glands. There is significant excretion via the gut and some via the kidneys. Gallium is also taken up by inflammatory sites, metabolically active bone and non-specifically by a variety of tumours.

^{67}Ga has a $T_{1/2}$ of 78 h and principal γ-emissions at 93, 185 and 300 keV, so image quality is fairly poor.

Equipment

1. Gamma camera, preferably with whole body and SPECT facilities
2. Medium- or high-energy collimator.

Patient preparation

If the abdomen is being investigated, laxatives may be given (if not contraindicated) for 2 days after injection of ^{67}Ga-citrate to clear bowel activity. Additionally, an enema or suppository may be given on the day of imaging.

Technique

1. ^{67}Ga-citrate is administered i.v.
2. Delayed images are acquired as below with energy windows about the lower two or all three of the main photopeaks.

Images

1. 48 and 72 h. Whole-body, spot views and SPECT as appropriate. SPECT can increase the sensitivity and specificity of the investigation.
2. Non-specific bowel activity can be discriminated by imaging on two separate occasions. Activity in bowel contents should move between scans and abnormal areas of accumulation will be stationary. If there is still any doubt at 72 h, later images at up to 7 days may prove helpful.

Additional techniques

1. A radionuclide bone scan may be performed prior to gallium imaging.
2. A radiocolloid scan may help to discriminate between lesions in the region of the liver or spleen and normal uptake in these organs. Image subtraction techniques may be used.

Aftercare

None.

Complications

None.

References

1. Bangerter, M., Griesshammer, M. & Bergmann, L. (1999) Progress in medical imaging of lymphoma and Hodgkin's disease. *Curr. Opin. Oncol.* **11**, 339–342.
2. Front, D., Bar-Shalom, R. & Israel, O. (1997) The continuing clinical role of gallium 67 scintigraphy in the age of receptor imaging. *Semin. Nucl. Med.* **27**, 68–74.
3. Suzuki, T., Honjo, I. & Hamamoto, K. (1971) Positive scintiphotography of cancer of the liver with 67 gallium citrate. *Am. J. Roentgenol.* **113**, 92–103.
4. Bekerman, C., Caride, V.J., Hoffer, P.B., et al. (1990) Noninvasive staging of lung cancer. Indications and limitations of gallium-67 citrate imaging. *Radiol. Clin. N. Am.* **28**, 497–510.
5. Waxman, A.D., Siemsen, J.K., Levine, A.M., et al. (1981) Radiographic and radionuclide imaging in multiple myeloma: the role of gallium scintigraphy: concise communication. *J. Nucl. Med.* **22**, 232–236.
6. Southee, A.E., Kaplan, W.D., Jochelson, M.S., et al. (1992) Gallium imaging in metastatic and recurrent soft tissue sarcoma. *J. Nucl. Med.* **33**, 1594–1599.

RADIOIODINE MIBG SCAN

Indications

1. Neuroblastoma[1-4]
2. Phaeochromocytoma[5,6]
3. Carcinoid tumours[7,8]
4. Medullary thyroid carcinoma[9,10]
5. Other neuroendocrine tumours.[11]

Contraindications

None.

Radiopharmaceuticals

[123]I-metaiodobenzylguanidine (MIBG), 250 MBq typical, 400 MBq max (6 mSv ED with thyroid blocked).

[131]I-labelled MIBG is also available, and is still in common use outside Europe where ^{123}I-MIBG is not made commercially. However, it is an inferior imaging agent and should only be considered where ^{123}I-MIBG cannot be obtained.

MIBG has a similar structure to noradrenaline, and localizes in the storage vesicles of catecholamine-secreting tumours. The 13-h half-life of ^{123}I allows imaging up to 48 h.

Equipment

1. Gamma-camera, preferably with whole-body imaging and SPECT capabilities
2. Low-energy general purpose collimator for [123]I.

Patient preparation

1. Where possible, stop medications that interfere with MIBG uptake.[12] These include tricyclic antidepressants, antihypertensives, cocaine, sympathomimetics, decongestants containing pseudoephedrine, phenylpropanolamine and phenylephrine (many available over the counter) and others.
2. Thyroid blockade, continuing for 24 h after ^{123}I-MIBG injection.
   a. *Adults* – either oral potassium perchlorate (400 mg, 1 h before MIBG injection, then 200 mg every 6 h) or oral potassium iodate (85 mg twice daily starting 24 h before MIBG injection).
   b. *Children* – Lugol's iodine 0.1–0.2 ml diluted with water or milk three times a day starting 48 h before MIBG injection.

Potassium iodate is more palatable – the tablets need splitting for paediatric dosage.

3. Children with neuroblastoma should also have a radionuclide bone scan to detect the 10% of skeletal metastases which would otherwise be missed.[1]

Technique

1. MIBG is administered slowly i.v. over 1–2 min (a fast injection may cause adrenergic side-effects).
2. Imaging at 24 h (sometimes additionally at 4 or 48 h), emptying bladder before pelvic views.

Images

1. Anterior and posterior abdomen, 10–20 min per view.
2. Whole-body imaging for comprehensive search for metastases.
3. SPECT may help to localize lesions, particularly in thorax and abdomen.

Additional techniques

1. If therapy with ^{131}I-MIBG is being considered, quantitative assessment is performed using geometric mean and attenuation correction to calculate percentage of administered dose residing in tumour at 24 h.[13]
2. ^{111}In-octreotide, which binds to somatostatin receptors frequently expressed in neuroendocrine and other tumours, is an alternative imaging agent to MIBG. It appears to be more sensitive for carcinoids, and may be useful in cases where the MIBG scan is negative.[14,15] It also has therapeutic analogues under development.[16]

Aftercare

Normal radiation safety precautions (see Chapter 1).

Complications

None.

References

1. Gilday, D.L. & Greenberg, M. (1990) Editorial. The controversy about the nuclear medicine investigation of neuroblastoma. *J. Nucl. Med.* **31**, 135.
2. Jacobs, A., Delree, M., Desprechins, B., et al. (1990) Consolidating the role of *I-MIBG-scintigraphy in childhood neuroblastoma: five years of clinical experience. *Pediatr. Radiol.* **20**, 157–159.
3. Troncone, L., Rufini, V., Danza, F.M., et al. (1990) Radioiodinated metaiodobenzylguanidine (*I-MIBG) scintigraphy in neuroblastoma: a review of 160 studies. *J. Nucl. Med. Allied Sci.* **34**, 279–288.

4. Gordon, I., Peters, A.M., Gutman, A., et al. (1990) Skeletal assessment in neuroblastoma – the pitfalls of iodine-123-MIBG scans. *J. Nucl. Med.* **31**, 129–134.
5. Warren, M.J., Shepstone, B.J. & Soper, N. (1989) Iodine-131 metaiodobenzylguanidine (^{131}I-MIBG) for the localization of suspected phaeochromocytoma. *Nucl. Med. Commun.* **10**, 467–475.
6. Hanson, M.W., Feldman, J.M., Beam, C.A., et al. (1991) Iodine 131-labeled metaiodobenzylguanidine scintigraphy and bio-chemical analyses in suspected pheochromocytoma. *Arch. Intern. Med.* **151**, 1397–1402.
7. Hoefnagel, C.A., Den Hartog Jager, F.C.A., Taal, B.G., et al. (1987) The role of I-131-MIBG in the diagnosis and therapy of carcinoids. *Eur. J. Nucl. Med.* **13**, 187–191.
8. Bomanji, J., Ur, E., Mather, S., et al. (1992) A scintigraphic comparison of iodine-123-metaiodobenzyl-guanidine and an iodine-labelled somatostatin analog (Tyr-3-octreotide) in metastatic carcinoid tumors. *J. Nucl. Med.* **33**, 1121–1124.
9. Guerra, U.P., Pizzocaro, C., Terzi, A., et al. (1989) New tracers for the imaging of the medullary thyroid carcinoma. *Nucl. Med. Commun.* **10**, 285–295.
10. Clarke, S.E.M., Lazarus, C.R., Edwards, S., et al. (1987) Scintigraphy and treatment of medullary carcinoma of the thyroid with iodine-131 metaiodobenzylguanidine. *J. Nucl. Med.* **28**, 1820–1825.
11. Von Moll, L., McEwan, A.J., Shapiro, B., et al. (1987) Iodine-131 MIBG scintigraphy of neuroendocrine tumors other than pheochromocytoma and neuroblastoma. *J. Nucl. Med.* **28**, 979–988.
12. Solanki, K.K., Bomanji, J., Moyes, J., et al. (1992) A pharmacological guide to medicines which interfere with the biodistribution of radiolabelled meta-iodobenzylguanidine (MIBG). *Nucl. Med. Commun.* **13**, 513–521.
13. Troncone, L. & Rufini, V. (1997) 131I-MIBG therapy of neural crest tumours (review). *Anticancer Res.* **17**, 1823–1831.
14. Krenning, E.P., Kwekkeboom, D.J., Bakker, W.H., et al. (1993) Somatostatin receptor scintigraphy with [111In-DTPA-D-Phe[1]]- and [123I-Tyr[3]]-octreotide: the Rotterdam experience with more than 1000 patients. *Eur. J. Nucl. Med.* **20**, 716–731.
15. Tenenbaum, F., Lumbroso, J., Schlumberger, M., et al. (1995) Comparison of radiolabeled octreotide and meta-iodobenzylguanidine (MIBG) scintigraphy in malignant pheochromocytoma. *J. Nucl. Med.* **36**, 1–6.
16. Buscombe, J.R. & Caplin, M.E. (1999) Editorial. Radiolabelled somatostatins: towards the magic bullet? *Nucl. Med. Commun.* **20**, 299–301.

POSITRON EMISSION TOMOGRAPHY (PET) IMAGING

Until recently, PET imaging was restricted to a small handful of centres in the UK due to high capital cost and logistics of radio-pharmaceutical supply. It uses short-lived cyclotron-produced radionuclides such as [18]Fluorine, [11]Carbon, [13]Nitrogen and [15]Oxygen with half-lives of 110, 20, 10 and 2 min respectively. [18]Fluorine is the only one of these that can realistically be produced off-site due to these short decay times.

The main advantages of PET are the ability to image physio-logically important molecules, and the higher image resolution and detector sensitivity compared to conventional single photon emission nuclear medicine.

Technological advances in the design of gamma cameras have recently enabled PET imaging to be performed on adapted dual-headed systems at a fraction of the cost of dedicated PET cameras. Although the image quality is inferior to dedicated PET systems due to poorer sensitivity and count rate capability, it is still better than SPECT, and will allow much wider access to PET scanning than hitherto. Transmission attenuation correction is now becoming available on these systems, which further enhances diagnostic efficacy.

This advance has been coupled with increasing interest in the main PET tracer, ^{18}F-Fluorodeoxyglucose (FDG), a glucose analogue that is taken up in tissue in proportion to cellular glucose metabolism. This is particularly useful for tumour imaging, since most tumours have increased glucose metabolism and will concentrate FDG. It also concentrates in the normal brain and heart. However, FDG is a non-specific tracer which is also taken up by sites of inflammation or infection, so patient selection is important to avoid false positive scans.

As the only PET tracer likely to be widely available in the near future, this section is restricted to FDG imaging.

^{18}F-FLUORODEOXYGLUCOSE (FDG) PET SCANNING
Indications (Oncology)[1,2]

1. Investigation of solitary pulmonary nodule.
2. Staging of lung cancer, melanoma, lymphoma.
3. Evaluation of postoperative recurrence in colorectal cancer.
4. Differential diagnosis of recurrent disease versus scar tissue.
5. As a general tool for staging and assessing extent of disease and monitoring therapy.

Contraindications

Contraindications associated with co-administered drugs such as buscopan and diazepam should be considered.

Patient preparation

1. Fasting for 4-6 h, with plenty of fluids (no sugary drinks).
2. Monitor blood glucose before injection to ensure it is normal to low.
3. To reduce normal intestinal uptake of FDG on abdominal

scans, the smooth muscle relaxant Buscopan (20 mg) may be given at the same time as the FDG.[3]

4. A muscle relaxant such as diazepam may be given to reduce normal muscle uptake in tense individuals.

Technique

1. Up to 400 MBq FDG i.v. (10 mSv ED) is administered. Current gamma-camera PET systems can only effectively handle a maximum of 60–120 MBq due to their lower count rate capability.

2. To reduce normal muscle uptake of FDG, patients should remain in a relaxed environment such as lying in a darkened room, without talking if head and neck area are being imaged, between injection and scan.

3. Image at 1 h or more post-injection. Later imaging may enhance tumour contrast, and greater activity may be administered to allow for the extra radioactive decay up to the recommended UK limit of 400 MBq. Most systems permit whole body imaging, but for gamma-camera systems, the area covered will be a compromise with longer imaging over particular sites, up to a maximum imaging time of 90 min or so before radioactive decay becomes too great.

4. Transmission attenuation imaging if available can enhance diagnostic accuracy particularly for deep-seated lesions, but extends the scan time.

Other applications[4]

Coronary artery disease

1. Assessment of myocardial viability.
   FDG is considered to be the gold standard for myocardial viability assessment. Good attenuation correction is required, which is still in its infancy on gamma-camera PET systems.

Neurology

1. Location of epileptic foci.
   Interictal FDG scanning shows reduced uptake at foci, but is probably not as sensitive as ictal SPECT if this is logistically possible.

2. Assessment of dementia.

3. Assessment of brain tumours.

Infection and inflammation

FDG is taken up by inflammatory cells by virtue of their increased metabolic requirements, and this is an area of increasing interest.

References

1. Rigo, P., Paulus, P., Kaschten, B.J., et al. (1996) Oncological applications of positron emission tomography with fluorine-18 fluorodeoxyglucose. *Eur. J. Nucl. Med.* **23**, 1641–1674.
2. Delbeke, D. (1999) Oncological applications of FDG PET imaging. *J. Nucl. Med.* **40**, 1706–1715.
3. Stahl, A., Weber, W., Avril, N., et al. (1999) The effect of n-butylscopolamine on intestinal uptake of F-18-fluorodeoxyglucose in PET imaging of the abdomen. *Eur. J. Nucl. Med.* **26**, 1017.
4. von Schulthess, G.K. (ed) (1999) *Clinical Positron Emission Tomography*. Philadelphia: Lippincott Williams & Wilkins.

12 Bones and joints

Methods of imaging joints

1. Plain films
2. Arthrography
3. Radionuclide imaging
   - ^{99m}Tc methylene diphosphonate
   - ^{67}gallium citrate.
4. US
5. CT
6. MRI.

MRI has replaced arthrography as the dominant imaging modality which is now largely reserved for situations in which MRI is not available, where metal prostheses prohibit MR scanning or the patient is otherwise unsuitable for insertion into a magnet. Because arthrography may still be required, the following sections have been retained.

Further reading

Freiberger, R. & Kaye, J. (1979) Arthrography. New York: Appleton-Century-Crofts.
Van Holsbeek, M.T. (ed) (1999) Musculoskeletal ultrasound. Radiol. Clin. N. Am. **37 (4)**.

MUSCULOSKELETAL MRI – GENERAL POINTS   MRI

1. A surface coil gives a better signal-to-noise ratio and improved resolution than the body coil. However, the latter may be necessary to allow a larger field of view for a whole bone so that skip lesions are not missed.
2. Cartilaginous structures are seen well with gradient recalled echo techniques, e.g. multiplanar gradient recalled echo (MPGR).
3. In young children the growth plate is well-shown using proton density spin-echo sequence with fat suppression; the growth

plate may be differentiated from epiphyseal cartilage using a T2-weighted spin-echo sequence with fat suppression.

4. Gradient echo sequences (with a flip angle of 20°) differentiate articular cartilage from effusion.

5. Spoiled gradient echo images with fat suppression can delineate the thickness of articular cartilage.

6. Bone marrow abnormalities are imaged with fast multiplanar inversion recovery (FMPIR) and fast spin-echo (FSE) T2-weighted sequences.

7. Intravenous gadolinium contrast agents are used for imaging:
   a. infections – to delineate fluid-filled or drainable collections
   b. tumours – to characterize the lesion, determine the amount of necrosis and the extent of peritumoural oedema
   c. vascular lesions
   d. synovial disease, e.g. rheumatoid arthritis
   e. avascular necrosis, e.g. Perthe's disease.

ARTHROGRAPHY – GENERAL POINTS

1. The plain films should always be reviewed prior to the procedure, as it may be necessary to take further views to demonstrate fully an abnormality that would otherwise be obscured by the presence of contrast medium.

2. Aspiration of an effusion should always be performed before contrast medium is injected. This is because an effusion will dilute the contrast medium, and can also lead to a 'foamy' appearance on the radiographs. The aspirate should be sent, where appropriate, for:
   a. microscopy, culture (aerobic and anaerobic) and sensitivity
   b. crystal analysis
   c. cytology
   d. biochemistry.

3. Although meglumine salts can be used safely for arthrography, LOCM are generally diluted more slowly and allow more time for the examination. In addition the large molecular size of ioxaglate delays absorption further than other low osmolar agents (e.g. iohexol). This is of particular benefit in those investigations that may take some time, e.g. knee arthrography or CT arthrography of the shoulder or ankle.

4. If a needle is correctly sited within a joint space, a test

injection of a small volume of contrast medium will stream around the joint. However, if it is incorrectly sited, the contrast medium will remain in a diffuse cloud around the tip of the needle.

5. In the investigation of a suspected loose body, delayed films should be taken after an interval of half an hour. These may show adsorption of contrast medium onto a cartilaginous loose body.

6. The positive contrast medium is absorbed from the joint and excreted from the body in a few hours. However, the air may take up to 4 days to be completely absorbed from the joint space.

DOUBLE CONTRAST KNEE ARTHROGRAPHY

Indications

1. Cartilage, capsular or ligamentous injuries
2. Loose body
3. Popliteal cyst.

Contraindications

Local sepsis.

Contrast medium

1. LOCM 320
2. Air 40 ml.

Equipment

1. Fluoroscopy unit with spot film device and fine focal spot (0.3 mm^2)
2. Overcouch tube.

Patient preparation

None.

Preliminary film

Knee

1. AP
2. Lateral.

Additional films

1. Axial view of the patella (skyline)
2. Intercondylar (tunnel) view.

Technique

1. The patient lies supine; either a medial or a lateral approach can be used and it is as well to be familiar with both.
2. Using a sterile technique, the skin and underlying soft tissue are anaesthetized at a point 1–2 cm posterior to the mid-point of the patella.
3. A 21-G needle is advanced into the joint space from this point by angling it slightly anteriorly so the tip comes to lie against the posterior surface of the patella. By virtue of the anatomy, the tip of the needle must be within the joint space (Fig. 12.1). A more horizontal approach may result in the needle penetrating the infrapatellar fat pad, resulting in an extra-articular injection of contrast.
4. Any effusion is aspirated. If there is any doubt about the position of the needle, the injection of a few millilitres of air will encounter little resistance if the needle is correctly sited. If incorrectly sited, then resistance will be met, and as soon as pressure is released from the plunger of the syringe it will be forced back into the syringe. This test is not infallible and occasionally air can be injected into soft tissue with little

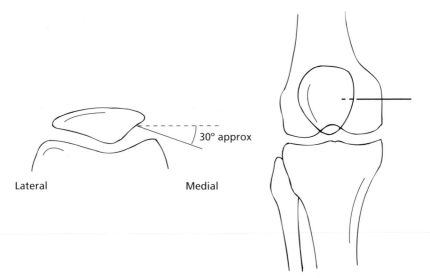

Figure 12.1   Technique of knee arthrography.

resistance. A test injection of a small volume of contrast medium can be made under fluoroscopic control to ensure the needle is correctly positioned and, if so, the contrast medium should be seen to flow rapidly away from the needle tip. If a satisfactory position is demonstrated, then the full volume of contrast medium and air may be injected.

5. The needle is then removed and the knee is manipulated to ensure even distribution of contrast medium within the joint; this is easily facilitated by asking the patient to walk around the room several times whilst bending the knee through as full a movement as is comfortable.

6. The patient is placed in the prone position with a pad or bolster under the thigh of the side to be examined. It is necessary to apply varus or valgus strain to the knee during the procedure and this is facilitated by applying a strap around the thigh and attaching this to the edge of the table top.

Films

1. Spot films:
   a. The knee joint is divided into quadrants for the purpose of the examination – an anterior and posterior quadrant for each of the medial and lateral compartments. The X-ray beam is collimated to the compartment being examined.
   b. Traction is applied to the joint and simultaneously valgus or varus strain is applied either with a lead glove or, as mentioned before, with the aid of a strap applied to the thigh. A variable degree of flexion may also be required to bring the tibial plateau and meniscus into profile.
   c. Four views of each quadrant are taken, rotating the leg approximately 20° between each spot view. This will result in eight views per meniscus.
2. Overcouch films: as for preliminary views.
3. In some instances when there is doubt it will be advisable to repeat the spot views. It is recognized that small meniscal tears may not be visible immediately and contrast may take time to adhere. Also meniscal cysts may be better seen on delayed films.

Aftercare

The patient is warned that there may be some discomfort in the joint for 1–2 days after the procedure. It is also necessary to refrain from strenuous exercise during this time.

Complications

Due to the contrast medium

1. Allergic reactions
2. Chemical synovitis.

Due to the technique

1. Pain
2. Infection
3. Capsular rupture
4. Trauma to adjacent structures.

Further reading

Coumas, J.M. & Palmer, W.E. (1998) Knee arthrography. Evolution and current status. *Radiol. Clin. N. Am.* **36 (4)**, 703–728.

HIP ARTHROGRAPHY

Indications

1. Congenital dislocation of the hip
2. Loose body
3. Trauma
4. Perthes' disease
5. Proximal focal femoral deficiency
6. Arthropathy
7. Painful hip prosthesis.

Contraindications

Local sepsis.

Contrast medium

LOCM 240.

1. *Child*: 1–2 ml.
2. *Adult*: 3–5 ml (in loose prostheses the false capsule may take 15–20 ml).

Equipment

1. Fluoroscopy unit
2. Overcouch tube
3. Lumbar puncture needle (7.5 cm, 20- or 22-G, short bevel).

Patient preparation

1. Nothing orally for 4 h prior to the procedure.
2. Children under 10 years may require general anaesthesia.

Preliminary film

Hip

1. AP
2. Lateral.

Additional films for children

Frog lateral.

Technique

1. The patient lies supine on the X-ray table, the leg is extended, internally rotated and the position maintained with sandbags so that the entire length of the femoral neck is visualized.
2. The position of the femoral vessels is marked to avoid inadvertent puncture.
3. The skin is prepared in a standard aseptic manner.
4. A metal marker (sterile needle) or a point on the skin is marked to show the position of entry (Fig. 12.2). The needle is then advanced vertically onto the femoral neck under fluoroscopic control; the capsule may be thick and a definite 'give' felt when the needle enters the joint.

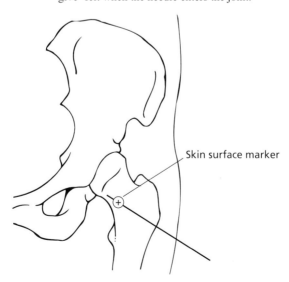

Skin surface marker

Figure 12.2   Technique of hip arthrography. x = site of entry into joint.

5. A test injection of contrast will demonstrate correct placement of the needle, the contrast will flow away from the needle tip. Any fluid in the joint should be aspirated at this stage and sent for analysis.

6. Approximately 3–5 ml (1–2 ml in children) of contrast medium are injected. The exact amount depends on the capacity of the joint capsule. If examining a prosthetic joint, larger volumes of contrast may be required (15–20 ml). By adding a radioactive tracer to the infusate (^{99m}Tc-colloid) and subsequent imaging with a gamma-camera, a more accurate assessment of loosening can be made, perhaps because the tracer is less viscous than the contrast medium and extends to a greater extent along the prosthesis.

7. After injection of the contrast medium the needle is removed and the joint is passively exercised to distribute the contrast medium evenly. Films are taken immediately.

Films

Adult

1. AP hip
2. AP in full internal rotation
3. AP in full external rotation
4. Lateral
5. Delayed films at 30 min if indicated.

Children

1. AP hip
2. Frog lateral
3. Abduction and internal rotation
4. Maximum abduction
5. Maximum adduction
6. Push/pull views to demonstrate instability.

Prosthetic joint

1. AP prior to injection of contrast
2. AP with limb immobilized after injection of contrast
3. Subtraction film using either digital or photographic method. This technique facilitates interpretation, as the metal prosthesis and the barium impregnated cement are subtracted out of the final image.

Aftercare

If the procedure was carried out under general anaesthetic the patient may require admission overnight. The patient should be warned of possible discomfort for 1–2 days and told to avoid strenuous exertion and driving for this time.

Complications

See 'Knee arthrography' (p. 265).

Further reading

Aliabadi, P., Baker, N.D. & Jaramillo, D. (1998) Hip arthrography, aspiration, block, and bursography. *Radiol. Clin. N. Am.* **36 (4)**, 673–690.

DOUBLE CONTRAST SHOULDER ARTHROGRAPHY

Indications

1. Rotator cuff tears
2. Loose body
3. Shoulder instability
4. Synovitis or capsulitis.

Contraindications

Local sepsis.

Contrast medium

1. LOCM 320
2. Air, approx. 8–10 ml.

Equipment

1. Fluoroscopy unit
2. Overcouch tube
3. Lumbar puncture needle (9 cm, 22-G, short bevel).

Patient preparation

None.

Preliminary film

Shoulder

1. AP in internal rotation
2. AP in external rotation
3. Axial.

Technique

1. The patient lies supine, with the arm of the side under investigation close to the body and the hand supinated. This is to rotate the long head of the biceps out of the path of the needle. The articular surface of the glenoid will face slightly forwards, which is important as it allows a vertically placed needle to enter the joint space without damaging the glenoid labrum.
2. The coracoid process is located by palpation. Using a sterile technique, the skin and soft tissues are anaesthetized at a point 1 cm inferior and 1 cm lateral to the coracoid process. Position is optimized by fluoroscopy.
3. A lumbar puncture needle (22-G) or a 21-G needle is inserted vertically down into the joint space (Fig. 12.3). The vertical direction allows precise control of the medial-lateral course of the needle. The position of the needle should be checked by intermittent screening. When it meets the resistance of the articular surface of the humeral head it is withdrawn by 1–2 mm to free the tip.

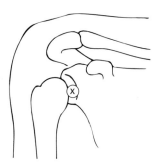

Figure 12.3   Technique of double contrast shoulder arthrography. x = site of entry into joint.

4. The intra-articular position of the needle is then confirmed by the injection of a few drops of the contrast medium under fluoroscopic control.
5. The remainder of the contrast medium and sufficient air to distend the synovial sac (8–10 ml) is injected. Patients with an adhesive capsulitis may experience pain after much smaller amounts. If this is severe then injection should be stopped. Resistance to injection is common, unlike injection into the knee, and more force is often required.
6. The needle is removed and the joint is gently manipulated to distribute the contrast medium.

Films

1. AP in neutral – erect
2. AP in external rotation – erect
3. AP in internal rotation – erect
4. Axial.

Additional films

1. Repeat steps 2 and 3 above with the tube angled caudad to bring the under surface of the acromion parallel to the beam.
2. AP in neutral with shoulder under load (5 kg) may help demonstrate supraspinatus tear.

Aftercare

The patient is warned of slight discomfort persisting for 1–2 days.

Complications

As for knee arthrography.

Further reading

Ghelman, B & Goldman, A.B. (1977) The double contrast shoulder arthrogram: evaluation of rotary cuff tears. *Radiology* **124**, 251–254.
Rafii, M. & Minkoff, J. (1998) Advanced arthrography of the shoulder with CT and MR imaging. *Radiol. Clin. N. Am.* **36 (4)**, 609–633.

CT SHOULDER ARTHROGRAPHY   CT

Indications

As for double contrast arthrography but particularly useful in joint instability.

Technique

1. Contrast medium is injected as outlined in the steps for double contrast arthrography. Too much contrast will flood the joint and so a smaller volume is all that is required (2.5–3 ml).
2. If any delay is anticipated in transfer to the CT scanner, then dilution of the contrast medium can be reduced by the addition of 0.2 ml of adrenaline 1:1000 to the injection.
3. CT examination is performed with the patient supine and positioned slightly eccentrically within the scanner to ensure that the shoulder is well within the scan field.
4. The contralateral arm can be elevated above the head to minimize image artefacts.

5. Scanning should be undertaken during arrested respiration to minimize motion artefact.

Films

1. Contiguous slices (3–4 mm) are obtained from the acromion to the axillary recess. Images should be targeted to the relevant shoulder with a magnification factor of 4.
2. Images should be viewed on both soft tissue and bone windows.
3. Additional information can occasionally be obtained by scanning prone. Direct sagittal scanning to better visualize the rotator cuff can also be employed, but it adds to time taken and the position may be difficult for the patient to maintain.

Further reading

Davies, A.M. (1991) The current role of computed tomographic arthrography of the shoulder. *Clin. Radiol.* **44**, 369–375.

ELBOW ARTHROGRAPHY

Indications

1. Loose body
2. Ligament injury
3. Capsular rupture.

Contraindications

Local sepsis.

Contrast medium

LOCM 240, 3–4 ml.

Equipment

1. Fluoroscopy unit
2. Overcouch tube.

Patient preparation

None.

Technique

Single contrast

1. The patient sits next to the table with his elbow flexed and resting on the table, the lateral aspect uppermost.

2. The radial head is located by palpation during gentle pronation and supination of the forearm. Using a sterile technique the skin and soft tissues are anaesthetized at a point just proximal to the radial head.

3. A 23-G needle is then inserted vertically down into the joint space between the radial head and the capitellum (Fig. 12.4).

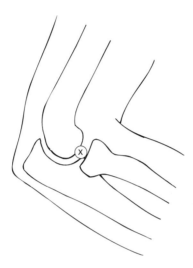

Figure 12.4   Technique of elbow arthrography. x = site of entry into joint.

4. An injection of a small volume of local anaesthetic will flow easily if the needle is correctly sited. This can be confirmed by the injection of a few drops of contrast medium under fluoroscopic control.

5. The remainder of the contrast medium is injected and the joint gently manipulated to distribute it evenly.

Double contrast

1. Position the patient as for single contrast technique and follow steps 1–4 above.

2. Inject 0.5 ml of contrast medium followed by 6–12 ml of air until the olecranon fossa is distended.

Films

1. AP
2. Lateral
3. Both 45° posterior obliques
4. Delayed films at 30 min, if indicated.

Aftercare

The patient is warned that there may be discomfort for 1–2 days afterwards.

Complications

As for knee arthrography.

Further reading

Steinbach, L.S. & Schwartz, M. (1998) Elbow arthrography. *Radiol. Clin. N. Am.* **36 (4)**, 635–649.

WRIST ARTHROGRAPHY

RADIOCARPAL JOINT

Indications

1. Ligament injury
2. Synovial swelling.

Contraindications

Local sepsis.

Contrast medium

LOCM 240, 2–4 ml.

Equipment

1. Overcouch tube
2. Fluoroscopy unit.

Patient preparation

None.

Preliminary films

1. PA
2. Lateral.

Technique

1. The patient is seated next to the screening table with the forearm resting in a neutral prone position. The wrist should be supported over a wedge with about 10–15° of flexion.
2. Using a sterile technique, the skin and soft tissues are anaesthetized on the dorsal aspect of the wrist at a point just distal to the mid-point of the lower end of the radius (Fig. 12.5).

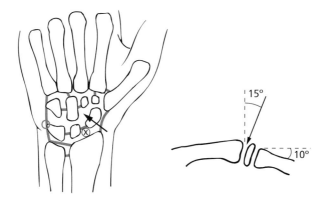

Figure 12.5   Technique of wrist arthrography. Arrow and x = site of entry into radiocarpal joint. Arrowhead = site of entry into midcarpal joint.

3. A 23-G needle is inserted into the joint by advancing it downwards and at an angle of about 15° proximally.
4. Contrast medium is injected under fluoroscopic control; if any leakage occurs into the midcarpal joint or distal radioulnar joints, then spot views should be taken. If this is not done, it is possible to miss small tears that later become obscured by the anterior and posterior extensions of the radiocarpal joint.

Films

1. PA
2. PA with ulnar deviation
3. PA with radial deviation
4. Lateral
5. 45° oblique.

MIDCARPAL JOINT

Indications

Ligamentous injury.

Contraindications

Local sepsis.

Contrast medium

LOCM 240, 3 ml.

Equipment

1. Overcouch tube
2. Fluoroscopy unit with video facility.

Preliminary film

1. PA
2. Lateral.

Technique

1. The wrist is positioned as for radiocarpal injection but with ulnar deviation, as this widens the joint space.
2. The skin and soft tissues are anaesthetized at point over the mid-point of the scaphocapitate joint (Fig. 12.5).
3. A 23-G needle is inserted vertically into the joint space under fluoroscopic control.
4. Contrast is injected under fluoroscopic control, ideally with video-recording facility, until the joint space is full. Without continuous monitoring it may not be possible to tell which of the ligaments separating the midcarpal from the radiocarpal joint are torn from the plain films alone.

Films

1. PA
2. PA with ulnar deviation
3. PA with radial deviation
4. Lateral
5. 45° oblique.

Aftercare

The patient should be warned of possible discomfort for 1–2 days after the procedure.

Complications

As for knee arthrography.

Further reading

Linkous, M.D. & Gilula, L.A. (1998) Wrist arthrography today. *Radiol. Clin. N. Am.* **36 (4)**, 651–672.

Robert, M., et al (1985) Midcarpal wrist arthrography for the detection of tears of the scapholunate and lunotriquetral ligaments. *Am. J. Roentgenol.* **144**, 107–108.

ANKLE ARTHROGRAPHY

Indications

1. Ligament injury
2. Loose body
3. Joint rupture
4. Osteochondral defect.

Contraindications

Local sepsis.

Contrast medium

LOCM 240, 6–8 ml.

Equipment

Overcouch tube.

Patient preparation

None.

Preliminary film

1. AP
2. Lateral.

Technique

1. The patient lies supine with the ankle slightly plantar-flexed. An anterior approach is used.
2. Using a sterile technique, the skin is anaesthetized at a point 1 cm above and 1 cm lateral to the tip of the medial malleolus (Fig. 12.6). Position is optimized by fluoroscopy.

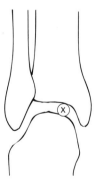

Figure 12.6   Technique of ankle arthrography. x = site of entry into joint.

3. A 21-G needle is inserted and advanced in an AP direction into the joint space.

Films

1. AP
2. Lateral
3. 45° obliques
4. Inversion and eversion stress films.

Additional films

AP and lateral tomography.

Aftercare

The patient should be warned of possible discomfort for 1–2 days following the procedure and to avoid strenuous activity and driving for this time.

Complications

As for knee arthrography.

CT ANKLE ARTHROGRAPHY

Indications

Osteochondral defects.

Technique

1. Contrast medium is introduced into the joint as outlined in the steps above for standard single contrast arthrography. Low osmolar contrast has the advantage of slower dilution in the event of delay prior to scanning. Adrenaline, 0.1 ml of 1:1000, can be used to delay absorption further.
2. The patient is positioned in the scanner, supine with the knee flexed and the foot placed sole-flat on the couch.
3. The scanner gantry is then tilted to obtain, as close as is possible, true coronal sections through the ankle joint.

Films

1. Contiguous thin sections are acquired (3–4 mm) through the joint from anterior to posterior.
2. Direct axial sections may also be acquired if necessary.

Further reading

Davies, A.M., & Cassar-Pullicino, V.N. (1989) Demonstration of osteochondritis dissecans of the talus by coronal computed tomography arthrography. *Br. J. Radiol.* **62 (744)**, 1050–1055.

TEMPOROMANDIBULAR JOINT ARTHROGRAPHY

Indications

Dysfunction, pain, clicking or failure of conservative management.

Contraindications

Local sepsis.

Contrast medium

LOCM 300, 2 ml.

Equipment

1. Fluoroscopy unit   2. Overcouch tube.

Patient preparation

None.

Technique

Two methods are described.

Single contrast

1. The patient lies on their side, with a pad under the lower shoulder, and the head resting on the table. The degree of lateral flexion of the head is adjusted using fluoroscopy to obtain the optimum visualization of the temporomandibular joint under investigation.
2. Using a sterile technique, the overlying skin and soft tissues are anaesthetized.
3. With the mouth a little open, a 25-G needle is advanced down onto the posterosuperior aspect of the condyle of the mandible (Fig. 12.7). If satisfactorily sited, it will move forwards with the condyle as the mouth is opened.

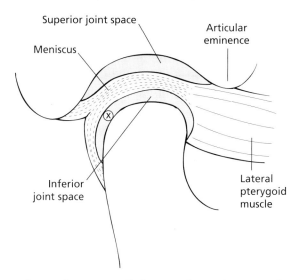

Figure 12.7   Technique of temporomandibular joint arthrography. x = site of entry into joint.

4. A small volume (0.3–0.6 ml) is injected under fluoroscopic control. It should flow freely forward to the anterior aspect of the head of the condyle.

Films

1. Lateral oblique-mouth open
2. Lateral oblique-mouth closed
3. Video full range of temporomandibular joint movement.

Double contrast

1. Position the patient as for single contrast technique (see above).
2. Using a 25-G needle, the lower joint is entered as described above. Approx. 0.5 ml of air is injected followed by 0.1 ml of contrast followed by a further 0.8 ml of air.
3. The needle is repositioned level with and 3 mm posterior to the upper tip of the condyle. The needle is advanced until it meets the articular eminence. It is then withdrawn slightly and 0.5 ml of air is injected followed by 0.15 ml of contrast and a further 1 ml of air. This should outline the superior joint compartment.

Films

AP and lateral tomography with the mouth closed.

Aftercare

The patient is warned of possible discomfort for 1–2 days after the procedure.

Complications

As for knee arthrography.

Further reading

Bell, K.A. & Walters, P.J. (1983) Videofluoroscopy during arthrography of the temporomandibular joint. *Radiology* **147**, 879.
Doyle, T. (1983) Arthrography of the temporomandibular joint: a simple technique. *Clin. Radiol.* **34**, 147–151.
Westesson, P.L., Omnell, K.A. & Rohlin, M. (1980) Double contrast tomography of the temporomandibular joint. *Acta. Radiol. Diagn.* **21**, 777–784.

TENOGRAPHY

Methods of imaging tendons

1. Tenography
2. US
3. CT
4. MRI.

General points

1. Tenography is used to detect abnormalities of tendons and their surrounding sheaths. With the advent of CT and MRI, the number of such procedures performed has declined.
2. Although MRI can show fluid within tendon sheaths, the resolution is not capable of detailing fine irregularity of tendons seen in minimal to moderate tenosynovitis or the scarring that develops in stenosing tenosynovitis.
3. Tenography can be used to identify with certainty the positioning of therapeutic injections of local anaesthetic and steroid.
4. Tenography can be used for any tendon that has an approachable sheath and one which has suitable anatomical surface landmarks. Commonly evaluated tendon sheaths around the ankle joint include personeal, posterior tibial, extensor hallucis longus, anterior tibial, flexor digitorum longus and flexor hallucis longus. In the wrist and hand, the carpal tunnel and abductor pollicis longus can be evaluated in this way.
5. The technique is essentially similar for any tendon sheath.

Indications

1. Tenosynovitis:
   a. acute
   b. chronic stenosing
2. Capsular or tendon sheath tears
3. Traumatic rupture
4. Extrinsic compression
5. Tendon displacement
6. Therapeutic placement of steroid.

Contraindications

Local sepsis.

Contrast medium

LOCM 240. Volume depends on the tendon to be evaluated.

Equipment

1. Fluoroscopy unit
2. Overcouch tube.

Technique

1. Before injection, the origin, course and insertion of the tendon should be familiarized.

2. By moving the joint passively the tendon of interest can be palpated. The point of insertion should be marked.
3. Using an aseptic technique the skin and soft tissue is anaesthetized with local infiltration with lignocaine 1%.
4. A 23- or 25-G needle is advanced into the tendon sheath until firm resistance is met from the tendon. The needle is slowly withdrawn, exerting gentle pressure to a syringe containing local anaesthetic. When this flows easily the needle is within the sheath. This is then confirmed by the injection of 1 ml of contrast under fluoroscopic control; contrast will be seen to flow away from the needle.
5. Sufficient contrast material is then injected to fill the sheath to its distal reflection.
6. Fluoroscopy during injection is advisable to identify filling defects or lobulations.

Films

1. Spot films during fluoroscopy
2. AP
3. Lateral
4. Both 45° obliques.

Additional films

1. Spot films after full range of movement of the tendon under evaluation
2. AP or lateral with skin marker to identify point of maximal tenderness.

Aftercare

Patient should be warned of discomfort lasting for 24–48 h.

Complications

As for arthrography.

Further reading

Baker, K.S. & Gilula, L.A. (1990) The current role of tenography and bursography. *Am. J. Roentgenol.* **154**, 129–133.

ULTRASOUND OF THE PAEDIATRIC HIP

Indications

1. Developmental hip dysplasia

2. Hip effusion
3. Slipped femoral capital epiphysis.

Equipment

5–7.5 MHz linear transducer.

Technique

Developmental hip dysplasia

With ultrasonography the unossified elements of the hip – femoral head, greater trochanter, labrum, triradiate cartilage – as well as the bony acetabular roof, can be identified in the first 6 months of life.[1] After 9–12 months the degree of ossification precludes adequate imaging by US and plain film radiography becomes superior. There are two main methods – static and dynamic, and both may be used during one examination.

Static (Graf) method

This assesses the morphology and geometry of the acetabulum. Although independent of the position of the infant, it is recommended that the infant be placed in the decubitus position. A single longitudinal image is obtained with the transducer placed over the greater trochanter and held at right angles to all the anatomical planes. The following landmarks are identified, and in the following sequence: chondroosseous boundary between femoral shaft and head, joint capsule, labrum, cartilaginous roof, superior bony rim of acetabulum. Although most images can be 'eyeballed', two angles can be measured from the image and form the basis for the Graf classification.[2]

Dynamic method

This assesses the stability of the hip when stressed. The hip is studied in the coronal and axial planes with the infant supine. With the hip flexed and adducted, the femur is pushed and pulled with a piston-like action.[3]

Hip joint effusion

Approximately 50% of children with acute hip pain have intra-articular fluid[4] and the sensitivity of US for detecting effusion approaches 100%. With the child supine, the hip is scanned anteriorly with the transducer parallel to the femoral neck. Bulging of the anterior portion of the joint capsule can be readily identified[5]. The normal distance between the bony femoral neck and the joint capsule is always less than 3 mm, and the difference between the affected and unaffected sides should not be greater than 2 mm.

Slipped femoral capital epiphysis

Although plain radiographs constitute the usual means of diagnosis, a mild posterior slip can be identified in the acute situation by longitudinal scanning along the femoral neck.

References

1. Youzefzadeh, D. & Ramilo J.L. (1987) Normal hip in children: correlation of U.S. with anatomic and cryomicrotome sections. *Radiology* **165**, 647–655.
2. Graf, R. (1987) *Guide to Sonography of the Infant Hip.* New York: Thième Medical.
3. Clark, N.M.P., Harcke, T.H., McHugh, P. et al. (1985) Real time ultrasound in the diagnosis of congenital dislocation and dysplasia of the hip. *J. Bone Joint Surg.* **67B**, 406–412.
4. Dörr, U., Zieger, M. & Hanke, H. (1988) Ultrasonography of the painful hip. Prospective studies in 204 patients. *Pediatr. Radiol.* **19**, 36–40.
5. Miralles, M., Gonzalea, G., Pulpeiro, J.R. et al. (1989) Sonography of the painful hip in children: 500 consecutive cases. *Am. J. Roentgenol.* **152**, 579–582.

RADIONUCLIDE BONE SCAN

Indications

1. Staging of cancer and response to therapy, especially breast, prostatic and bronchial carcinoma
2. Assessment of primary bone tumours
3. Bone infections
4. Metabolic bone disease
5. Bone pain
6. Painful hip and knee prosthesis
7. Avascular necrosis and bone infarction
8. Trauma not obvious on X-ray, e.g. stress fractures
9. Osteoarthritis
10. Assessment of non-accidental injury.

Contraindications

None.

Radiopharmaceuticals

^{99m}Tc-methylene diphosphonate (MDP) or other ^{99m}Tc-labelled diphosphonate, 500 MBq typical, 600 MBq max (3 mSv ED), 800 MBq SPECT (5 mSv ED).

These compounds are phosphate analogues which are stable in vivo and rapidly excreted by the kidneys, so giving a good contrast between bone and soft tissue.

Equipment

1. Gamma-camera, preferably with SPECT and whole body imaging
2. Low-energy high-resolution collimator.

Patient preparation

The patient must be well hydrated.

Technique

1. ^{99m}Tc-diphosphonate is injected i.v. When infection is suspected or blood flow to bone or primary bone tumour is to be assessed, a bolus injection is given with the patient in position on the camera. A three-phase study is then performed with arterial, blood-pool and delayed static imaging.
2. The patient should be encouraged to drink plenty and empty the bladder frequently.
3. The bladder is emptied immediately prior to imaging.
4. Delayed static imaging is performed 2 or more hours after injection: up to 4 h for imaging of extremities and up to 6 h for those on dialysis or in renal failure.

Films

Standard

High-resolution images are acquired with a pixel size of 1–2 mm.

1. The whole skeleton. The number of views will depend upon the field of view of the camera and whether a whole-body imaging facility is available. A point to consider is that whole-body images will have lower resolution than spot views over parts of the skeleton where the camera is some distance from the patient (unless a body-contour tracking facility is available), since resolution falls off with distance. Spot views should be overlapping.
2. Anterior oblique views of the thorax are useful to separate sternum and spine uptake.
3. For examination of the posterior ribs, scapula or shoulder, an extra posterior thorax view with arms above the head should be taken to move the scapula away from the ribs.
4. For imaging small bones and joints, magnified views should be taken, with a pinhole collimator if necessary.
5. SPECT can be useful for lesion localization, e.g. in vertebrae and joints, and to detect avascular necrosis.[1]

Three-phase

1. *Arterial phase 1*: 1–2 s frames of the area of interest for 1 min post-injection.
2. *Blood pool phase 2*: 3-min image of the same area 5 min post-injection.
3. *Delayed phase 3*: views 2 or more hours post-injection, as for standard imaging.

Analysis

1. For the arterial phase, time–activity curves are created for regions of interest symmetrical about the mid-line.
2. For SPECT, reconstruction of transaxial, coronal, sagittal and possibly oblique slices to demonstrate the lesion.

Additional techniques

1. SPECT can be useful for improved lesion detection and localization in complex bony structures, e.g. spine and knees.[2]
2. Additional information about renal function may be obtained with dynamic imaging during the first 20–30 min post-injection, e.g. in prostatic carcinoma.[3]

Aftercare

Normal radiation safety precautions (see Chapter 1).

Complications

None.

References

1. Murray, I.P.C. & Dixon, J. (1989) The role of single photon emission computed tomography in bone scintigraphy. *Skeletal Radiol.* **18**, 493–505.
2. Ryan, P.J. & Fogelman, I. (1995) The bone scan: where are we now? *Semin. Nucl. Med.* **25**, 76–91.
3. Narayan, P., Lillian, D., Hellstrom, W., et al. (1988) The benefits of combining early radionuclide renal scintigraphy with routine bone scans in patients with prostate cancer. *J. Urol.* **140**, 1448–1451.

Further reading

Freeman, L.M. & Blaufox, M.D. (eds) (1988) Nuclear orthopedics. *Semin. Nucl. Med.* **18 (2)**.
Krasnow, A.Z., Hellman, R.S., Timins, M.E. et al. (1997) Diagnostic bone scanning in oncology. *Semin. Nucl. Med.* **27**, 107–141.

13 Brain

Methods of imaging the brain

Although imaging has explored the brain from the beginnings of radiology, many of the earlier methods are now only of historical interest, or of very restricted usefulness:

1. Plain films. These are of little value except in cases of head injury.
2. Tomography (obsolete). In departments where neither CT nor MRI are available, tomography could be said to have uses, but in practical terms it is unlikely that such departments will have the resources to deal with any pathology discovered.
3. Angiography. This is still important in intracranial haemorrhage, especially subarachnoid haemorrhage, but in centres with MRI it is of diminishing value in other clinical situations. It is, however, still often requested for preoperative assessment of tumours. Angiographic expertise is nevertheless vital for the practice of many interventional radiological techniques in the nervous system.
4. Computed tomography (CT). This is the technique of choice in most centres for the investigation of serious head injury, for suspected intracranial haemorrhage, stroke, infection, and for other acute neurological emergencies. Diagnostically highly effective, and in practice much easier and safer to use in the emergency situation than MRI.
5. Magnetic resonance imaging (MRI). This is the best and most versatile imaging modality for the brain, constrained only by availability, patient acceptability, and the logistics and safety of patient handling in emergency situations. New protocols have raised the sensitivity of MRI in subarachnoid haemorrhage, acute stroke and aneurysm detection. It is the only effective way of diagnosing multiple sclerosis, which is the commonest chronic neurological disease.
6. Radionuclide imaging. This is practised by three principal methods. Firstly there is conventional brain scanning, using

blood–brain barrier damage detection. This is obsolete where CT or MRI are available, but is nevertheless quite sensitive in the detection of metastases and meningioma. Secondly, there is regional cerebral blood flow scan scanning, still more used in research than in clinical management, especially in the dementias and in parkinsonism. Finally, there is positron emission tomography (PET). By this method focal hypermetabolism may be shown using 18F-fluoro-deoxyglucose, for example in some case of epilepsy, and cell turnover may be shown using 11C-methionine, for example in tumour studies.

7. Ultrasound (US). This is particularly of use in infants, via the fontanelles, and is of value in the study of haemorrhagic and ischaemic syndromes, developmental malformations, and hydrocephalus in the neonate, and for the first year of life. In adults, transcranial Doppler may be used for intracerebral arterial velocity studies.

Further reading

MacLaren, R.E., Ghoorahoo, H.I. & Kirby, N.G. (1993) Skull X-ray after head injury: the recommendations of the Royal College of Surgeons Working Party report in practice. Arch. Emerg. Med. **10**, 138–144.

CT OF THE BRAIN

Indications

The best indications are all emergency situations. Apart from these, CT is second best, but widely used in order to conserve the scarce MRI resource for the case in which it is most important.

1. Following major head injury (if the patient has lost consciousness, has impaired consciousness, or has a neurological deficit). The presence of a skull fracture also justifies the use of CT.
2. In suspected intracranial infection (the use of contrast enhancement is mandatory).
3. In suspected intracranial haemorrhage (sensitive in the detection of subarachnoid haemorrhage for several days after the ictus, dependent on the amount of blood extravasated).
4. In suspected raised intracranial pressure, and as a precaution before lumbar puncture (the evidence that CT is helpful in this situation is very slender indeed, but the practice is now so

widespread that it is very difficult to avoid compliance with the clinicians request).

5. In cases of stroke, both ischaemic and haemorrhagic.

6. In other situations, such as seizures, migraine, suspected tumour, demyelination, dementia and psychosis CT is a poor tool, and if imaging can be justified, MRI is greatly preferable. However, in practice, CT will often be used for these indications.

Technique

1. Most clinical indications are adequately covered by a series of 5-mm sections parallel to the floor of the anterior cranial fossa, from the foramen magnum to the lower third ventricle, with 10-mm sections to the vertex. In trauma cases, hard copy should include both soft tissue and bone windowed images.

2. In suspected infection, tumours, vascular malformations and subacute infarction, the sections should be repeated following intravenous contrast enhancement (using the equivalent of 15 g iodine, any of the modern non-ionic monomeric contrast media is suitable. Standard precautions with regard to a possible adverse response to contrast medium should be taken).

MRI OF THE BRAIN   MRI

Indications

All cases of suspected intracranial pathology in which imaging is likely to be helpful, except for those listed 1–5 in the CT section above. Techniques in use vary widely, and continue to change with the development of new imaging sequences, and the continuing exploration of the usefulness of MRI. The techniques described below are therefore only a guide to basic methods in use. The most single useful precept in the planning of any study is the knowledge that the versatility of MRI lies in the differing information content of images weighted for different signal characteristics, and obtained in a variety of imaging planes.

Technique

1. Long TR sequences. Such sequences may be used with conventional or fast spin-echo methods to produce images weighted for proton density and for T2 relaxation time. Formerly such dual-echo techniques were very time

consuming, but it is now possible to cover the whole brain with a sequence of twenty 5-mm sections with a 1 mm interspace, obtaining both proton density and T2-weighted images, in less than 4 min. Many standard brain protocols in everyday use routinely employ fast spin echo sequences of this type in transverse and coronal planes.

2. Short TR sequences. T1-weighted sections are anatomically rich, but as a broad generalization they less helpful for disease detection except in conjunction with intravenous gadolinium contrast enhancement. However, it is common practice to obtain a sagittal T1-weighted sequence as part of a standard brain study.

3. Gradient-echo (field-echo) T2-weighted sequences. Although suffering from various artefacts, the sensitivity of these sequences to susceptibility effects makes them very sensitive to the presence of the sequelae of cerebral haemorrhage, such as in cases of previous head injury. Residual haemosiderin produces marked focal loss of signal in such cases, and all patients with a history of head injury or other cause of haemorrhage should be imaged by this method. Use of the coronal plane simplifies the recognition of susceptibility artefacts arising from the skull base and air sinuses.

4. FLAIR sequences (*FL*uid *A*ttenuated *I*nversion *R*ecovery) provide great sensitivity in the detection of demyelination and infarction, and have the advantage that juxta-ventricular pathology contrasts with dark cerebrospinal fluid (CSF), and is not lost by proximity to the intense brightness of the ventricular CSF, as is sometimes the case in spin-echo T2-weighted studies.

5. Angiographic sequences. There are many possible methods, of which 'time-of flight' is one of the more commonly used. This is a very short TR, T1-weighted gradient echo 3D sequence, with sequential presaturation of each partition so that only non-presaturated inflowing blood gives a high signal. Image display is by so-called 'MIP' or maximum intensity projection, giving a 3D model of the intracranial vessels.

IMAGING OF ACOUSTIC NEUROMAS

The older methods, using plain films of the internal auditory meatus, evoked brain stem responses and caloric testing are now largely obsolete. MRI is the definitive diagnostic method, and is in effect the only investigation necessary. Although expensive, newer systems are able to carry out large numbers of acoustic neuroma studies in a short space of time, without the use of contrast material. As a result the net cost-effectiveness is high, and the need for the older methods is eliminated. The neurophysiological methods, although quite sensitive, tended to produce a large number of false positives, which required confirmation by MRI.

COMPUTERIZED TOMOGRAPHY

Intravenous contrast-enhanced axial CT with bone and soft-tissue-windowed images was the standard method of diagnosis of acoustic neuroma prior to the introduction of MRI. Most departments used 5-mm axial sections, though some authors recommended 2-mm sections. It was unusual to show tumours less than 1 cm in size by this method, and intracanalicular tumours could not be shown. CT-air meatography enjoyed a brief vogue as a high sensitivity method when MRI was less widely available. The requirement for the introduction of a small amount of air by lumbar puncture, and some temporary resulting morbidity were its main disadvantages, together with a small number of false positive studies (there were virtually no false negatives).

MAGNETIC RESONANCE IMAGING

The quality of thin T2-weighted sections with older 0.5-T MRI systems is insufficiently good to allow their effective use as a screening method, and accordingly on such systems it is necessary to obtain T1-weighted sections before and after gadolinium enhancement, in transverse and coronal planes. If only post-contrast studies are obtained, it will occasionally be necessary to recall the patient in apparently positive cases to ensure that the rare lipoma has not been mistaken for an enhancing tumour. Sections should be 3–4-mm thick, with minimal interspace.

On modern 1.0- or 1.5-T systems, the spatial and contrast resolution is such that acoustic neuroma may be diagnosed on high-resolution (512 matrix) T2-weighted images without the need for intravenous contrast. Three-mm, near-contiguous sections are required in transverse and coronal planes.

Further reading
Daniels, R.L., Shelton, C. & Harnsberger, H.R. (1998) Ultra high resolution nonenhanced fast spin echo magnetic resonance imaging: cost-effective screening for acoustic neuroma in patients with sudden sensori-neural hearing loss. *Otolaryngol. Head Neck Surg.* **119**, 364–369.

Robson, A.K., Leighton, S.E., Anslow, P. & Milford, C.A. (1993) MRI as a single screening procedure for acoustic neuroma: a cost effective protocol. *J. Roy. Soc. Med.* **86**, 455–457.

IMAGING THE PITUITARY

The older methods, consisting of plain films, pituitary fossa tomography, air encephalography, CT cisternography, and cavernous sinus venography are now only of historical interest.

COMPUTERIZED TOMOGRAPHY

CT is still used for the demonstration of pituitary disease, but is less sensitive than MRI because of lower contrast resolution, beam-hardening artefacts and restricted imaging planes (axial and coronal). In addition the coronal imaging plane requires uncomfortable neck extension, which may be impossible in older patients, and in the presence of cervical spondylosis. For these reasons MRI is preferable where available, but since MRI is still a limited resource, the technique for the use of CT is described:

1. The patient is positioned for coronal imaging. Most patients seem to prefer the supine position, but an equivalent position can also be achieved with the patient prone, and there is no difference in the images obtained. Maximum neck extension is supplemented by gantry angulation, to achieve as near as possible to a true coronal image, perpendicular to the radiographic baseline.
2. Intravenous contrast medium (the equivalent of 30 g of iodine; any of the current non-ionic monomers is suitable) is given immediately prior to imaging, since blood pool imaging gives better tumour to gland contrast. If a very slow CT scanner is in use, a continuous i.v. infusion of contrast medium during the study is preferable.
3. Contiguous 2-mm sections through the whole pituitary gland are obtained, using a 16-cm field of view.
4. The images are viewed and hard copied on soft tissue window settings.

MAGNETIC RESONANCE IMAGING

MRI is more comfortable for the patient, has better contrast resolution and spatial resolution, which is generally at least as good as CT and on modern high field scanners is substantially better.

1. Imaging may be performed in any plane, but generally sagittal and coronal planes are used.
2. Spin-echo T1-weighted sections are widely used, before and after gadolinium enhancement. T2-weighted coronal sections are of occasional use. Susceptibility effects close to the skull base make gradient echo sequences less effective.
3. 3-mm sections are optimal on most equipment, though some modern scanners allow 2-mm sections with good signal to noise ratio. A 16-cm field of view is appropriate, any wrap around artefact not intruding into area of interest.

PETROSAL SINUS SAMPLING

The blood draining from the pituitary into the two inferior petrosal sinuses is sampled. Catheters are introduced into the femoral veins and advanced through the venous system, into the jugular bulbs. The inferior petrosal sinuses drain into the jugular bulb, and the catheters are placed in their ostia (headhunter 1-shaped catheters are suitable).

After obtaining peripheral and baseline readings, cortico-trophin releasing hormone is injected, and the ACTH level assayed on each side at intervals for 30 min. Lateralization of a functioning tumour may be determined by identifying the side on which the higher level of ACTH is found.

RADIONUCLIDE IMAGING   RN

There are three main modalities: conventional radionuclide brain scanning (blood–brain barrier imaging), regional cerebral blood flow imaging and positron emission tomography (PET imaging).

CONVENTIONAL RADIONUCLIDE BRAIN SCANNING (BLOOD–BRAIN BARRIER IMAGING)

Indications

None if CT and/or MRI are available. Otherwise there is reason-able sensitivity in the detection of cerebral metastases, meningioma and high-grade glioma.

Contraindications

None.

Radiopharmaceuticals

1. ^{99m}Tc-DTPA. Crosses the damaged blood–brain barrier and demonstrates areas of increased vascularity. Higher lesion-to-background ratio than pertechnetate because of faster plasma clearance.
2. ^{99m}Tc-pertechnetate. Crosses the damaged blood–brain barrier, but accumulates in the choroid plexus, thyroid and salivary glands, so requires prior blocking with potassium perchlorate. Considered inferior to DTPA.[1]
3. ^{99m}Tc-glucoheptonate. Similar efficacy to DTPA, but no longer available in the UK.

500 MBq max for static imaging (3 mSv ED), 800 MBq max for dynamic imaging and SPECT (5 mSv ED).

Equipment

1. Gamma-camera
2. Low-energy general purpose collimator.

Patient preparation

Pertechnetate only: blockade with 200–400 mg potassium perchlorate orally 30–90 min before study or 50–100 mg sodium perchlorate i.v. at the time of radiopharmaceutical injection.

Technique

The study consists of a dynamic or vascular phase followed by static imaging.

1. The patient lies supine with the camera centred over head and neck to include the carotid arteries. If information about intracranial arterial flow alone is required, the camera is positioned over the vertex of the skull.
2. A rapid i.v. injection of radiopharmaceutical in a small volume is given, starting computer acquisition at the same time.
3. Dynamic images are acquired for 1 min following injection to assess flow in the major arteries.
4. Static views 1–2 h after injection.
5. Delayed images at 3–5 h can improve the sensitivity.

Images

1. *Dynamic.* Anterior, 60 × 1-s frames on computer. Hard copy:

2-s images from first arrival of bolus generated from computer images, or 2–6 s analogue images for 1 min post-injection.
2. *Static*. Patient sitting if capable; 300–500 kilocounts per view:
   a. anterior, forehead and nose in contact with camera
   b. posterior, head well flexed to separate posterior fossa from nasal mucosa
   c. left and right lateral
   d. a vertex view may be taken to improve demonstration of lesions high in the cerebral hemispheres.

Analysis

Dynamic. Time–activity curves are produced from regions over the carotid arteries and cerebral hemispheres.

Aftercare

Normal radiation safety precautions (see General Notes).

Complications

None.

Reference

1. Banzo, J.I., Banzo, J., Abós, M.D., et al. (1982) ^{99m}Tc-DTPA and ^{99m}Tc-GH cerebral imaging: a comparative analysis. *Nucl. Med. Commun.* **3**, 304–308.

Further reading

Nisbet, A.P., Ratcliffe, G.E., Ellam, S.V., et al. (1983) Clinical indications for optimal use of the radionuclide brain scan. *Br. J. Radiol.* **56**, 377–381.
Smith, F.W. (1998) The central nervous system. In: Sharp, P.F., Gemmell, H.G. & Smith, F.W. (eds) *Practical Nuclear Medicine*, pp. 119–134. Oxford: Oxford University Press.

REGIONAL CEREBRAL BLOOD FLOW IMAGING   RN

Indications

1. Localization of epileptic foci
2. Mapping of cerebrovascular disease
3. Investigation of dementias including Huntington's and Alzheimer's disease
4. Assessment of effects of treatment regimes
5. Confirmation of brain death.

Contraindications

None.

Radiopharmaceuticals[1]

1. ^{99m}Tc-hexamethylpropyleneamineoxime (HMPAO or exametazime), 500 MBq (5 mSv ED).

   The most commonly used agent, HMPAO is a lipophilic complex that crosses the blood–brain barrier and localizes roughly in proportion to cerebral blood flow. It is rapidly extracted by the brain, reaching a peak of 5–6% of injected activity within a minute or so, with minimal redistribution (about 86% remains in the brain at 24 h). It has the disadvantage of a short shelf life once reconstituted, and the manufacturer advises use within 30 min. However, efforts have been made to stabilize the product,[2] and a commercial kit which is stable for up to 6 h or so may soon be available.

2. ^{99m}Tc-ethyl cysteinate dimer (ECD), 500 MBq (5 mSv ED).

   Also localizes rapidly in proportion to cerebral blood flow, but the distribution has some differences to that of HMPAO which may need to be taken into consideration for clinical diagnosis.[3,4] It currently has the advantage of greater stability than HMPAO and can be used for up to 6 h after reconstitution, which is of particular benefit for ictal epilepsy studies where an injection is only given once a seizure occurs.

Equipment

1. SPECT gamma camera, preferably dual-headed
2. SPECT imaging couch with head extension
3. Low-energy high-resolution collimator (or more specialized slant-hole or fan-beam collimator).

Patient preparation

Since cerebral blood flow is continuously varying with motor activity, sensory stimulation, emotional arousal, etc., it is important to standardize the conditions under which the tracer is administered, especially if serial studies are to be undertaken in the same individual. Familiarization with the procedure to reduce anxiety and injection in a relaxing environment through a previously positioned i.v. cannula should be considered.

For localization of epileptic foci, ictal studies are much more sensitive than interictal, and if feasible the patient should be admitted under constant monitoring, with injection as soon as a seizure starts.

Technique

1. Administer 500 MBq of tracer

2. SPECT imaging is performed any time from 5 min to 2 h or so after injection with the patient supine. Ensure that the head is not rotated and care is taken to obtain the smallest orbit possible – a 12 cm radius orbit should be feasible on most heads, with the shoulders moved down as far as possible to avoid coming into contact with the camera.

Images

The acquisition protocol will depend upon the system available. Suitable parameters for a modern single-headed gamma-camera might be:

1. 360° circular orbit.
2. 60–90 projections or continuous rotation over a 30-min acquisition.
3. Combination of matrix size and zoom to give a pixel size of 3–4 mm.

Analysis

A cine film of the projections is looked at before the patient leaves to detect any movement. If significant movement has occurred and cannot be corrected by computer motion correction algorithms available, the patient must be re-scanned. Transverse, coronal and sagittal slices parallel and orthogonal to the orbitomeatal plane with a thickness of approximately 8 mm are reconstructed.

Additional techniques

1. If blood flow in the carotid and major cerebral arteries is of interest, a dynamic study during injection is performed. The patient lies supine with the camera anterior. If information about intracranial arterial blood flow alone is required, the camera is positioned over the vertex of the skull. The tracer is administered rapidly in a small volume, and dynamic imaging commenced with 60×1-s frames. Time-activity curves are then produced from regions over the carotid arteries and cerebral hemispheres.
2. Three-dimensional mapping of activity distributions onto standard brain atlases, image registration with MRI, CT and quantitative analysis are areas of increasing interest, but these are still complex procedures and are not yet in routine use.[5]

Aftercare

Radiation dose may be reduced by administration of a mild laxative on the day after the study and maintenance of good hydration to promote urine output.

Complications

None.

References

1. Saha, G.P., Macintyre, W.J., & Go, R.T. (1994) Radiopharmaceuticals for brain imaging. *Semin. Nucl. Med.* **24**, 324–349.
2. Solanki, C., Wraight, E.P., Barber, R.W., et al. (1998) Seven-hour stabilization of $^{99}Tc^{m}$-exametazime (HMPAO) for cerebral perfusion. *Nucl. Med. Commun.* **19**, 567–572.
3. Asenbaum, S., Brucke, T., Pirker, W., et al. (1998) Imaging of cerebral blood flow with technetium-99m-HMPAO and technetium-99m-ECD: a comparison. *J. Nucl. Med.* **39**, 613–618.
4. Koyama, M., Kawashima, R., Ito, H., et al. (1997) SPECT imaging of normal subjects with technetium-99m-HMPAO and technetium-99m-ECD. *J. Nucl. Med.* **38**, 587–592.
5. Costa, D.C., Pilowsky, L.S. & Ell, P.J. (1999) Nuclear medicine in neurology and psychiatry. *Lancet* **354**, 1107–1111.

Further reading

Costa, D.C. & Ell, P.J. (1991) *Clinician's Guide to Nuclear Medicine: Brain Blood Flow in Neurology and Psychiatry.* Edinburgh: Churchill Livingstone.
Messa, C., Fazio, F., Costa, D.C., et al (1995) Clinical brain radionuclide imaging studies. *Semin. Nucl. Med.* **25**, 111–143.

ULTRASOUND OF THE INFANT BRAIN

Indications

Any suspected intracranial pathology, particularly suspected haemorrhage or ischaemia, developmental malformations, and hydrocephalus.

Equipment

5-MHz, sector transducer. Occasionally a 3.5-MHz transducer may be needed for larger brains and a 7.5- or 10-MHz transducer may be necessary to visualize superficial structures.

Patient preparation

None is generally required, though a recently fed infant is more likely to submit to examination without protest. A fractious child should be calmed by the mother or other carer by any appropriate method.

Methods

1. Via the anterior fontanelle (method described below)
2. Through the squamosal portion of the temporal bone to

visualize extracerebral collections and the region of the circle of Willis and to obtain Doppler signals of the middle cerebral arteries

3. Via the posterior fontanelle, for the posterior fossa.

Technique

Six coronal and six sagittal images are obtained and supplemented with other images of specific areas of interest. The base of the skull must be perfectly symmetrical on coronal scans. The first image is obtained with the transducer angled forward and subsequent images obtained by angling progressively more posteriorly. The anatomical landmarks that define each view are:

Coronal

1. The orbital roofs and cribriform plate (these combine to produce a 'steer's head' appearance); anterior interhemispheric fissure; frontal lobes.
2. Greater wings, lesser wings and body of sphenoid (these produce a 'mask' appearance); the cingulate sulcus; frontal horns of lateral ventricles.
3. Pentagon view: five-sided star formed by the internal carotid, middle cerebral and anterior cerebral arteries (these may be observed to pulsate and Doppler interrogation is possible).
4. Frontal horns of lateral ventricles; cavum septum pellucidum; basal ganglia. Bilateral C-shaped echoes from the parahippocampal gyri; thalami.
5. Trigones of lateral ventricles containing choroid plexus; echogenic inverted V from the tentorium cerebelli; cerebellum.
6. Occipital horns of lateral ventricles; parietal and occipital cortex; cerebellum.

Sagittal

For the sagittal images, the reference plane should be a mid-line image with the third ventricle, septum pellucidum and fourth ventricle all on the same image. The more lateral parasagittal images are obtained with the transducer angled laterally and slightly oblique because the occipital horn of the lateral ventricle is more lateral than the frontal horn.

1. Two views of the mid-line.
2. Parasagittal scan of the left lateral ventricle. This is angled approximately 15° from the mid-line.
3. Steep parasagittal scan, approximately 30° from the mid-line, of the left frontal, temporal and parietal cortex.

4. Parasagittal scan of the right lateral ventricle.
5. Steep parasagittal scan of the right frontal, temporal and parietal cortex.

CEREBRAL ANGIOGRAPHY

Indications

1. Intracerebral and subarachnoid haemorrhage (in the investigation of suspected intracranial aneurysms and arteriovenous malformations)
2. Aneurysms presenting as space occupying lesions
3. Cavernous sinus syndromes
4. Carotico-cavernous fistula
5. Cerebral ischaemia both of extracranial and intracranial origin
6. Preoperative assessment of cerebral tumours
7. Suspected venous sinus thrombosis.

NB: All these indications are in a state of regular review with the continuing advancement in the capabilities of MRI.

Contraindications

1. Patients with unstable neurology (usually following subarachnoid haemorrhage or stroke)
2. Patients unsuitable for surgery
3. Patients in whom vascular access would be impossible or excessively risky.

Equipment

Single or biplane digital subtraction angiography apparatus, with a C-arm allowing unlimited imaging planes, high quality fluoroscopy, and preferably a road mapping facility. There should be good access for the radiologist and anaesthetist to the patient and appropriate head immobilization facilities.

Preparation

When the patient is able to understand what is proposed, a clear explanation should be given, together with a fair presentation of the risks and benefits. Most patients can be examined using mild oral sedation, e.g. 5–10 mg of diazepam. Children, patients who are excessively anxious, those who cannot cooperate because of confusion, or who would be managed better during the procedure with full ventilation control are examined under general anaesthesia. Most interventional studies are better done under general anaesthesia. Groin shaving is now regarded as unnecessary in many departments, but may be used if this is local practice. Patients should not be starved unless general anaesthesia is to be used, but should nevertheless be restricted to fluid intake and only very light food intake.

Technique

Catheter flushing solutions should consist of heparinized saline (2500 IU l^{-1} of normal saline). Using standard percutaneous catheter introduction technique, the femoral artery (usually the right side for convenience) is catheterized. There is a wide range of catheters available and there are proponents of many types. In patients up to middle age without major hypertension, there will be little difficulty with any standard catheter, and a simple 5-F polythene catheter with a slightly curved tip will suffice in the great majority. Older patients and arteriopaths will need catheters offering greater torque control, the headhunter (Fig. 13.1) and sidewinder (Fig. 13.2)

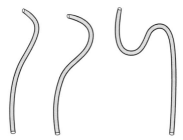

End holes: 1   Side holes: 0

Figure 13.1   Headhunter catheters.

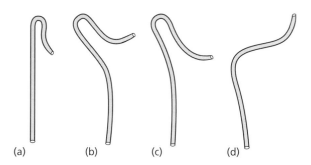

(a)   (b)   (c)   (d)

End holes: 1   Side holes: 0

Figure 13.2   Simmons (sidewinder) catheters. (a) For narrow aorta. (b) For moderately narrow aorta. (c) For wide aorta. (d) For elongated aorta.

shapes are appropriate; 6-F may be preferred for greater stability. If the patient has a large amount of subcutaneous fat in the puncture area, catheter control will be better if passed through an introducer set, and this is also indicated where it is anticipated that catheter exchange may be required. The detail of the selection of individual vessels is beyond the scope of this book, but the following points should be noted:

1. The hazards of cerebral angiography are very largely avoidable; they consist of the complications common to all forms of angiography (see Chapter 9) and those which are particularly related to cerebral angiography.
2. Any on-table ischaemic event has an explanation. Cerebral angiography does not possess an inherently unavoidable complication rate as has been suggested in the past. If an event occurs there has been a mistake, and its cause must be identified so that it will not happen again.
3. The most significant complications are embolic in origin, and the most important emboli are particulate. Air bubbles should be avoided as part of good angiographic practice, but are unlikely to cause a neurological complication. In contrast, an injection of a solid particle may well cause a neurological deficit.
4. Emboli may come from the injected solutions. Avoid contamination from glove powder, and dried blood or clot on gloves. Take care to avoid blood contamination of the saline which may sometimes be dangerous, or contamination of the contrast medium which is always dangerous. Avoid exposure of solutions to air. Contrast medium or heparin/saline in an open bowl is bad practice.
5. Emboli may arise from dislodgement of plaque or thrombus. Never pass a catheter or guide-wire through a vessel that has not been visualized by preliminary injection of contrast medium. Use appropriate guide-wires: if there is any resistance to the passage of a standard wire use a more flexible or a hydrophilic wire. Do not try to negotiate excessively acute bends in vessels. The splinting effect of the catheter will cause spasm and arrest the flow in the artery. Also dissection may occur which may lead to occlusion. Sharp curves can only be safely negotiated with microcatheters, which have interventional rather than diagnostic applications for the most part.
6. Emboli may arise from the formation of thrombus within a catheterized vessel. Always ensure that there is free blood flow

past the catheter, and avoid forceful or impatient passage of a guide-wire or catheter in such a way as may damage the intima of the vessel and cause thrombus formation.

7. Emboli may arise within the catheter. Do not allow blood to flow back into the catheter, flush regularly or by continuous infusion. Never allow a guide-wire to remain within a catheter for more than 1 min without withdrawal and flushing, and never introduce a guide-wire into a contrast filled catheter, but fill the catheter with heparinized saline first.

8. Keep study time to a minimum, but not at the expense of curtailing the study, thus necessitating a repeat examination.

Contrast medium

Nonionic monomer e.g. iohexol, iopamidol. The concentration required is equipment-dependent, but with a good DSA set, about $150 \, \mathrm{mg \, I \, ml^{-1}}$ will be suitable, i.e. 50% dilution of a standard $300 \, \mathrm{mg \, I \, ml^{-1}}$ solution.

Contrast medium volume

1. Into the common carotid – about 10 ml by hand in about 1.5–2 s.
2. Into the internal carotid – about 7 ml by hand in about 1.5 s.
3. Into the vertebral artery – about 6 ml by hand in about 1.5 s.

Projections

As required, but basically AP, Townes, lateral, occipitomental, submento-vertical and oblique views as indicated. Multiple projections are especially needed for aneurysm studies to open loops and profile aneurysms.

Films

From early arterial to late venous, about 8 s in total in most cases, at about 2–4 frames $\mathrm{s^{-1}}$ depending on the type of study.

Aftercare

1. Standard nursing care for the arterial puncture site.
2. Most departments adopt the practice of maintaining neurological observation for a period of 4 h or so after the procedure.
3. Good hydration should be maintained.

14 Spine

Methods of imaging the spine

As with the brain, many of the earlier methods are now only of historical interest.

1. Plain films. These are of little management value in chronic back pain because of the prevalence of degenerative changes in both symptomatic and asymptomatic individuals of all ages beyond the second decade. They are, however, indicated in suspected spinal injury, in developmental malformations and for the demonstration of spondylolisthesis.

2. Tomography (obsolete except where CT or MRI are unavailable).

3. Myelography/radiculography. This is used for the lumbar spine where neither CT or MRI are available, or for the cervical spine where MRI is unavailable. There is an occasional requirement where MRI is contraindicated or unacceptable to the patient.

4. Discography is not widely practised in the UK, though advocates still regard it as the only technique able to verify the presence and source of discogenic pain, and it is widely accepted by American radiologists.

5. Facet joint arthrography. This is a technique for the verification of pain of facet joint origin, and for injection of local anaesthetic. The radiological appearances of the arthrogram are not helpful for the most part.

6. Epidurography (obsolete).

7. Lumbar epidural venography (obsolete).

8. Arteriography. This is used for further study of vascular malformations shown by other methods, usually MRI, and for assessment for potential embolotherapy. It is not appropriate for the primary diagnosis of spinal vascular malformations.

9. CT with CSF opacification by intrathecal contrast medium, or CT myelography. This is a sensitive technique for cervical

radiculopathy studies, but declining in usage with improving MR instrumentation. CT with intravenous contrast medium is now obsolete.

10. Radionuclide imaging. This is largely performed for suspected bone metastases, for which it is a sensitive and cost-effective technique. Plain films are required in addition to tracer images as focal high activity may result from associated degenerative disease.

11. Magnetic resonance imaging, if necessary with intravenous gadolinium enhancement. This is the preferred technique for most spinal pathology. It is the only technique for diagnosing spinal multiple sclerosis, and by far the best technique for the acute management of spinal compression.

12. Ultrasound is of use as an intraoperative method, and has uses in the infant spine.

IMAGING APPROACH TO BACK PAIN AND SCIATICA: THE USE OF CT AND MRI

There are many ways to image the spine, many of which are expensive. The role of the radiologist is to ensure that diagnostic algorithms are selected for diagnostic accuracy, clinical relevance and cost-effectiveness. Each diagnostic imaging procedure has a different degree of sensitivity and specificity when applied to a particular diagnostic problem. A combination of imaging techniques can be used in a complementary way to enhance diagnostic accuracy. The appropriate use of the available methods of investigating the spine is essential, requiring a sensible sequence and timing of the procedures to ensure cost-effectiveness, maximal diagnostic accuracy and minimum discomfort to the patient.

The philosophy underlying the management of low back pain and sciatica encompasses the following fundamental points:

1. Radiological investigation is essential if surgery is proposed.
2. Radiological findings should be compatible with the clinical picture before surgery can be advised.
3. It is vital for the surgeon and radiologist to identify those patients who will and who will not benefit from surgery.
4. In those patients judged to be in need of surgical intervention, success is very dependent on precise identification of the site, nature and extent of disease by the radiologist.

The need for radiological investigation of the lumbosacral spine is based on the results of a thorough clinical examination. A useful and basic preliminary step, which will avoid unnecessary investigations, is to determine whether the predominant symptom is back pain or leg pain. Leg pain extending to the foot is indicative of nerve root compression and imaging needs to be directed towards the demonstration of a compressive lesion, typically disc prolapse. This is most commonly seen at the L4/5 or L5/S1 levels (90–95%), and the non-invasive techniques, CT and MRI, should be employed as the primary modes of imaging. If the predominant symptom is back pain with or without proximal lower limb radiation, then invasive techniques may be required, including discography and facet joint arthrography. The presence of degenerative disc and facet disease demonstrated by plain films, CT or MRI bears no direct correlation with the incidence of clinical symptomatology. The annulus fibrosus of the intervertebral disc and the facet joints are richly innervated, and only direct injection can assess them as a potential pain source. However unless there are therapeutic implications, there is no indication to proceed to these lengths, as many of patients can be managed by physical methods and mild analgesics.

PLAIN RADIOGRAPHY

Routine plain radiographic evaluation at the initial assessment of a patient with acute low back pain does not usually provide clinically useful information. Eighty-five per cent of such patients will return to work within 2 months having received only conservative therapy, indicating the potential for non-contributory plain films. Despite the known limitations of plain films, it is often helpful to obtain routine radiographs of the lumbar spine before other investigation is requested. The role of plain radiographs can be summarized in the following points:

1. They assist in the diagnosis of conditions that can mimic mechanical or discogenic pain, e.g. infection, spondylolysis, ankylosing spondylitis and bone tumours, though in most circumstances ^{99m}Tc scintigraphy, CT and MRI are more sensitive.

2. They serve as a technical aid to survey the vertebral column and spinal canal prior to myelography, CT and MRI, particularly in the sense of providing basic anatomical data regarding segmentation. Failure to do this may lead to errors in

interpreting correctly the vertebral level of abnormalities prior to surgery.

3. Correlation of CT or MRI data with plain film appearances is often helpful in interpretation.

CT AND MRI

The advent of CT and MRI has rendered invasive techniques such as epidurography and lumbar epidural venography obsolete. They should replace myelography as the first method for investigating suspected disc prolapse. High quality axial imaging by CT is an accurate means of demonstration of disc herniation, but in practice, many studies are less than optimal due to obesity, scoliosis and beam-hardening effects due to dense bone sclerosis. For these reasons, and because of better contrast resolution, MRI is the preferred technique. It alone has the capacity to show the morphology of the intervertebral disc, and can show ageing changes, typically dehydration, in the disc nucleus. It provides sagittal sections, which have major advantages for the demonstration of the spinal cord and cauda equina, vertebral alignment, stenosis of the spinal canal, and for showing the neural foramina. Far lateral disc herniation cannot be shown by myelography, but is readily demonstrated by CT or MRI. CT may be preferred to MRI where there is a suspected bone injury, for the assessment of tumours of bony origin, and in the study of spondylolysis. MRI in spinal stenosis provides all the required information: it shows all the relevant levels on a single image, it shows the degree of stenosis and the secondary effects such as the distension of the vertebral venous plexus. The relative contributions of bone, osteophyte, ligament or disc, while better evaluated by CT, are relatively unimportant in the management decisions. Furthermore, MRI will show conditions which may mimic spinal stenosis such as prolapsed dorsal disc, ependymoma of the conus medullaris and dural arteriovenous fistula.

Apart from the diagnosis of prolapsed intervertebral disc, CT and MRI differentiate the contained disc, where the herniated portion remains in continuity with the main body of the disc, from the sequestrated disc where there is a free migratory disc fragment. This distinction may be crucial in the choice of conservative or surgical therapy, and percutaneous rather than open surgical techniques. Despite the presence of nerve root compression, a disc prolapse can be entirely asymptomatic. Gadolinium enhancement of compressed lumbar nerve roots is seen in *symptomatic* disc prolapse with a specificity of 95.9%.[1]

Finally in the decision as to whether to choose CT or MRI it should not be forgotten that lumbar spine CT delivers a substantial radiation dose, which is important, particularly in younger patients.

The main remaining uses of myelography are in patients with claustrophobia and those who are pacemaker-dependent. There are two remaining clinical indications: first, it is necessary for the assessment of some cases of infantile spinal dysraphism, particularly suspected diastematomyelia, and there are advocates for the use of CT myelography in the investigation of MRI negative cervical radiculopathy. Myelography also allows a dynamic assessment of the spinal canal in instances of spinal stenosis and instability.

The problems of the 'post-laminectomy' patient or 'failed back surgery syndrome' are well known. Accurate preoperative assessment should limit the number of cases resulting from inappropriate surgery and surgery at the wrong level. The investigation of the postoperative lumbar spine is difficult, and re-operation has a poor outcome in many cases. Although the investigation of the postoperative lumbar spine is difficult, it is vital to make the distinction between residual or recurrent disc prolapse at the operated level and epidural fibrosis, in order to minimize the risk of a negative exploration. The best available technique is gadolinium-enhanced MRI, although success has been achieved by CT using a large volume of intravenous contrast medium for blood pool enhancement.

Arachnoiditis is a cause of postoperative symptoms and its features are shown on myelography, CT myelography and MRI. In the past, many cases were caused by the use of myodil (Pantopaque) as a myelographic contrast medium. It is likely that the use of myodil as an intrathecal contrast agent caused arachnoiditis in most cases, but this became symptomatic in only a minority. The potentiating effects of blood in the CSF, particularly as a result of surgery, have been evident in many cases. New cases of arachnoiditis are no longer seen, but there is residue of chronic disease still presenting from time to time.

Conclusions

MRI has revolutionized the imaging of spinal disease. Advantages include non-invasiveness, multiple imaging planes and lack of radiation exposure. Its superior soft tissue contrast enables the distinction of nucleus pulposus from annulus fibrosus of the healthy disc and enables the early diagnosis of degenerative changes. However, up to 35% of asymptomatic individuals before 40 years of age have significant intervertebral disc disease at one or more levels on MRI images. Correlation with the clinical evidence is therefore essential before any relevance is attached to their presence and surgery undertaken. MRI is, at present, not as accurate as discography in the diagnosis and delineation of annular disease and has stimulated a resurgence of interest in discography. MRI should be used as a predictor of the causative levels contributing to the back pain with discography having a significant role in the investigation of discogenic pain prior to surgical fusion.[2]

References

1. Tyrrell, P.N.M., Cassar-Pullicino, V.N. & McCall, I.W. (1998) Gadolinium-DTPA enhancement of symptomatic nerve roots in MRI of the lumbar spine. *Eur. Radiol.* **8**, 116–122.
2. Cassar-Pullicino, V. (1998) MRI of the ageing and herniating intervertebral disc. *Eur. J. Radiol.* **27**, 206–214.

Further Reading

Boden, S., Davis, D.O., Dina, T.S., et al. (1990) Abnormal magnetic resonance scans of the lumbar spine in asymptomatic subjects. *J. Bone Joint Surg. Am.* **72**, 403–408.

Butt, W.P. (1989) Radiology for back pain. *Clin. Radiol.* **40**, 6–10.

Du Boulay, G.H., Hawkes, S., Lee, C.C., et al. (1990) Comparing the cost of spinal MR with conventional myelography and radiculography. *Neuroradiology* **32**, 124–136.

Heuftle, M.G., Modic, M.T., Ross, J.S., et al. (1988) Lumbar spine: post-operative MR imaging with gadolinium-DTPA. *Radiology* **167**, 817–824.

Horton, W.C. & Daftari, T.K. (1992) Which disc as visualised by magnetic resonance imaging is actually a source of pain? A correlation between magnetic resonance imaging and discography. *Spine* **17**, 164–171.

Powell, M.C., Szypryt, P., Wilson, M., et al. (1986) Prevalence of lumbar disc degeneration observed by magnetic resonance in symptomless women. *Lancet* **2**, 1366–1367.

MYELOGRAPHY AND RADICULOGRAPHY

CONTRAST MEDIA

Historically the contrast media that have been used for myelography include gas (CO_2, air), lipiodol, abrodil, myodil, (Pantopaque, iodophenylate), meglumine iothalamate (Conray), meglumine iocarmate (Dimer X), metrizamide (Amipaque), iopamidol (Niopam), iohexol (Omnipaque) and iotrolan (Isovist). The early oil-based media were diagnostically poor and led to arachnoiditis. The early water-soluble media were very toxic and also led to arachnoiditis, and the first intrathecal contrast medium with acceptably low toxicity was metrizamide. This was a non-ionic dimer. Only iohexol, iopamidol and iotrolan are currently available and licensed for use in the thecal sac. Iohexol and iopamidol are non-ionic monomers, and iotrolan is a non-ionic dimer. All are well tolerated with some slight advantage in favour of iotrolan, and all are sufficiently safe to allow the use of myelography in outpatients. The slightly greater viscosity of iotrolan is also a slight advantage in controlling the flow of contrast medium.

CERVICAL MYELOGRAPHY

This may be performed by introduction of contrast medium into the thecal sac by lumbar puncture or by cervical canal puncture at C1/2. Suboccipital puncture can also be used, but is unpopular. It requires flexion of the neck to tense the ligamentum flavum, in order to permit safe puncture of the cisterna magna, but injection must then be performed after repositioning of the head with the neck in extension, to avoid contrast entry into the cranial cavity. The lateral C1/2 technique does not require head repositioning after needle placement.

Indications

Suspected spinal cord pathology or root compression in patients unable or unwilling to undergo MRI imaging.

Lateral cervical or C1/2 puncture vs. lumbar injection

Cervical puncture is quick, simple, safe and reliable, but is contra-indicated in patients with suspected high cervical or cranio-cervical pathology, and where the normal bony anatomy and landmarks are distorted or lost by anomalous development or rheumatoid disease. Complications are rare but include vertebral artery damage and inadvertent cord puncture. Cervical puncture is particularly indicated where there is severe lumbar disease, which may restrict the flow of contrast medium, and which may make lumbar puncture difficult, and when there is thoracic spinal canal stenosis. It is also required for the demonstration of the upper end of a spinal block. It is not a good technique for whole spine myelography; after completion of a cervical myelogram, the contrast medium is too dilute for effective use in the remainder of the spinal canal. When lumbar injection is used, a good lumbar study is possible without dilution, following which a cervical and thoracic study is entirely feasible. Lumbar injection for cervical myelography is as effective as cervical injection when nothing restricts the upward flow of contrast medium. The post-procedural morbidity, mainly consisting of headache is rather less after cervical puncture.

Equipment

Tilting X-ray table with a C-arm fluoroscopic facility for screening and radiography in multiple planes.

Patient preparation

Mild sedation with oral diazepam is appropriate in anxious patients, but is no longer essential to counter contrast medium toxicity. The skin puncture point is outside the hair line and no hair removal is generally needed, though the hair should be gathered into a paper cap.

Technique

1. The patient lies prone with arms at the sides and chin resting on a soft pad so that the neck is in a neutral position or in slight extension. Marked hyperextension is undesirable as it accentuates patient discomfort, particularly in those with spondylosis, who comprise the majority of patients referred for this procedure. In such cases it will further compromise a narrowed canal and may produce symptoms of cord compression. The patient must be comfortable and able to breathe easily.

2. Using lateral fluoroscopy the C1/2 space is identified. The beam should be centred at this level to minimize errors due to parallax. Head and neck adjustments may be needed to ensure a true lateral position. The aim is to puncture the subarachnoid space between the laminae of C1 and C2, at the junction of the middle and posterior thirds of the spinal canal, i.e. posterior to the spinal cord. A 20-G spinal needle is used. There is better control with the relatively stiff 20-G needle, and the requirement for a small needle size to minimize CSF loss does not apply in the cervical region, where CSF pressure is very low.

3. Using aseptic technique, the skin and subcutaneous tissues are anaesthetized with 1% lignocaine. The spinal needle is introduced with the stilette bevel parallel to the long axis of the spine, i.e. to split rather than cut the fibres of the interlaminar ligaments. Lateral fluoroscopy is used to adjust the direction of the needle, and ensure the maintenance of a perfect lateral position as the needle is advanced. It is very helpful if a nurse steadies the patient's head.

4. The sensation of the needle penetrating the dura is similar to that experienced during a lumbar puncture and the patient may experience slight discomfort at this stage. A feature that indicates that the needle tip is close to the dura is the appearance of venous blood at the needle hub as the epidural space is traversed. If the needle trajectory is too far posterior, tenting of the dura may occur, with failure to puncture the CSF space, even though AP screening may show that the needle tip has crossed the midline. Repositioning may be needed in such cases. Severe acute neck or radicular pain indicates that the needle has been directed too far anteriorly and has come into contact with an exiting nerve root. Clumsy technique is known to have caused cord puncture, but permanent neurological damage as a result is unlikely.

5. Following removal of the stilette, CSF will drip from the end of the needle, and a sample may be collected if required.

6. Under fluoroscopy a small amount of contrast medium is injected to verify correct needle tip placement. This will flow away from the needle tip and gravitate anteriorly to layer behind the vertebral bodies. Transient visualization of the dentate ligaments is obtained.

7. Injection is continued slowly until the required dose has been delivered. The cervical canal should be opacified anteriorly from the foramen magnum to C7/T1. If contrast tends to flow into the head before filling the lower cervical canal, tilt the table feet down slightly, and vice-versa if contrast is flowing into the thoracic region without filling the upper cervical canal. The total dose should not exceed 3 g of iodine, i.e. 10 ml of contrast medium with a concentration of 300 mg ml^{-1}. Adequate filling usually only requires 7–8 ml, or even less when the canal is narrow.

Aftercare

Although many centres request the patient to remain sitting or semi-recumbent for about 6 h, allowing the patient to remain ambulant does not increase the incidence of side-effects. A high fluid intake is generally encouraged, though evidence for its usefulness is lacking.

LUMBAR RADICULOGRAPHY

This may be performed by injection of contrast medium into the lumbar thecal sac. If for any reason lumbar puncture is not possible, e.g. because of lumbar spine deformity or arachnoiditis, it is possible to introduce the contrast medium from above by cervical injection. Dilution of the contrast as it passes downwards is a major disadvantage. The contrast medium is the same as that used for cervical myelography. The maximum dose is again the equivalent of 3 g of iodine, and may be given as 10 ml of contrast medium of 300 mg ml^{-1} concentration, or 12.5 ml of 240 mg ml^{-1}.

Indications

Suspected lumbar root or cauda equina compression, spinal stenosis and conus medullaris lesions in patients in whom CT is inconclusive, and who are unable or unwilling to undergo MRI.

Contraindications

Lumbar puncture is potentially hazardous in the presence of raised intracranial pressure. It may be difficult to achieve satisfactory intrathecal injection in patients who have had a recent lumbar puncture, since subdural CSF accumulates temporarily, and this space may be entered rather than the subarachnoid space. Accordingly an interval of a week or so is advisable.

Equipment

Tilting fluoroscopic table.

Patient preparation

As for cervical myelography.

Preliminary film

1. AP and lateral projections of the region under study.
   Preliminary examination of plain films is helpful to assess the anatomy of the spine, in order to facilitate the lumbar puncture, and to assist in interpretation of the images. It is important to draw the surgeon's attention to any question of ambiguous segmentation, either lumbarization or sacralization. There is a potential danger of operating at the wrong level if this is not made absolutely clear in the report. A clear description of any anomaly is required, together with a statement of how the vertebrae have been numbered in the report.

Technique

1. The lumbar thecal sac is punctured at L2/3, L3/4 or L4/5. The higher levels tend away from the most common sites of disc herniation and stenosis, and puncture may therefore be easier.
2. Lumbar puncture can technically be performed in the lateral

decubitus position, in the sitting position, or even in the prone position. The latter is unsatisfactory as the spinous processes are approximated, rendering puncture more difficult. In addition the spinal extension produces a relatively narrow thecal sac. The sitting position allows easy lumbar puncture but is unsatisfactory for two reasons. First, the injected contrast medium drops through a large volume of CSF to accumulate in the sacral sac, and becomes diluted as it descends. Second, patients may faint in this position, a complication that can be very dangerous, since the radiologist is on the wrong side of the table to help in preventing the patient from coming to any harm.

3. Accordingly, lumbar puncture should be carried out in the lateral decubitus position. Moderate spinal flexion is desirable, but there is no need for the extreme flexion sometimes demanded of the patient. The relevant interspace is one or two spinous processes above the plane of the iliac crest. If the spinous process cannot be felt, lateral fluoroscopy may help.

4. In obese patients the apparent soft tissue midline gravitates below the spinal midline. The midline position may be verified while introducing local anaesthetic (1% lignocaine) into the skin and subcutaneous tissue, though there is no need to infiltrate the interspinous ligament. A 22-G spinal needle should be used. It should be introduced with only a 10–15° cranial angulation. The passage of the needle through the interspinous ligament has a very characteristic sensation of moderate smooth resistance. Lack of resistance implies passage in the fatty tissues lateral to the midline, and a gritty sensation means impingement on the bone of the spinous process.

5. There is a tendency in inexperienced operators to introduce the needle at too steep a cranial angle, which a casual inspection of the spinous process anatomy can be shown to be incorrect. While traversing the interspinous ligament the bevel should be in the coronal plane to avoid deflection to one side or the other, but once well established in the ligament may be turned to penetrate the thecal sac parallel to its long axis.

6. There is a characteristic sudden loss of resistance as the needle enters the thecal sac, and at this time the stilette should be withdrawn to verify CSF flow out of the needle. It should then be reintroduced and the needle advanced about 2 mm to ensure that the whole of the bevel has entered the thecal sac. A flexible connector is attached, taking care not to disturb the needle position.

7. Most difficulties are technical, arising from non-midline positioning of the needle, but in the presence of canal stenosis it may be difficult to find a position among the crowded roots where good CSF flow will take place. In most cases, radiologists will prefer to observe the entry of contrast medium into the thecal sac on the fluoroscopic screen, and this is especially important if there has been any difficulty in achieving a good needle position.

8. After the contrast medium has been injected, the patient turns to lie prone, and a series of films is obtained. Before taking films ensure that the relevant segment of the spinal canal is adequately filled with contrast medium. This usually requires some degree of feet down tilt of the table, and a footrest should be in place to support the patient.

Films

1. AP and oblique views are obtained. (About 25° of obliquity is usual, but tailored in the individual case to profile the exit sleeves of the nerve roots of the cauda equina.)

2. A lateral view with a horizontal beam is useful, but further laterals in the erect or semi-erect position on flexion and extension are very useful, adding a dynamic dimension to the study not available on CT or MRI.

3. Some radiologists advocate lateral decubitus frontal oblique views, to allow full entry of contrast medium into the dependent root sleeves of the whole lumbar and lower thoracic thecal sac. When turning patients from one side to the other ensure that they turn through the prone position, as turning supine will produce irretrievable contrast medium dilution.

At this stage the study will be complete as far as the question of root compression is concerned. The films should be carefully reviewed at this stage to ensure that all areas are fully covered, as the next manoeuvre will make any return to this area impossible. If the study is good, the patient should be screened in the lateral decubitus position, and tilted level or slightly head down until the contrast medium flows up to lie across the thoraco-lumbar junction. The patient may then be turned to lie supine and films of the conus and lower thoracic area obtained in the AP projection.

Additional technique

Post-myelographic CT may be required for good visualization of the conus.

THORACIC MYELOGRAPHY

If the thoracic spine is the primary region of interest the injection is made with the patient lying on one side, with the head of the table lowered and the patient's head supported on a bolster or pad to prevent contrast medium from running up into the head. If an obstruction to flow is anticipated, about half the volume of contrast medium may be injected and observed as it flows upwards. If an obstruction is encountered, the contrast medium is allowed to accumulate against it, and the remainder of the contrast medium is then injected slowly (this may cause some discomfort or pain and patience must be used.) This manoeuvre will, in some cases, cause a little of the contrast medium to flow past the obstructing lesion and demonstrate its superior extent. If there is no obstruction, the full volume is injected. When the injection is complete, lateral films may be taken and the patient then turned to lie supine. Further AP films are then taken.

CERVICAL MYELOGRAPHY BY LUMBAR INJECTION

The technique proceeds as for thoracic myelography, but the patient remains in the lateral decubitus position until the contrast medium has entered the neck. With the head raised on a pad or bolster it will not flow past the foramen magnum. When all the contrast has reached the neck the patient is turned to lie prone, and the study then completed as for a cervical injection study.

CT MYELOGRAPHY (CTM)

CT myelography should be delayed for up to 4 h to allow dilution of the contrast medium. A very high concentration may cause difficulty in resolving the cervical nerve roots. Turning the patient a few times prior to CT ensures even distribution and reduces layering effects. In studying the spinal cord a delay is not required, though again good mixing of the CSF with contrast medium is essential. The superior contrast resolution of CT allows the definition of very dilute contrast medium, e.g. beyond a spinal block, thus avoiding the need for a cervical puncture. Nerve root exit foramina may be studied by CTM in both the lumbar and cervical region, and has been shown to be a sensitive technique, though it fails to demonstrate far lateral discs.

PAEDIATRIC MYELOGRAPHY

A few points need to be borne in mind when carrying out myelography in the paediatric age group.

1. General anaesthetic is essential for all children aged 6 years or younger, and for many children up to the age of 12 years.
2. Lumbar puncture in cases of spinal dysraphism carries the risk of damaging a low-lying cord due to tethering. The thecal sac is usually wide in these conditions and the needle should be placed laterally in the thecal sac. In addition, as low a puncture as possible will minimize the risk, though in practice spinal cord injury is very uncommon or masked by the neurologic deficit already present.
3. In dysraphism, the frequent association of cerebellar tonsillar herniation precludes lateral C1/2 puncture.

Aftercare

Most patients may be discharged home after being allowed to rest for a few hours after the study. The practice of automatic hospitalization for myelography can no longer be justified in the light of improved contrast media with very low rates of serious morbidity. The patient may remain ambulant. A good fluid intake is generally advised though its value is unproven.

Complications

1. Headache occurs in about 25% of cases, and is a little more frequent in females.
2. Nausea and vomiting in about 5%.
3. Modern contrast media do not produce seizures, and hallucinations do not occur.
4. Subdural injection of contrast medium. This occurs when only part of the needle bevel is within the subarachnoid space. Contrast medium initially remains loculated near the end of the needle, but can track freely in the subdural space to simulate intrathecal flow. When in doubt, the injection should be stopped and AP and lateral views obtained with the needle in situ. The temptation of interpreting such an examination should be resisted and the patient re-booked.
5. Extradural injection of contrast medium outlines the nerve roots well beyond the exit foramina.
6. Intramedullary injection of contrast medium. This is a complication of lateral cervical puncture and is recognized as a slit-like collection of contrast medium in the spinal canal. Small collections are without clinical significance.

LUMBAR DISCOGRAPHY

Aims

1. To opacify the disc with contrast medium in order to demonstrate degeneration and herniation.
2. To provoke and reproduce the pain for which the patient is being investigated and to assess its response to anaesthetic injection.

Indications

Given the present status of MRI, any request for discography must be considered with great care, as it is not without risk and if infection occurs the disc will be permanently damaged.

1. Suspected discogenic pain without radicular signs.
2. Confirmation of normal discs above or below a proposed surgical fusion.

Contraindications

1. None absolute.
2. Any local or distant sepsis will add to the risk of infective discitis.

Contrast medium

Non-ionic contrast media such as iopamidol or iohexol. A normal disc will usually allow up to 1.0 ml to be injected.

Equipment

1. Radiographic equipment as for myelography.
2. Discography needles – a set of two needles are used for each level
   a. outer needle, 21-G, 12.5 cm
   b. inner needle, 26-G, 15.8 cm.

Patient preparation

The procedure and its aim are explained to the patient. It is important (1) that patients are asked to describe what pain they experience and (2) that patients should not be told that they may get symptomatic pain. This precaution reduces the chance of obtaining a programmed response from the patient. No other preparation is needed. The procedure is done under local anaesthesia. Premedication and analgesia may alter the patient's subjective response to discography, diminishing its efficacy and usefulness. Diazepam may, however, be required in very anxious patients. Some authors recommend broad-spectrum antibiotic cover (e.g. cephalosporins) given immediately before the examination to minimize the risk of infection.

Preliminary film

AP and lateral films should be available or obtained.

Technique

1. There are two possible needle approaches:
   a. The posterior approach, which traverses the spinal canal
   b. The lateral oblique extradural approach, which avoids puncture of the dura and the vulnerable part of the posterior annulus. This is the preferred approach and can be carried out with the patient in the prone or left lateral decubitus position. The left lateral decubitus position is preferred, with the patient's head resting on a pillow and a pad placed in the lumbar angle to maintain a straight spine. Moderate spinal flexion is useful, especially at L5/S1.
2. Full aseptic technique is mandatory; there should be no compromise on this point. The operator and any assistant should be gowned, masked, capped and gloved, and the patient should be draped. The level to be examined is determined by fluoroscopy, and the skin is anaesthetized, usually a hand's breadth from the spinous processes.
3. The outer 21-G needle is then directed towards the posterior aspect of the disc under intermittent fluoroscopic control, at an angle of 45–60° to the vertical. An additional caudal tilt may be necessary for the L5/S1 level. This needle should reach but not traverse the annulus fibrosus. This point is recognized by a distinct feeling of resistance when the outer fibres are encountered. The 26-G needle is then introduced through the 21-G needle and the entry of its tip into the nucleus pulposus confirmed in two planes with the aid of the image intensifier prior to contrast medium injection.
4. Contrast medium is injected slowly using a 1-ml syringe. This is done under intermittent fluoroscopic control, while the pain response, the disc volume and its radiographic morphology are monitored. The resistance to flow will gradually increase in a normal disc during the 0.5–1.0-ml stage.

Films

1. AP and lateral films are obtained at each level examined.

2. At the end of the procedure after needle removal, AP and lateral films are taken in the standing position.
3. Films in flexion and extension may be useful.

Patient interrogation

Normal discs and some abnormal discs are asymptomatic. In the symptomatic abnormal discs, the pattern and distribution of pain are noted, together with any similarity to the usual symptomatology. At each symptomatic level local anaesthetic (bupivacaine hydrochloride 0.5%) may be injected to test its efficacy in producing symptomatic relief.

Aftercare

Simple analgesia may be required, and overnight admission is usually advised.

Complications

1. Discitis is the most important complication. Pain with or without pyrexia after a few days indicates this development. Narrowing of the disc space with a variable degree of endplate sclerosis is seen after a few weeks. Most cases are due to low-grade infection and require treatment with antibiotics.
2. With the transdural approach, post-lumbar puncture headache and/or vomiting may occur.

Further reading

Calhoun, W., McCall, I.W., Williams, W. & Cassar-Pullicino, V.N. (1988) Provocation discography as a guide to planning operations on the spine. *J. Bone Joint Surg. Br.* **70**, 267–271.

McCulloch, J.A. & Waddell, G. (1978) Lateral lumbar discography. *Br. J. Radiol.* **51**, 498–502.

Tehranzadeh, J. (1998) Discography 2000. *Radiol. Clin. N. Am.* **36 (3)**, 463–495.

INTRADISCAL THERAPY

The ability to carry out successful discography will enable the radiologist, in cooperation with interested clinicians, to carry out therapeutic procedures such as chemonucleolysis, mechanical percutaneous disc removal and laser therapy. While each has advocates, none is widely utilized, and the practice of such methods should be subject to very strict selection criteria and rigorous audit of the outcomes.

FACET JOINT ARTHROGRAPHY

Indications

This is performed for diagnostic and therapeutic purposes, primarily at the lumbar level. Intra-articular injection is the only effective means for assessing the facet joints as a source of back pain. The only indication therefore is suspected pain of facet joint origin. Such pain may strongly resemble radicular pain, and patients have often been managed on this basis over a long period of time without success.

Affected facets are usually degenerate as visualized on plain radiographs, CT or MRI. The facet joint capsule is richly innervated by the dorsal ramus of the lumbar spinal nerves. The procedure is valid in that many patients with degenerate facets do not have facet joint pain, and the role of the facet cannot therefore be determined without facet joint injection. The arthrogram is not therefore a study of pathological anatomy; the visualization of the joint is important only to verify the needle position. Having visualized the joint, local anaesthetic can be injected to judge the patient's response. In cases obtaining good relief of symptoms, further management will then consist either of a programme of regular injection therapy, or spinal fusion to prevent facet movement.

Equipment

1. As for myelography.
2. A 22-G spinal needle is appropriate for the study.

Contrast medium

Non-ionic contrast medium 0.1–0.2 ml should be used.

Technique

1. This is an outpatient procedure which involves the simultaneous injection of both joints at each level to be studied. More than one level should not be examined in each session to avoid diagnostic confusion.
2. The joint space is profiled by slowly rotating the patient from a prone position into a prone oblique orientation with the relevant side raised.
3. Sterile procedures are required.
4. The spinal needle is inserted and advanced perpendicularly to the facet joint, under fluoroscopic control. Caudal needle

angulation is sometimes needed if the iliac crest overlies the L5/S1 facet joints.

5. In the majority of cases a noticeable 'give' indicates that the capsule is penetrated.

6. Contrast medium injection confirms correct needle placement by demonstrating immediate opacification of a superior and inferior recess.

7. Films are taken to document intra-articular injection. The arthrographic appearances are not of any diagnostic consequence.

8. For diagnostic purposes up to 1 ml of 0.5% bupivacaine hydrochloride (Marcaine) is injected in the facet joint and the response over the ensuing 24-h period documented. For therapeutic injection, 0.5 ml of 0.5% Marcaine mixed with 0.5 ml of Depo-Medrone (methylprednisolone 40 mg ml^{-1}) is injected after arthrography.

Further reading

Fairbank, J.C.T., Park, W.M., McCall, I.W., et al. (1981) Apophyseal injection of local anaesthetic as a diagnostic aid in primary low back syndromes. *Spine* **6**, 598–605.

McCall, I.W., Park, W.M. & O'Brien, J.P. (1979) Induced pain referral from posterior lumbar elements in normal subjects. *Spine* **4**, 441–446.

Maldague, B., Mathurin, P. & Malghem, J. (1981) Facet joint arthrography in lumbar spondylolysis. *Radiology* **140**, 29–36.

Mooney, V. & Robertson, J. (1976) The facet syndrome. *Clin. Orthopaed.* **115**, 149–156.

PERCUTANEOUS VERTEBRAL BIOPSY

The percutaneous approach to obtaining a representative sample of tissue for diagnosis prior to therapy is both easy and safe, avoiding the morbidity associated with open surgery. It has a success rate of around 90%. Accurate lesion localization prior to and during the procedure is required. Vertebral body lesions may be biopsied under either CT or fluoroscopic control. Small lesions, especially those located in the posterior neural arch, are best done under CT control. A preliminary CT scan is helpful, whatever method is finally chosen to control the procedure.

Indications

Suspected vertebral or disc infection and vertebral neoplasia. Note that the presence of a more accessible lesion in the appendicular skeleton should be sought by radionuclide bone scanning before vertebral biopsy is undertaken.

Contraindications

1. Biopsy should not be attempted under any circumstances in the presence of abnormal and uncorrected bleeding or clotting time or if there is a low platelet count.
2. Lesions suspected of being highly vascular, e.g. aneurysmal bone cyst or renal tumour metastasis are relatively dangerous, and a fine-needle aspiration should be used instead of a trephine needle for these cases.

Equipment

1. Numerous types of biopsy needle are available. The commonest types used are the Jamshidi and Ackerman sets. A trephine needle with an internal diameter of 2 mm or more is required, minimizing histological distortion and reducing sampling error without increasing the complication rate. Specimen quality is higher with the Jamshidi type.

Patient preparation

Sedation/analgesia and, where necessary, general anaesthesia are required, preferably administered and monitored by an anaesthetist.

Technique

1. For a fluoroscopy-guided procedure the lateral decubitus position is used. For CT control the prone position is preferable.
2. The skin entry point distance from the mid-line is about 8 cm for the lumbar region and 5 cm in the thoracic region.
3. The aim of the procedure is to enter the vertebral body at about 4 o'clock or 8 o'clock (visualizing the body with the spinous process at 6 o'clock). Local anaesthetic may be injected via a 21-G spinal needle to allow deep infiltration of the soft tissues into close proximity to the periosteum.
4. The biopsy needle is advanced at between 30 and 45° to the sagittal plane in the thoracic and lumbar spine, respectively.
5. When the biopsy needle impinges on the cortex of the vertebral body its position is confirmed fluoroscopically in both AP and lateral planes, or on a single CT section. The trocar and cannula are then advanced through the cortex and the trocar is then withdrawn.
6. Using alternate clockwise and anticlockwise rotation the biopsy cannula is advanced approximately 1 cm.
7. By twisting the needle firmly several times in the same direction the specimen is severed.

8. At least two cores of bone may be obtained by withdrawing the needle back to the cortex, angulating and re-entering the vertebral body.

9. The needle is then withdrawn while simultaneous suction is applied by a syringe attached to the hub.

10. To remove the specimen, the trocar is re-inserted and the tissue is pushed out. Any blood clot should be included as part of the specimen.

11. In suspected infection the end-plate rather than the disc is biopsied. Most cases are due to osteomyelitis extending to the disc space. If there is a paravertebral abscess, aspiration and culture of its contents is preferable to vertebral biopsy.

Aftercare

1. Overnight stay with routine nursing observation and analgesia if needed.

2. The approach to a thoracic lesion should be extra-pleural, but if any doubt exists, a chest X-ray should be obtained after the procedure, as there is a small risk of pneumothorax or haemothorax.

Complications

These are rare, but there are potential risks to nearby structures in poorly controlled procedures, including the lung and pleura, aorta, nerve roots and spinal cord. Local bleeding is an occasional problem.

Further reading

Shaltot, A., Michell, P.A., Betts, J.A., et al. (1982) Jamshidi needle biopsy of bone lesions. *Clin. Radiol.* **33**, 193–196.

Stoker, D.J. & Kissin, C.M. (1985) Percutaneous vertebral biopsy: a review of 135 cases. *Clin. Radiol.* **36**, 569–573.

NERVE ROOT SLEEVE/PERINEURAL INJECTION IN THE LUMBAR SPINE

This is undertaken in difficult diagnostic cases, usually in the presence of multilevel pathology especially in postoperative situations. More recently, the instillation of local anaesthetic and betamethasone (Celestone Soluspan) has proved successful as a means of treating sciatica in patients with disc prolapse, especially in a foraminal location. The objective is to place the needle *outside* the nerve root sleeve so that the injected substances diffuse between the disc prolapse and the compressed nerve. Reduction of the inflammatory response induced by the herniated disc can be slow and improvement of symptoms can take up to 8–12 weeks.

The accurate placement of the tip of a spinal needle is confirmed by the injection of a small amount of contrast medium. Under local anaesthetic control, the needle is advanced using fluoroscopic or CT guidance, to a point inferior and lateral to the ipsilateral pedicle. The extra-foraminal nerve roots are outlined by contrast medium and a small amount of 0.5% bupivacaine is instilled as a means of assessing the correct level responsible for the patient's sciatica.

Further reading

Heron, L.D. (1989) Selective nerve root block in patient selection for lumbar surgery: surgical results. *J. Spinal Disord.* **2**, 75–79.

Van Akkerveeken, P.F. (1996) Pain patterns and diagnostic blocks. In: Weisel, S.W., Weinstein, J.N., Herkowitz, H., et al. (eds) *The Lumbar Spine*, pp 105–127. Philadelphia: WB Saunders.

Weiner, B.K, & Fraser, R.D. (1997) Foraminal injection for lateral lumbar disc herniation. *J. Bone Joint Surg. Br.* **79**, 804–807.

15 Lacrimal system

DACRYOCYSTOGRAPHY

Methods

1. Fluoroscopy
2. CT.[1]

Indications

Epiphora – to demonstrate the site and degree of obstruction.

Contraindications

None.

Contrast medium

Lipiodol, 0.5–2.0 ml per side.

Equipment

1. Skull unit (using macroradiography technique)
2. Silver dilator and cannula, or 18-G blunt needle with polythene catheter (the catheter technique has the advantage that the examination can be performed on both sides simultaneously, and films can be taken during the injection).

Patient preparation

None.

Preliminary film

Skull

1. Occipitomental
2. Lateral (centred to the inferior orbital margin).

Technique

1. The lacrimal sac is massaged to express its contents prior to injection of the contrast medium. The lower eyelid is everted

to locate the lower canaliculus at the medial end of the lid. The lower canaliculus is dilated and the cannula or catheter is inserted. The lower lid should be drawn laterally during insertion to straighten the bend in the canaliculus, and so avoid perforation by the cannula.

2. The contrast medium is injected, and radiographs are taken immediately afterwards (or during the injection if a catheter is used).

Films

The preliminary views are repeated.

Aftercare

None.

Complications

Perforation of the canaliculus.

Reference

1. Waite, D.W., Whitlet, H.B. & Shun-Shin, G.A. (1993) Technical note: computed tomographic dacryocystography. *Br. J. Radiol.* **66**, 711–713.

16 Salivary glands

Methods of imaging the salivary glands

1. Plain films
2. Sialography
3. CT ± enhancement by sialographic or i.v. contrast medium
4. US
5. MRI
6. Radionuclide imaging (sialoscintigraphy)
   a. ^{99m}Tc-pertechnetate (40 MBq max.) i.v. followed by dynamic imaging during uptake and oral stimulation of saliva secretion
   b. incidental visualization also occurs with:
      - ^{123}I- or ^{131}I-iodide
      - ^{123}I- or ^{131}I-MIBG
      - ^{67}Ga-citrate, especially in radiation sialitis and sarcoidosis
      - unstable or poor ^{99m}Tc radiopharmaceutical preparations resulting in significant amounts of free pertechnetate.

Further reading

Pilbrow, W.J., Brownless, S.M., Cawood, J.I., et al. (1990) Salivary gland scintigraphy – a suitable substitute for sialography? *Br. J. Radiol.* **63**, 190–196.

Silvers, A.R. & Som, P.M. (1998) Salivary glands. *Radiol. Clin. N. Am.* **36 (5)**, 941–966.

Weissman, J.L. (1995) Imaging of the salivary glands. *Semin. US, CT MRI* **6**, 546–568

Yasumoto, M., Shibuyu, H., Suzuki, S., et al. (1992) Computed tomography and ultrasonography in submandibular tumours. *Clin. Radiol.* **46**, 114–120.

SIALOGRAPHY

Indications

1. Pain
2. Swelling
3. Sicca syndrome.

Contraindications

Acute infection or inflammation.

Contrast medium

1. HOCM or LOCM 240–300
2. Lipiodol Ultra Fluid.

Neither contrast medium has a clear advantage over the other.

Equipment

1. Skull unit (using macroradiography technique)
2. Silver lachrymal dilator
3. Silver cannula or 18G blunt needle and polythene catheter.

Patient preparation

Any radio-opaque artefacts are removed (e.g. false teeth).

Preliminary film

Parotid gland

1. AP with the head rotated 5% away from the side under investigation. Centre to the mid-line of the lower lip.
2. Lateral, centred to the angle of the mandible.
3. Lateral oblique, centred to the angle of the mandible, and with the tube angled 20% cephalad.

Submandibular gland

1. Inferosuperior using an occlusal film. This is a useful view to show calculi.
2. Lateral, with the floor of the mouth depressed by a wooden spatula.
3. Lateral oblique, centred 1 cm anterior to the angle of the mandible, and with the tube angled 20% cephalad.

Technique

1. The orifice of the parotid duct is adjacent to the crown of the second upper molar, and that of the submandibular duct is at the base of the frenulum of the tongue. If they are not visible, a sialogogue (e.g. citric acid) is placed in the mouth to promote secretion from the gland, and so render the orifice visible.
2. The orifice of the duct is dilated with the silver wire probe and the cannula or polythene catheter is introduced into the duct. The catheter can be held in place by the patient gently biting on it.
3. Up to 2 ml of contrast medium are injected. The injection is

terminated immediately any pain is experienced. The duct must not be overfilled.
4. If the cannula method is used, films are taken immediately after the injection. The catheter method has the advantage that films can be taken during the injection, with the catheter in situ, and that both sides can be examined simultaneously.

Films

1. *Immediate* – the same views as for the preliminary films are repeated. The occlusal film for the submandibular gland may be omitted, as this is only to demonstrate calculi.
2. *Post-secretory* – the same views are repeated 5 min after the administration of a sialogogue. The purpose of this is to demonstrate sialectasis.

Aftercare

None.

Complications

1. Pain
2. Damage to the duct orifice
3. Rupture of the ducts
4. Infection.

Further reading

Nicholson, D.A. (1990) Contrast media in sialography: a comparison of lipiodol, ultra fluid and urografin. *Clin. Radiol.* **42**, 423–426.

MR SIALOGRAPHY

MR is increasingly used in the diagnosis of lesions of the salivary glands.

Non–contrast studies can be useful in differentiating benign or low-grade malignant from high-grade malignant tumours. Contrast enhancement is useful in the differential diagnosis of cystic from solid lesions, and when determining the degree of perineural spread of malignant disease.[1]

Pulse sequences

T1-weighted and T2-weighted unenhanced images are taken with a slice thickness of 3 mm and interslice gap of 1 mm. Fast spin-echo T2-weighted images may require fat suppression.

Gadolinium-enhanced scans with T1 weighting and fat suppression are obtained in the axial plane; sagittal and coronal images may be obtained at the radiologist's discretion.[2,3]

References

1. Parker, G.D. & Harnsberger, H.R. (1991) Clinical–radiologic issues in perineural tumour spread of malignant diseases of the extracranial head and neck. *Radiographics* **11**, 383–399.
2. Chaudhuri, R., Bingham, J.B., Crossman, J.E., et al. (1992) Magnetic resonance imaging of the parotid gland using the STIR sequence. *Clin. Otolaryngol.* **17**, 211–217.
3. Tabor, E.K. & Curtin, H.D. (1989) MR of the salivary glands. *Radiol. Clin. N. Am.* **27**, 379–392.

Further reading

Silvers, A.R. & Som, P.M. (1998) Salivary glands. *Radiol. Clin. North. Am.* **36**, 941–966.

SIALOSCINTIGRAPHY   RN

Indications

1. Assessment of xerostomia
2. Assessment of salivary duct patency
3. Assessment of salivary gland function.

Contraindications

None.

Radiopharmaceuticals

^{99m}Tc-pertechnetate (40 MBq max, 0.5 mSv ED).

Pertechnetate is chemically similar to other negatively charged ions produced in saliva. It is accumulated by gland cells and then secreted into saliva.

Equipment

1. Gamma-camera
2. Low-energy general purpose or high sensitivity collimator.

Patient preparation

Remove dentures.

Technique

1. The patient is sat in front of the camera with the head tilted back slightly to give good separation of sub-mandibular and parotid glands.

2. Administer 40 MBq ^{99m}Tc-pertechnetate i.v.
3. Simultaneously start a 64 × 64 dynamic study with 20-s frames for 30 min.
4. At 20 min, administer salivary stimulation by asking the patient to suck a slice of lemon, acid drop or similar.
5. Throughout the study, the patient should not talk or chew.
6. Anterior and lateral static images may be taken at 30 min as required.

Analysis

1. Regions of interest are drawn round each gland and background areas.
2. Time–activity curves are plotted.
3. Quantitative parameters may be calculated, e.g. maximum gland-to-background ratio and percentage secretion.[1]

Aftercare

None.

Complications

None.

Reference

1. Umehara, I., Yamada, I., Murata, Y., et al. (1999) Quantitative evaluation of salivary gland scintigraphy in Sjögren's syndrome. *J. Nucl. Med.* **40**, 64–69.

Further reading

Pilbrow, W.J., Brownless, S.M., Cawood, J.I., et al. (1990) Salivary gland scintigraphy – a suitable substitute for sialography? *Br. J. Radiol.* **63**, 190–196.

Smith, F.W. (1998) 99m-Technetium pertechnetate. In: Sharp, P.F., Gemmell, H.G. & Smith, F.W. (eds) *Practical Nuclear Medicine*, pp. 318–320. Oxford: Oxford University Press.

17 Thyroid and parathyroids

Methods of imaging the thyroid gland

1. Plain film
2. US
3. Radionuclide imaging
4. CT
5. MRI.

ULTRASOUND OF THE THYROID   US

Indications

1. Palpable thyroid mass
2. Suspected thyroid tumour
3. 'Cold spot' on radionuclide imaging
4. Suspected retrosternal extension of thyroid
5. Guided aspiration or biopsy.

Contraindications

None.

Patient preparation

None.

Equipment

5–10-MHz transducer. Linear array for optimum imaging.

Technique

Patient supine with the neck extended. Longitudinal and transverse scans of both lobes of the thyroid. The isthmus is imaged in a transverse scan as it crosses anterior to the trachea. If there is retrosternal extension, angling downwards and scanning during swallowing may enable the lowest extent of the thyroid to be visualized.

Further reading

Solbiati, L., Cioffi, V. & Ballarati, E. (1992) Ultrasonography of the neck. *Radiol. Clin. N. Am.* **30**, 941–954.

RADIONUCLIDE THYROID IMAGING

Indications[1]

1. Investigation of thyroid nodules
2. Assessment of goitre
3. Assessment of thyroid uptake prior to radio-iodine therapy
4. Assessment of neonatal hypothyroidism.[2]

Contraindications

None.

Radiopharmaceuticals

1. *^{99m}Tc-pertechnetate*, 80 MBq max (1 mSv ED). Pertechnetate ions are trapped in the thyroid by an active transport mechanism, but are not organified. Cheap and readily available. Inferior to ^{123}I, but is considered an acceptable alternative.
2. *^{123}I-sodium iodide*, 20 MBq max (4 mSv ED). Iodide ions are trapped by the thyroid in the same way as pertechnetate, but are also organified, allowing overall assessment of thyroid function. The agent of choice, but ^{123}I is a cyclotron product and is therefore relatively expensive with limited availability.

Equipment

1. Gamma-camera
2. Pinhole, converging or high-resolution parallel hole collimator.

Patient preparation

None, but uptake may be reduced by antithyroid drugs and iodine-based preparations and contrast media.

Technique

^{99m}Tc-pertechnetate

1. Intravenous injection of pertechnetate.
2. After 15 min, immediately before imaging, the patient is given a drink of water to wash away pertechnetate secreted into saliva.

3. Start imaging 20 min post-injection when the target-to-background ratio is maximum.

4. The patient lies supine with the neck slightly extended and the camera anterior. For a pinhole collimator, the pinhole should be positioned to give the maximum magnification for the camera field of view (usually 7–10 cm from the neck).

5. The patient should be asked not to swallow or talk during imaging.

6. An image is acquired with markers on the suprasternal notch, clavicles, edges of neck and any palpable nodules.

^{123}I-sodium iodide

The technique is similar to that for pertechnetate except:

1. Sodium iodide may be given i.v. or orally.

2. Imaging is performed 3–4 h after i.v. administration or 24 h after an oral dose.

3. A drink of water is not necessary, since ^{123}I is not secreted into saliva in any significant quantity.

Films

200 kilocounts or 15 min maximum:

1. Anterior

2. Left and right anterior oblique views as required, especially for assessment of multinodular disease

3. Take large field of view image if retrosternal extension or ectopic thyroid tissue is suspected.

Analysis

The percentage thyroid uptake may be estimated by comparing the background-subtracted attenuation-corrected organ counts with the full syringe counts measured under standard conditions before injection.

Additional techniques

1. Whole-body ^{131}I imaging is often performed after thyroidectomy and ^{131}I ablation for thyroid cancer to locate sites of metastasis.[3]

2. Perchlorate discharge tests can be performed to assess possible organification defects, particularly in congenital hypothyroidism.[2]

Aftercare

None.

Complications

None.

Reference

1. Freitas, J.E. & Freitas, A.E. (1994) Thyroid and parathyroid imaging. *Semin. Nucl. Med.* **24**, 234–245.
2. El-Desouki, M., Al-Jurayyan, N., Al-Nuaim, A., et al. (1995) Thyroid scintigraphy and perchlorate discharge test in the diagnosis of congenital hypothyroidism. *Eur. J. Nucl. Med.* **22**, 1005–1008.
3. Lind, P. (1999) [131]I whole body scintigraphy in thyroid cancer patients. *Q. J. Nucl. Med.* **43**, 188–194.

Further reading

Naik, K.S. & Bury, R.F. (1998) Imaging the thyroid. *Clin. Radiol.* **53**, 630–639.
Martin, W.H., Sandler, M.P., Shapiro, B., et al. (1998) Thyroid, parathyroid, and adrenal gland imaging. In: Sharp, P.F., Gemmell, H.G. & Smith, F.W. (eds) *Practical Nuclear Medicine*, 2nd edn, pp. 253–259. Oxford: Oxford University Press.

RADIONUCLIDE PARATHYROID IMAGING

Indications

Preoperative localization of parathyroid adenomas and hyperplastic glands, usually before second-look surgery.[1,2]

Contraindications

None.

Radiopharmaceuticals

1. ^{99m}Tc-*methoxyisobutylisonitrile (MIBI or sestamibi)*, 500 MBq typical, 900 MBq max (11 mSv ED) and ^{99m}Tc-*pertechnetate*, 80 MBq max (1 mSv ED). Both MIBI and pertechnetate are trapped by the thyroid, but only MIBI accumulates in hyperactive parathyroid tissue. With computer subtraction of pertechnetate from MIBI images, abnormal accumulation of MIBI may be seen. MIBI also washes out of normal thyroid tissue faster than parathyroid, so delayed images (1–4 h) can highlight abnormal parathyroid activity.

2. ^{99m}Tc-*tetrofosmin (Myoview)* can be used as an alternative to MIBI, and is as effective if the subtraction technique is used, but not as good for delayed imaging since differential washout is not as great as for MIBI.[3]

3. ^{201}Tl-*thallous chloride* (80 MBq max, 18 mSv ED) was previously used in conjunction with ^{99m}Tc-pertechnetate, but is

increasingly being replaced by the technetium agents due to their superior imaging quality and lower radiation dose.[4,5]

Equipment

1. Gamma-camera (small field of view preferable for thyroid images, large field of view for chest images)
2. High-resolution parallel hole collimator. A pinhole collimator can also be used, but may result in repositioning magnification errors that compromise subtraction techniques
3. Imaging computer capable of image registration and subtraction.

Patient preparation

None, but uptake may be modified by antithyroid drugs and iodine-based medications, skin preparations and contrast media.

Technique

A variety of imaging protocols have been used, with either pertechnetate or MIBI administered first, with subtraction and possibly additional delayed imaging, and using MIBI alone with early and delayed imaging.[4,6] Subtraction techniques are most sensitive, but additional delayed imaging may increase sensitivity slightly and improve confidence in the result. The advantage of administering pertechnetate first is that MIBI injection can follow within 30 min with the patient still in position to minimize movement, and if subtraction shows a clearly positive result, the patient does not need to stay for delayed imaging. With MIBI injected first, pertechnetate can only be administered after several hours when washout has occurred.

1. 80 MBq ^{99m}Tc-pertechnetate is administered i.v. through a cannula which is left in place for the second injection.
2. After 15 min the patient is given a drink of water immediately before imaging, to wash away pertechnetate secreted into saliva.
3. The patient lies supine with the neck slightly extended.
4. The camera is positioned anteriorly over the thyroid.
5. The patient should be asked not to move during imaging. Head immobilizing devices may be useful, and marker sources may aid repositioning.
6. 20 min post-injection, a 10-min 128×128 image is acquired.
7. Without moving the patient, 500 MBq ^{99m}Tc-MIBI is injected i.v. through the previously positioned cannula

(to avoid a second venepuncture which might cause patient movement).

8. 10 min post-injection, a further 10-min 128×128 image is acquired.

9. A chest and neck image should then be acquired on a large field of view camera to detect ectopic parathyroid tissue.

10. Computer image registration and normalization is performed and the pertechnetate image subtracted from the 10-min MIBI image.

11. If a lesion is clearly visible in the subtracted image, the patient can leave.

12. If the lesion is not obvious, late MIBI imaging can be performed at hourly intervals up to 4 h if necessary to look for differential washout.

Additional techniques

1. In patients in whom pertechnetate thyroid uptake is suppressed, e.g. with use of iodine-containing contrast media or skin preparations, oral [123]I (20 MBq) administered several hours before MIBI may be considered.

2. SPECT may be used to improve localization and small lesion detection.[7]

3. Dynamic imaging with motion correction may reduce motion artefact.

Aftercare

None.

Complications

None.

References

1. Pattou, F., Huglo, D. & Proye, C. (1998) Radionuclide scanning in parathyroid diseases. *Br. J. Surg.* **85**, 1605–1616.

2. O'Doherty, M.J. (1997) Editorial: Radionuclide parathyroid imaging. *J. Nucl. Med.* **38**, 840–841.

3. Fjeld, J.G., Erichsen, K., Pfeffer, P.F., et al. (1997) Technetium-99m-tetrofosmin for parathyroid scintigraphy: a comparison with sestamibi. *J. Nucl. Med.* **38**, 831–834.

4. Lind, P. (1997) Editorial: Parathyroid imaging with technetium-99m labelled cationic complexes: which tracer and which technique should be used? Eur. *J. Nucl. Med.* **24**, 243–245.

5. Giordano, A., Marozzi, P., Meduri, G., et al. (1999) Quantitative comparison of technetium-99m tetrofosmin and thallium-201 images of the thyroid and abnormal parathyroid glands. *Eur. J. Nucl. Med.* **26**, 907–911.

6. Chen, C.C., Holder, L.E., Scovill, W.A., et al. (1997) Comparison of parathyroid imaging with technetium-99m-pertechnetate/sestamibi subtraction, double-phase technetium-99m-sestamibi and technetium-99m-sestamibi SPECT. *J. Nucl. Med.* **38**, 834–839.

7. Geatti, O. (1999) Parathyroid scintigraphy. *Q. J. Nucl. Med.* **43**, 207–216.

Further reading

Greenspan, B.S., Brown, M.L., Dillehay, G.L., et al. (1998) Procedure guideline for parathyroid scintigraphy. Society of Nuclear Medicine. *J. Nucl. Med.* **39**, 1111–1114.

Appendix I
Emergency equipment for the X-ray department

Equipment

Oxygen – piped or in a cylinder
Suction and catheters
Face mask – adult and paediatric sizes
Airway – adult and paediatric sizes
Laryngoscope
Endotracheal tubes
Ventilation bag
Needles and syringes
I.V. giving set
Scalpel, blade and French's needle
Stethoscope and sphygmomanometer

Drug	Route	Adult dose	Paediatric dose
Adrenaline 1:1000	s.c.	0.5 ml	0–1 year : 0.01 ml kg^{-1} 1 year : 0.12 ml 7 years: 0.25 ml
Aminophyline 250 mg in 10 ml	i.v.	250 mg over 5 min	4 mg kg^{-1} over 10 min
Atropine 600 μg in 1 ml	i.v.	600 mg	0–1 year : 15 mg kg^{-1} 1 year : 150 mg 7 years: 300 mg
Sodium bicarbonate, 8.4%, 200 ml	i.v.		
Calcium gluconate 10%, 10 ml	i.v., slowly	10 ml	30 mg kg^{-1} 10% solution diluted to 2.5%
Chlorpheniramine10 mg in 1 ml	i.v. diluted with blood over 1 min	10 mg	0–1 year : 0.25 mg kg^{-1} 1 year : 2.5 mg 7 years: 5 mg
Dextrose 5%, 500 ml	i.v.		
Dextrose 50% w.v	i.v.	50 ml	1 ml kg^{-1}
Diazepam 10 mg in 2 ml	i.v.	10–20 mg at a rate of 0.5 ml per 30 s. Repeat after 30 min if necessary	200–300 μg kg^{-1}
Dopamine 800 mg in 5 ml to be diluted in 500 ml N saline or 5% dextrose	i.v. infusion	2.5 μg kg^{-1} min^{-1} initially; increase if necessary	
Frusemide 10 mg ml^{-1} 2 ml, 5 ml and 25 ml ampoules	i.v.	20–50 mg	0.5–1.5 mg kg^{-1}
Hydrocortisone 100 mg	i.v. slowly	100–500 mg	4 mg kg^{-1}
Lignocaine 100 mg in 10 ml	i.v.	100 mg over a few mins	
N saline 500 ml	i.v.		
Naloxone 400 μg in 1 ml	i.v.	0.8–2 mg	10 μg kg^{-1}
Protamine sulphate 10 mg ml^{-1}	i.v. slowly	1 mg for each 100 U of heparin up to 50 mg. If more than 15 min has elapsed since heparin was given, then give less, as heparin is rapidly excreted.	
Water for injection			

Appendix II
Treatment of emergencies

The flow charts on the following pages outline the steps to be taken during the most frequently occurring emergencies in the X-ray department. Drug dosages are given in Appendix I.

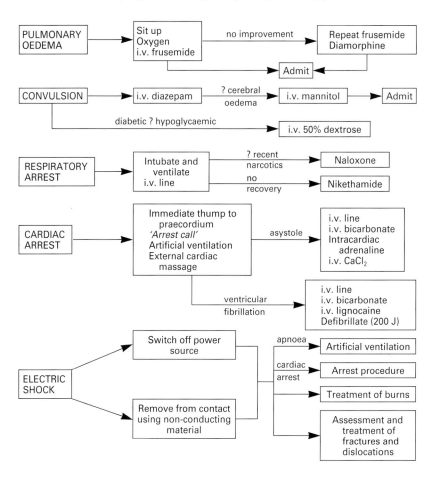

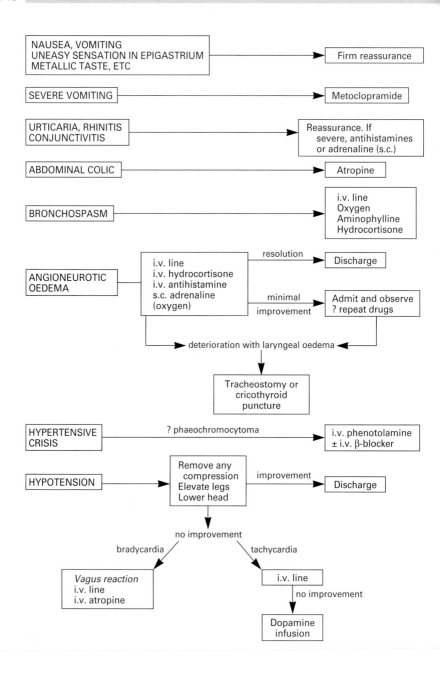

Appendix III
Dose limits – the Ionising
Radiations Regulations (1999)[1]

Body part etc	Dose limit (mSv)			
	Employees 18 years or over	Special circumstances#	Trainees aged under 18 years	Other persons (including any person below 16 years)
Effective dose in any calendar year	20	50 (not more than 100 mSv averaged over 5 years)	6	1 (5*)
Equivalent dose for the skin in a calendar year as applied to the dose averaged over any area of 1 cm^2, regardless of the area exposed. Equivalent dose for hands, forearms, feet and ankles in a calendar year	500	500	150	50
Equivalent dose for the lens of the eye in a calendar year	150	150	50	15
Equivalent dose for the abdomen of a woman of reproductive capacity at work, being the equivalent dose from exposure to ionizing radiation averaged throughout the abdomen in any consecutive 3-monthly period	13	13	n/a	n/a

\# If an employer demonstrates to the Health and Safety Executive (HSE) that it cannot meet the 20 mSv/calendar year limit. It may apply this limit after notifying HSE, the employees concerned and the approved dosimetry service.

* The dose limit for persons who are exposed to ionizing radiation from a medical exposure of another person but are not 'comforters or carers,[2] is 5 mSv in any period of 5 consecutive calendar years.

References

1. Crown copyright 1999 with the permission of the Controller of Her Majesty's Stationery Office.
2. A 'comforter and carer' is defined in IRR 99 as an individual who (other than as part of his occupation) knowingly and willingly incurs an exposure to ionizing radiation resulting from the support and comfort of another person who is undergoing or who has undergone any medical exposure.

Appendix IV
Average effective dose equivalents for some common examinations

Examination	Effective dose equivalent (mSv)	Miles travelled by car*	Equivalent period of natural background radiation	Probability of radiation effect occurring ($\times 10^{-6}$) (fatal somatic)	
				Male	Female
Chest (PA)	0.02	50	3 days	0.27	0.47
Skull	0.1	250	2 weeks	1.7	1.7
Cervical spine	0.1	250	2 weeks		
Thoracic spine	1.0	2 500	6 months	7.0	11
Lumbar spine	2.4	5 000	14 months	25	26
Hip (1 only)	0.3	750	2 months		
Pelvis	1.0	2 500	6 months	3.9	3.9
Abdomen	1.5	3 750	9 months	9.4	9.5
Extremity (e.g. hand, foot)	< 0.01	< 25	< 1.5 days		
Barium:					
Meal	5.0	12 500	2.5 years	26	31
Small bowel	6.0	15 000	3 years		
Large bowel	9.0	22 500	4.5 years	37	38
I.V. Urography	4.6	11 500	2.5 years	26	37
CT					
Head	2.0	5 000	1 year	62	69
Chest	8.0	20 000	4 years	330	370
Abdomen	8.0	20 000	4 years	330	370

* ICRP 60.

Appendix V
The Ionising Radiation (Medical Exposure) Regulations 2000[1]

These Regulations, together with the Ionising Radiations Regulations 1999 (S.I. 1999/3232) partially implement, as respects Great Britain, Council Directive 97/43/Euratom (OJ No. L180, 9.7.97, p. 22) laying down basic measures for the health protection of individuals against dangers of ionizing radiation in relation to medical exposure. The Regulations impose duties on those responsible for administering ionizing radiation to protect persons undergoing medical exposure whether as part of their own medical diagnosis or treatment or as part of occupational health surveillance, health screening, voluntary participation in research or medico-legal procedures.

They replace The Ionising Radiation (Protection of Persons Undergoing Medical Examination or Treatment) Regulations 1988.

1. Commencement

These regulations come into force –

a. except for regulation 4(1) and 4(2) on 13 May 2000;
b. as regards regulation 4(1) and 4(2) on 1 January 2001.

2. Glossary of [some of the] terms

adequate training means training which satisfies the requirements of Schedule 2; and the expression *adequately trained* shall be similarly construed;

appropriate authority means the Secretary of State as regards England, the National Assembly for Wales as regards Wales, or the Scottish Ministers as regards Scotland;

child means a person under the age of 18 in England and Wales or a person under the age of 16 in Scotland;

clinical audit means a systematic examination or review of medical radiological procedures which seeks to improve the quality and the outcome of patient care through structured review whereby radiological practices, procedures and results are examined against agreed standards for good medical radiological procedures, intended to lead to modification of practices where indicated and the application of new standards if necessary;

diagnostic reference levels means dose levels in medical radio-diagnostic practices or, in the case of radioactive medicinal products, levels of activity, for typical examinations for groups of standard-sized patients or standard phantoms for broadly defined types of equipment;

dose constraint means a restriction on the prospective doses to individuals which may result from a defined source;

the Directive means Council Directive 97/43/Euratom laying down measures on health protection of individuals against the dangers of ionizing radiation in relation to medical exposure;

employer means any natural or legal person who, in the course of a trade, business or other undertaking, carries out (other than as an employee), or engages others to carry out, medical exposures or practical aspects, at a given radiological installation;

employer's procedures means the procedures established by an employer pursuant to regulation 4(1);

equipment means equipment which delivers ionizing radiation to a person undergoing a medical exposure and equipment which directly controls or influences the extent of such exposure;

individual detriment means clinically observable deleterious effects that are expressed in individuals or their descendants the appearance of which is either immediate or delayed and, in the latter case, implies a probability rather than a certainty of appearance;

ionizing radiation means the transfer of energy in the form of particles or electromagnetic waves of a wavelength of 100 nanometres or less or a frequency of 3×10^{15} hertz or more capable of producing ions directly or indirectly;

medical exposure means any exposure to which regulation 3 applies and which involves an individual being exposed to ionizing radiation;

medical physics expert means a person who holds a science degree or its equivalent and who is experienced in the application of physics to the diagnostic and therapeutic uses of ionizing radiation;

medico-legal procedure means a procedure performed for insurance or legal purposes without a medical indication;

operator means any person who is entitled, in accordance with the employer's procedures, to carry out practical aspects including those to whom practical aspects have been allocated pursuant to regulation 5(3), medical physics experts as referred to in regulation 9 and, except where they do so under the direct supervision of a person who is adequately trained, persons participating in practical aspects as part of practical training as referred to in regulation 11(3);

patient dose means the dose concerning patients or other individuals undergoing medical exposure;

practical aspect means the physical conduct of any of the exposures referred to in regulation 3 and any supporting aspects including handling and use of radiological equipment, and the assessment of technical and physical parameters including radiation doses, calibration and maintenance of equipment, preparation and administration of radioactive medicinal products and the development of films;

practitioner means a registered medical practitioner, dental practitioner or other health professional who is entitled in accordance with the employer's procedures to take responsibility for an individual medical exposure;

quality assurance means any planned and systematic action necessary to provide adequate confidence that a structure, system, component or procedure will perform satisfactorily and safely complying with agreed standards and includes quality control;

quality control means the set of operations (programming, coordinating, implementing) intended to maintain or to improve quality and includes monitoring, evaluation and maintenance at required levels of performance;

radioactive medicinal product has the meaning given in the Medicines (Administration of Radioactive Substances) Regulations 1978;

referrer means a registered medical practitioner, dental practitioner or other health professional who is entitled in accordance with the employer's procedures to refer individuals for medical exposure to a practitioner.

3. These Regulations apply to the following medical exposures:

    a. the exposure of patients as part of their own medical diagnosis or treatment;

    b. the exposure of individuals as part of occupational health surveillance;

    c. the exposure of individuals as part of health screening programmes;

    d. the exposure of patients or other persons voluntarily participating in medical or biomedical, diagnostic or therapeutic, research programmes;

    e. the exposure of individuals as part of medico-legal procedures.

4. Duties of the Employer

1. The employer shall ensure that written procedures for medical exposures including the procedures set out in Schedule 1 are in place and

    a. shall take steps to ensure that they are complied with by the practitioner and operator; or

    b. where the employer is concurrently practitioner or operator, he shall comply with these procedures himself.

2. The employer shall ensure that written protocols are in place for every type of standard radiological practice for each equipment.

3. The employer shall establish

    a. recommendations concerning referral criteria for medical exposures, including radiation doses, and shall ensure that these are available to the referrer;

    b. quality assurance programmes for standard operating procedures;

    c. diagnostic reference levels for radiodiagnostic examinations falling within regulation 3(a), (b), (c) and (e) having regard to European diagnostic reference levels where available;

    d. dose constraints for biomedical and medical research programmes falling within regulation 3(d) where no direct medical benefit for the individual is expected from the exposure.

4. The employer shall take steps to ensure that every practitioner or operator engaged by the employer to carry out medical exposures or any practical aspect of such exposures:

    a. complies with the provisions of regulation 11(1); and

    b. undertakes continuing education and training after

qualification including, in the case of clinical use of new techniques, training related to these techniques and the relevant radiation protection requirements; or

c. where the employer is concurrently practitioner or operator, he shall himself ensure that he undertakes such continuing education and training as may be appropriate.

5. Where the employer knows or has reason to believe that an incident has or may have occurred in which a person, while undergoing a medical exposure was, otherwise than as a result of a malfunction or defect in equipment, exposed to ionizing radiation to an extent much greater than intended, he shall make an immediate preliminary investigation of the incident and, unless that investigation shows beyond a reasonable doubt that no such overexposure has occurred, he shall forthwith notify the appropriate authority and make or arrange for a detailed investigation of the circumstances of the exposure and an assessment of the dose received.

6. The employer shall undertake appropriate reviews whenever diagnostic reference levels are consistently exceeded and ensure that corrective action is taken where appropriate.

5. Duties of the Practitioner, Operator and Referrer

1. The practitioner and the operator shall comply with the employer's procedures.

2. The practitioner shall be responsible for the justification of a medical exposure and such other aspects of a medical exposure as is provided for in these Regulations.

3. Practical aspects of a medical exposure or part of it may be allocated in accordance with the employer's procedures by the employer or the practitioner, as appropriate, to one or more individuals entitled to act in this respect in a recognized field of specialization.

4. The operator shall be responsible for each and every practical aspect which he carries out as well as for any authorization given pursuant to regulation 6(5) where such authorization is not made in accordance with the guidelines referred to in regulation 6(5).

5. The referrer shall supply the practitioner with sufficient medical data (such as previous diagnostic information or medical records) relevant to the medical exposure requested by the referrer to enable the practitioner to decide on whether there is a sufficient net benefit as required by regulation 6(1)(a).

6. The practitioner and the operator shall cooperate, regarding practical aspects, with other specialists and staff involved in a medical exposure, as appropriate.

7. For the avoidance of doubt, where a person acts as employer, referrer, practitioner and operator concurrently (or in any combination of these roles) he shall comply with all the duties placed on employers, referrers, practitioners or operators under these Regulations accordingly.

6. Justification of Individual Medical Exposures

1. No person shall carry out a medical exposure unless:
   a. it has been justified by the practitioner as showing a sufficient net benefit giving appropriate weight to the matters set out in paragraph (2); and
   b. it has been authorized by the practitioner or, where paragraph (5) applies, the operator; and
   c. in the case of a medical or biomedical exposure as referred to in regulation 3(d), it has been approved by a Local Research Ethics Committee; and
   d. in the case of an exposure falling within regulation 3(e), it complies with the employer's procedures for such exposures; and
   e. in the case of a female of child-bearing age, he has enquired whether she is pregnant or breast feeding, if relevant.

2. The matters referred to in paragraph (1)(a) are
   a. the specific objectives of the exposure and the characteristics of the individual involved;
   b. the total potential diagnostic or therapeutic benefits, including the direct health benefits to the individual and the benefits to society, of the exposure;
   c. the individual detriment that the exposure may cause; and
   d. the efficacy, benefits and risk of available alternative techniques having the same objective but involving no or less exposure to ionizing radiation.

3. In considering the weight to be given to the matters referred to in paragraph (2), the practitioner justifying an exposure pursuant to paragraph (1)(a) shall pay special attention to
   a. exposures on medico-legal grounds;
   b. exposures that have no direct health benefit for the individuals undergoing the exposure; and
   c. the urgency of the exposure, where appropriate, in cases involving:
      i. a female where pregnancy cannot be excluded, in

particular if abdominal and pelvic regions are involved, taking into account the exposure of both the expectant mother and the unborn child; and

ii. a female who is breast feeding and who undergoes a nuclear medicine exposure, taking into account the exposure of both the female and the child.

4. In deciding whether to justify an exposure under paragraph (1)(a) the practitioner shall take account of any data supplied by the referrer pursuant to regulation 5(5) and shall consider such data in order to avoid unnecessary exposure.

5. Where it is not practicable for the practitioner to authorize an exposure as required by paragraph (1)(b), the operator shall do so in accordance with guidelines issued by the practitioner.

7. Optimization

1. In relation to all medical exposures to which these Regulations apply except radiotherapeutic procedures, the practitioner and the operator, to the extent of their respective involvement in a medical exposure, shall ensure that doses arising from the exposure are kept as low as reasonably practicable consistent with the intended purpose.

2. In relation to all medical exposures for radiotherapeutic purposes the practitioner shall ensure that exposures of target volumes are individually planned, taking into account that doses of non-target volumes and tissues shall be as low as reasonably practicable and consistent with the intended radiotherapeutic purpose of the exposure.

3. Without prejudice to paragraphs (1) and (2), the operator shall select equipment and methods to ensure that for each medical exposure the dose of ionizing radiation to the individual undergoing the exposure is as low as reasonably practicable and consistent with the intended diagnostic or therapeutic purpose and in doing so shall pay special attention to

   a. quality assurance;

   b. assessment of patient dose or administered activity; and

   c. adherence to diagnostic reference levels for radiodiagnostic examinations falling within regulation 3(a), (b), (c) and (e) as set out in the employer's procedures.

4. For each medical or biomedical research programme falling within regulation 3(d), the employer's procedures shall provide that

   a. the individuals concerned participate voluntarily in the research programme;

    b. the individuals concerned are informed in advance about the risks of the exposure;

    c. the dose constraint set down in the employer's procedures for individuals for whom no direct medical benefit is expected from the exposure is adhered to; and

    d. individual target levels of doses are planned by the practitioner for patients who voluntarily undergo an experimental diagnostic or therapeutic practice from which the patients are expected to receive a diagnostic or therapeutic benefit.

5. In the case of patients undergoing treatment or diagnosis with radioactive medicinal products, the employer's procedures shall provide that, where appropriate, written instructions and information are provided to

    a. the patient, where he has capacity to consent to the treatment or diagnostic procedure; or

    b. where the patient is a child who lacks capacity so to consent, the person with parental responsibility for the child; or

    c. where the patient is an adult who lacks capacity so to consent, the person who appears to the practitioner to be the most appropriate person.

6. The instructions and information referred to in paragraph (5) shall

    a. specify how doses resulting from the patient's exposure can be restricted as far as reasonably possible so as to protect persons in contact with the patient;

    b. set out the risks associated with ionizing radiation; and

    c. be provided to the patient or other person specified in paragraph (5) as appropriate prior to the patient leaving the hospital or other place where the medical exposure was carried out.

7. In complying with the obligations under this regulation, the practitioner and the operator shall pay special attention to

    a. the need to keep doses arising from medico-legal exposures as low as reasonably practicable;

    b. medical exposures of children;

    c. medical exposures as part of a health screening programme;

    d. medical exposures involving high doses to the patient;

    e. where appropriate, females in whom pregnancy cannot be excluded and who are undergoing a medical exposure, in particular if abdominal and pelvic regions are involved, taking into account the exposure of both the expectant mother and the unborn child; and

    f. where appropriate, females who are breast feeding and who are undergoing exposures in nuclear medicine, taking into account the exposure of both the female and the child.

8. The employer shall take steps to ensure that a clinical evaluation of the outcome of each medical exposure, is recorded in accordance with the employer's procedures or, where the employer is concurrently practitioner or operator, shall so record a clinical evaluation, including, where appropriate, factors relevant to patient dose.

9. In the case of fluoroscopy:

    a. the operator shall ensure that examinations without devices to control the dose rate are limited to justified circumstances; and

    b. no person shall carry out an examination without an image intensification or equivalent technique.

8. Clinical Audit

The employer's procedures shall include provision for the carrying out of clinical audit as appropriate.

9. Expert advice

1. The employer shall ensure that a medical physics expert shall be involved in every medical exposure to which these Regulations apply in accordance with paragraph (2).

2. A medical physics expert shall be:

    a. closely involved in every radiotherapeutic practice other than standardized therapeutic nuclear medicine practices;

    b. available in standardized therapeutic nuclear medicine practices and in diagnostic nuclear medicine practices;

    c. involved as appropriate for consultation on optimization, including patient dosimetry and quality assurance, and to give advice on matters relating to radiation protection concerning medical exposure, as required, in all other radiological practices.

10. Equipment

1. The employer shall draw up, keep up-to-date and preserve at each radiological installation an inventory of equipment at that installation and, when so requested, shall furnish it to the appropriate authority.

2. The inventory referred to in paragraph (1) shall contain the following information:

    a. name of manufacturer,

    b. model number,

    c. serial number or other unique identifier,

    d. year of manufacture, and

    e. year of installation.

3. The employer shall ensure that equipment at each radiological installation is limited to the amount necessary for the proper carrying out of medical exposures at that installation.

11. Training

1. Subject to the following provisions of this regulation no practitioner or operator shall carry out a medical exposure or any practical aspect without having been adequately trained.

2. A certificate issued by an institute or person competent to award degrees or diplomas or to provide other evidence of training shall, if such certificate so attests, be sufficient proof that the person to whom it has been issued has been adequately trained.

3. Nothing in paragraph (1) above shall prevent a person from participating in practical aspects of the procedure as part of practical training if this is done under the supervision of a person who himself is adequately trained.

4. The employer shall keep and have available for inspection by the appropriate authority an up-to-date record of all practitioners and operators engaged by him to carry out medical exposures or any practical aspect of such exposures or, where the employer is concurrently practitioner or operator, of his own training, showing the date or dates on which training qualifying as adequate training was completed and the nature of the training.

5. Where the employer enters into a contract with another to engage a practitioner or operator otherwise employed by that other, the latter shall be responsible for keeping the records required by paragraph (4) and shall supply such records to the employer forthwith upon request.

12. Enforcement

1. The provisions of these Regulations shall be enforced as if they were health and safety regulations made under section 15 of the Health and Safety at Work etc. Act 1974 and, except as provided in paragraph (2), the provisions of that Act, as regards enforcement and offences, shall apply for the purposes of these Regulations.

2. The enforcing authority for the purposes of these Regulations shall be the appropriate authority.

13. Defence of due diligence

In any proceedings against any person for an offence consisting of the contravention of these Regulations it shall be a defence for that person to show that he took all reasonable steps and exercised all due diligence to avoid committing the offence.

SCHEDULE 1

Regulation 4(1)

Employer's Procedures

The written procedures for medical exposures shall include:

a. procedures to identify correctly the individual to be exposed to ionizing radiation;

b. procedures to identify individuals entitled to act as referrer or practitioner or operator;

c. procedures to be observed in the case of medico-legal exposures;

d. procedures for making enquiries of females of child-bearing age to establish whether the individual is or may be pregnant or breast feeding;

e. procedures to ensure that quality assurance programmes are followed;

f. procedures for the assessment of patient dose and administered activity;

g. procedures for the use of diagnostic reference levels established by the employer for radiodiagnostic examinations falling within regulation 3(a), (b), (c) and (e), specifying that these are expected not to be exceeded for standard procedures when good and normal practice regarding diagnostic and technical performance is applied;

h. procedures for determining whether the practitioner or operator is required to effect one or more of the matters set out in regulation 7(4) including criteria on how to effect those matters and in particular procedures for the use of dose constraints established by the employer for biomedical and medical research programmes falling within regulation 3(d) where no direct medical benefit for the individual is expected from the exposure;

i. procedures for the giving of information and written instructions as referred to in regulation 7(5);

j. procedures for the carrying out and recording of an evaluation for each medical exposure including, where appropriate, factors relevant to patient dose;

k. procedures to ensure that the probability and magnitude of accidental or unintended doses to patients from radiological practices are reduced so far as reasonably practicable.

SCHEDULE 2

Regulation 2(1)

Adequate Training

Practitioners and operators shall have successfully completed training, including theoretical knowledge and practical experience, in:

i. such of the subjects detailed in section A as are relevant to their functions as practitioner or operator; and

ii. such of the subjects detailed in section B as are relevant to their specific area of practice.

A. Radiation production, radiation protection and statutory obligations relating to ionizing radiations

1. Fundamental Physics of Radiation

    1.1 Properties of radiation
         Attenuation of ionizing radiation
         Scattering and absorption

    1.2 Radiation hazards and dosimetry
         Biological effects of radiation
         Risks/benefits of radiation
         Dose optimization
         Absorbed dose, dose equivalent, effective dose and their units

    1.3 Special attention areas
         Pregnancy and potential pregnancy
         Infants and children
         Medical and biomedical research
         Health screening
         High dose techniques

2. Management and Radiation Protection of the Patient

    2.1 Patient selection
         Justification of the individual exposure
         Patient identification and consent
         Use of existing appropriate radiological information
         Alternative techniques
         Clinical evaluation of outcome
         Medico-legal issues

2.2   Radiation protection
General radiation protection
Use of radiation protection devices
– patient
– personal
Procedures for untoward incidents involving
overexposure to ionizing radiation

3.   Statutory Requirements and Advisory Aspects
3.1   Statutory requirements and non-statutory
recommendations
Regulations
Local rules and procedures
Individual responsibilities relating to medical
exposures
Responsibility for radiation safety
Routine inspection and testing of equipment
Notification of faults and Health Department hazard
warnings
Clinical audit

B. Diagnostic radiology, radiotherapy and nuclear medicine

4.   Diagnostic Radiology
4.1   General
Fundamentals of radiological anatomy
Fundamentals of radiological techniques
Production of X-rays
Equipment selection and use
Factors affecting radiation dose
Dosimetry
Quality assurance and quality control
4.2   Specialized techniques
Image intensification/fluoroscopy
Digital fluoroscopy
Computed tomography scanning
Interventional procedures
Vascular imaging
4.3   Fundamentals of image acquisition etc.
Image quality vs. radiation dose
Conventional film processing
Additional image formats, acquisition, storage and
display
4.4   Contrast media
Non-ionic and ionic

Use and preparation
Contra-indications to the use of contrast media
Use of automatic injection devices
5. Radiotherapy
   5.1 General
      Production of ionizing radiations
      Use of radiotherapy
      – benign disease
      – malignant disease
      – external beam
      – brachytherapy
   5.2 Radiobiological aspects for radiotherapy
      Fractionation
      Dose rate
      Radiosensitization
      Target volumes
   5.3 Practical aspects for radiotherapy
      Equipment
      Treatment planning
   5.4 Radiation protection specific to radiotherapy
      Side-effects – early and late
      Toxicity
      Assessment of efficacy
6. Nuclear Medicine
   6.1 General
      Atomic structure and radioactivity
      Radioactive decay
      The tracer principle
      Fundamentals of diagnostic use
      Fundamentals of therapeutic use
      – dose rate
      – fractionation
      – radiobiology aspects
   6.2 Principles of radiation detection, instrumentation and
      equipment
      Types of systems
      Image acquisition, storage and display
      Quality assurance and quality control
   6.3 Radiopharmaceuticals
      Calibration
      Working practices in the radiopharmacy
      Preparation of individual doses
      Documentation

6.4   Radiation protection specific to nuclear medicine
       Conception, pregnancy and breast feeding
       Arrangements for radioactive patients
       Disposal procedures for radioactive waste

Reference

1. Crown copyright 2000. With the permission of the Controller of Her Majesty's Stationery Office

Appendix VI
MRI signal intensities

Substance	T1-weighted	T2-weighted
Water	Dark grey	Light grey or white
Fat	White	Light grey
Muscle	Grey	Grey
Air	Black	Black
Cortical bone	Black	Black
Fatty bone marrow	White	Light grey
Liver	Grey	Grey
Spleen	Grey	Grey
Flowing blood*	Black	Black
Brain		
White matter	Light grey	Grey
Grey matter	Grey	Very light grey
CSF in ventricle	Dark grey	Light grey or white
CSF 'fast' flow	Dark grey or black	Dark grey or black

*Depends on signal sequence and velocity of flow.

Appendix VII
Artefacts in MRI

Chemical shift

This is the most noticeable of the artefacts.

Protons in fat and water have different resonant frequencies. Signal arising from protons in fat will be interpreted as arriving from a different point along the frequency encoded read-out axis relative to signal from water. This difference will depend on the strength of the main magnetic field and will be more apparent at higher field strengths. Shift artefact will also be greater when the field gradient is less. Chemical shift artefact is most noticeable around the bladder, kidneys and vertebral endplates (regions with fat/water interfaces).

Motion

All motion – cardiac, CSF pulsation, gastrointestinal, respiratory and that due to blood vessel pulsation – causes artefact. This increases noise, edge blurring and streaking. Respiratory and cardiac artefact can be minimized by gating or compensation, but this adds significantly to the scan time. Peristalsis can be minimized by using relaxants such as glucagon. Blood flow produces signal loss as protons in arterial blood are moving rapidly and phase mismatches occur. Ghosting can occur, particularly noticeable in axial sections, in which faint images of blood vessels are seen at points distant from their true location in the phase encoded readout axis. Saturation radiofrequency (RF) pulses applied to tissue outside the region of interest can help reduce motion artefact.

Ferromagnetic

Ferromagnetic objects alter the T1 and T2 decay characteristics of the local magnetic environment and usually result in a signal void around the object. Non-ferromagnetic metals can induce similar though less marked artefact due to induced eddy currents.

Radiofrequency

RF noise degrades MR images. Patient generated noise can occur due to eddy currents from thermal movement of ions. System-generated noise from coils or amplifiers may produce specific patterns such as herringbone artefact. Extrinsic RF may produce linear streaking and can arise from any malfunctioning electrical device, e.g. light bulb or leaking RF door seals.

Aliasing

If the field of view is smaller than the area of tissue excited, structures that are peripheral to the field of view will wrap around the image and be seen on the opposite edge.

Partial volume averaging

This is analogous to similar artefact occurring in CT. The signal intensity of any particular voxel is determined by the average signal intensity within it. Artefact due to partial volume averaging increases with the section thickness.

Further reading

Bellon, E.M., Haacke, E.M., Coleman, P.E., et al. (1986) MR artifacts; a review. *Am. J. Roentgenol.* **147**, 1271–1281.

Edelmann, R.R. & Hesselink, J.R. (eds) (1990) Artefacts in MR imaging. *Clinical Magnetic Resonance Imaging*, Ch. 3. Philadelphia: WB Saunders.

Ludeke, K.M., Roschmann, A. & Tischler, R. (1985) Susceptibility artefacts in MR imaging. *Magn. Reason. Imaging* **3**, 327–343.

Index